DISEASE *free*

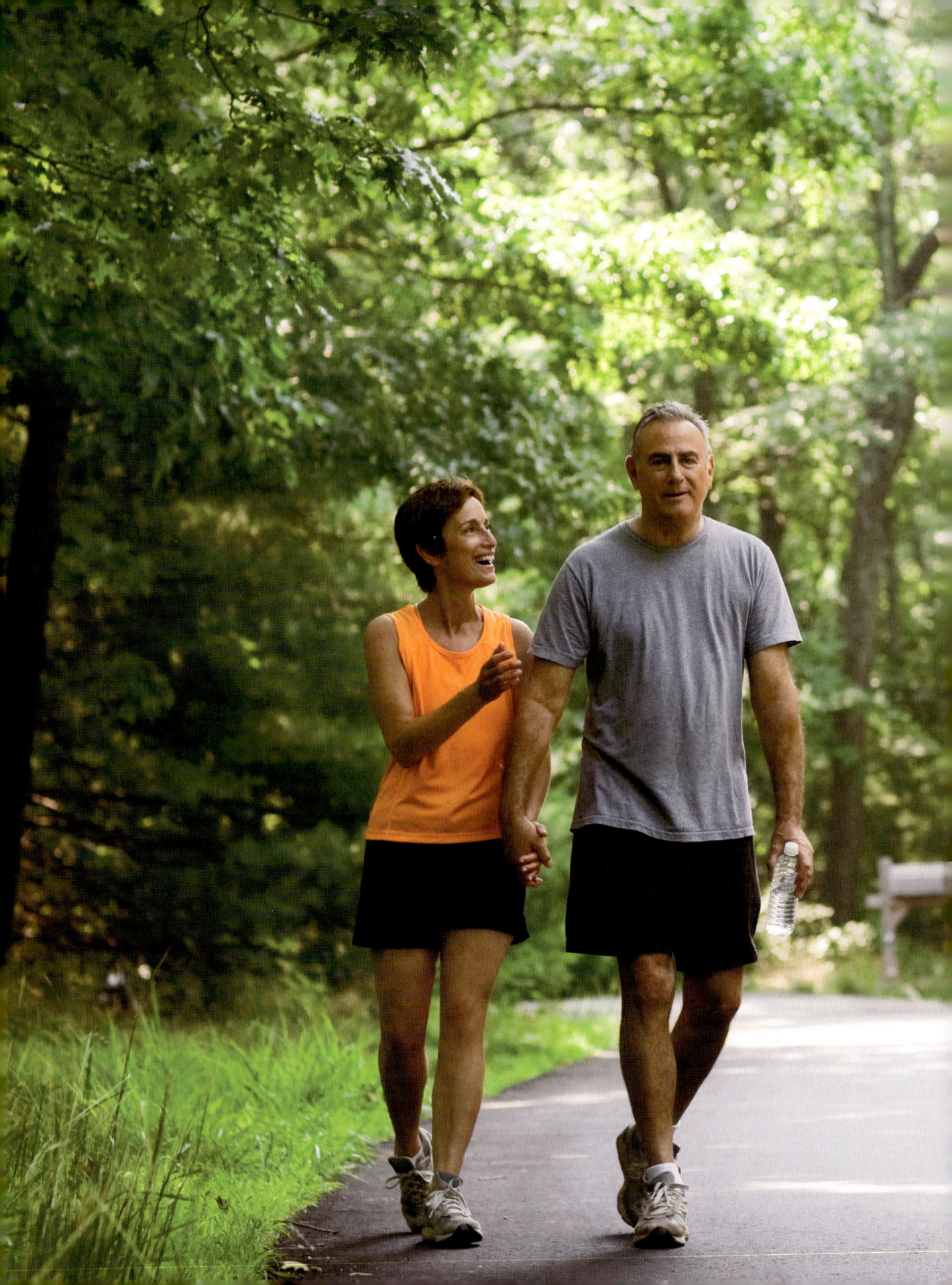

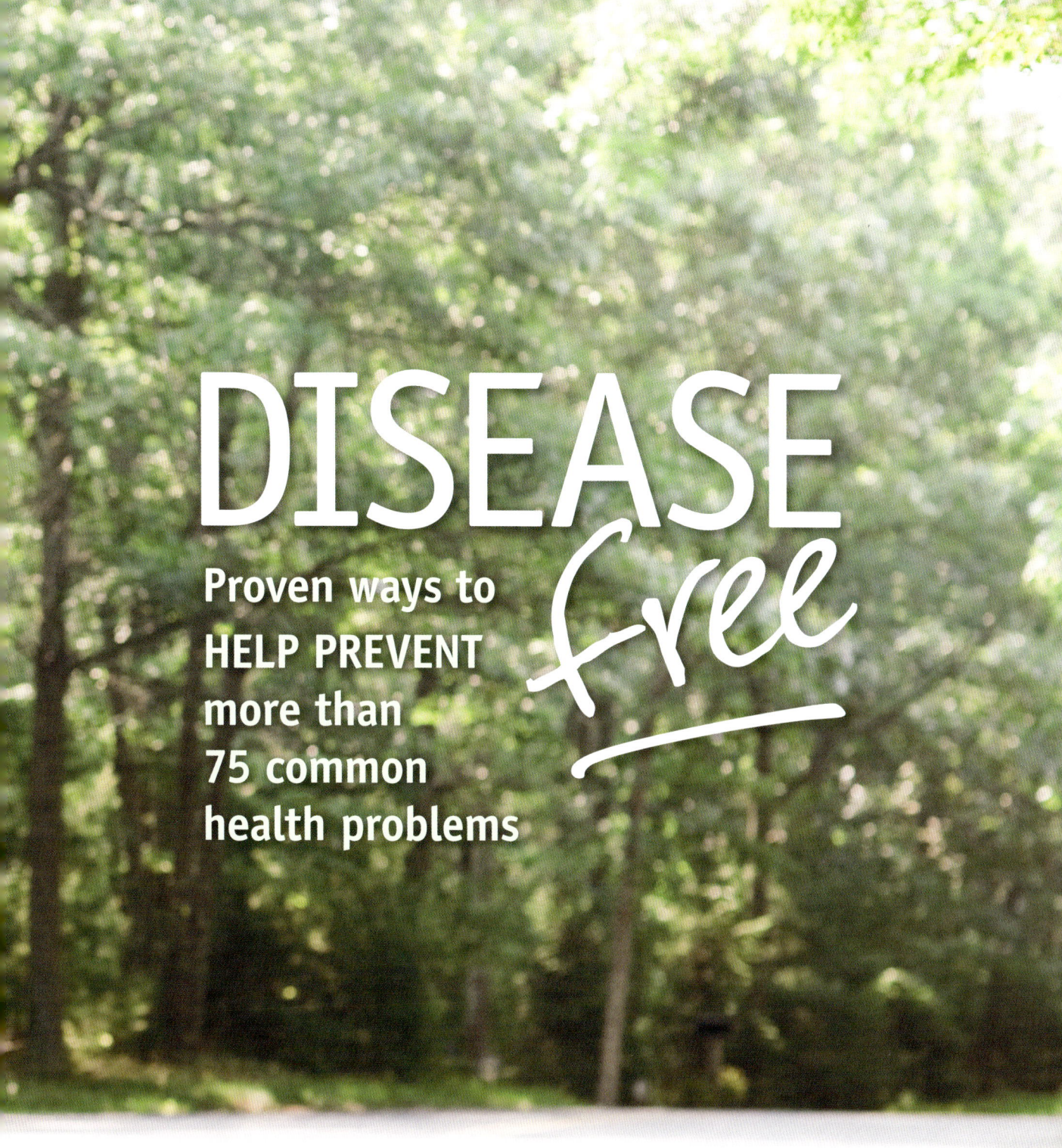

DISEASE *free*

Proven ways to **HELP PREVENT** more than 75 common health problems

Reader's Digest

DISEASE FREE

Writers Debra Gordon, Timothy Gower, Sari Harrar, Alice Kelly

Project Editor Liz Connolly

Recipe Editor Zoe Harpham

Project Designer Clare Forte

Proofreader Kevin Diletti

Indexer Diane Harriman

Senior Production Controller Monique Tesoriero

READER'S DIGEST GENERAL BOOKS

Editorial Director Elaine Russell

Managing Editor Rosemary McDonald

Art Director Carole Orbell

NOTE TO READERS
The information in this book should not be substituted for, or used to alter, medical therapy without your doctor's advice. For a specific health problem, consult your doctor for guidance. The mention of any products, retail businesses or websites in this book does not imply or constitute an endorsement by the authors or by The Reader's Digest (Australia) Pty Limited.

Disease Free is published by Reader's Digest (Australia) Pty Limited, 80 Bay Street, Ultimo, NSW 2007

www.readersdigest.com.au;
www.readersdigest.co.nz;
www.readersdigest.co.za

This book was originated by the editorial team of The Reader's Digest Association, Inc, USA in 2009

This edition first published 2010

Copyright © Reader's Digest (Australia) Pty Limited 2010
Copyright © Reader's Digest Association Far East Limited 2010
Phillippines Copyright © Reader's Digest Association Far East Limited 2010

All rights reserved. Unauthorised reproduction, in any manner, is prohibited. No part of this book may be reproduced, stored in a retrieval system, or transmitted in any form or by any means, electronic, electrostatic, magnetic tape, mechanical photocopying, recording or otherwise, without permission in writing from the publishers.

Reader's Digest and The Digest are registered trademarks of The Reader's Digest Association, Inc.

National Library of Australia Cataloguing-in-publication data:
Disease Free: proven ways to help prevent more than 75 common health problems.
Includes index
ISBN: 9781921569609 (h/b)
ISBN: 9781921743184 (p/b)
1. Medicine, preventive.
613

Prepress by Sinnott Bros, Sydney
Printed and bound by Leo Paper, China

We are interested in receiving your comments on the content of this book. Write to:

The Editor, General Books Editorial,
Reader's Digest (Australia) Pty Limited,
GPO Box 4353, Sydney, NSW 2001,
or email us at bookeditors.au@readersdigest.com

To order additional copies of *Disease Free* call 1300 300 030 (Australia), 0800 400 060 (New Zealand) or 0800 980 572 (South Africa) or email us at customerservice@au.readersdigest.com

Picture credits
Exercise Photography Jill Wachter
Food Photography Tara Donne
Additional Photography courtesy of Jupiter Images, RD Publications, Veer, Getty Images, iStockphoto and Shutterstock
Illustrations Bryan Christie Design

CHIEF CONSULTANT FOR AUSTRALIA AND NEW ZEALAND

Kathy Kramer MBBS, BSc (Med) (Hons), BA

CONSULTANT FOR SOUTH AFRICA

Judy Beyer

CONSULTANTS AND CONTRIBUTORS

Graham Colditz MD, DrPH, Niess-Gain Professor in the School of Medicine, Department of Surgery; Associate Director Prevention and Control, Alvin J Siteman Cancer Center, Washington University School of Medicine

Andrea Fagiolini MD, Associate Professor of Psychiatry, University of Pittsburgh School of Medicine

Steven R Feldman MD, PhD, Professor of Dermatology, Pathology and Public Health Sciences, Wake Forest University Health Sciences

David R Friedland MD, PhD, Associate Professor, Otology and Neuro-otologic Skull Base Surgery, Department of Otolaryngology and Communication Sciences, Medical College of Wisconsin

Leonard G Gomella MD, FACS, The Bernard W Godwin Professor of Prostate Cancer; Chairman, Department of Urology; Associate Director of Clinical Affairs, Jefferson Kimmel Cancer Center, Thomas Jefferson University

David L Katz MD, Associate Clinical Professor, Public Health and Medicine, Yale University School of Medicine

Robert B Kelly MD, MS, Associate Professor of Family Medicine, Case Western Reserve University School of Medicine

Wendy Klein MD, FACP, Associate Professor Emeritus of Medicine, Obstetrics and Gynecology, Virginia Commonwealth University School of Medicine; Senior Deputy Director, VCU Institute for Women's Health

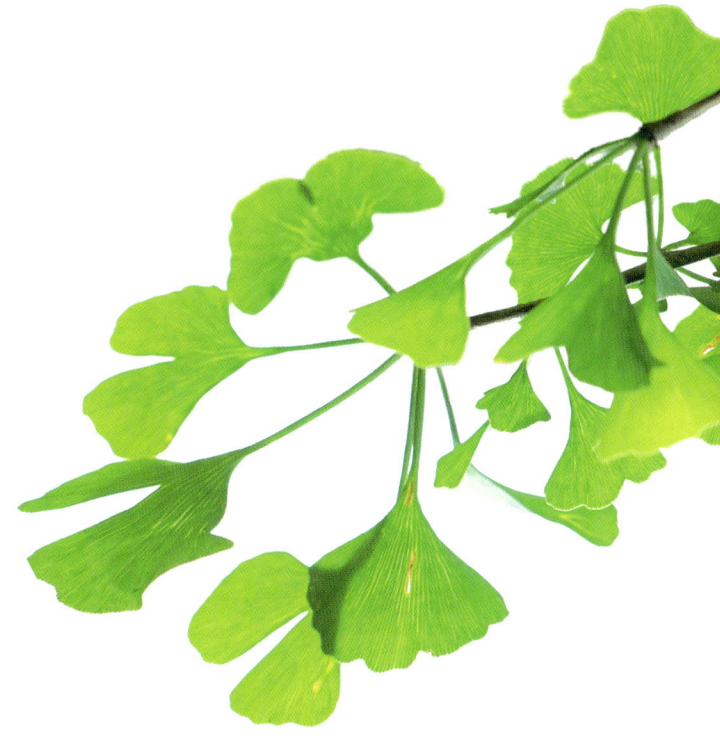

Michelle Lee MD, Assistant Professor of Clinical Medicine, Columbia University

JoAnn E Manson MD, DrPH, Chief, Division of Preventive Medicine, Brigham and Women's Hospital; Professor of Medicine and the Elizabeth F Brigham Professor of Women's Health, Harvard Medical School

Daniel Muller MD, PhD, Associate Professor of Medicine, University Wisconsin-Madison

Gerard E Mullin MD, Division of Gastroenterology and Liver Disease, Johns Hopkins Hospital

Donald L Price MD, Professor of Pathology, Neurology and Neuroscience Director, Division of Neuropathology, Director, Alzheimer's Disease Research Center, The Johns Hopkins University School of Medicine

Christopher Randolph MD, Associate Clinical Professor at Yale Division of Allergy

Elizabeth A Stewart MD, Professor of Obstetrics and Gynecology, Division of Reproductive Endocrinology, Mayo Clinic and Mayo Medical School

Contents

Disease-free living

Healthy choices for a longer life **10**

   Quiz: is your health on track? **18**

What causes disease? **20**

   Symptoms you should never ignore **34**

Key steps to disease prevention **60**

Safeguarding your health **80**

Disease and major symptom prevention

Acne **94**
Allergies **96**
Alzheimer's disease **100**
Anxiety **104**
Arthritis **106**
Asthma **114**
Back pain **118**
Benign prostatic hyperplasia **128**
Bladder cancer **130**
Breast cancer **132**
Bursitis and tendonitis **134**
Carpal tunnel syndrome **136**
Cataracts **142**
Cervical cancer **144**
Colds **146**
Colorectal cancer **148**
Congestive heart failure **152**
Constipation **154**
Coronary artery disease **156**
Depression **160**
Diabetes **164**

Diverticular disease **168**
Dry eyes **172**
Eczema **174**
Emphysema and chronic bronchitis **178**
Erectile dysfunction **180**
Fatigue **182**
Flatulence **184**
Flu **186**
Gallstones **188**
Glaucoma **190**
Gout **192**
Gum disease **194**
Haemorrhoids **196**
Headaches **198**
Hearing loss **200**
Heartburn and GORD **202**
Hepatitis **206**
Herpes simplex **208**
High blood pressure **210**
High cholesterol **214**
Hot flushes **218**

Incontinence 220
Infertility 222
Inflammatory bowel disease 224
Insomnia 228
Irritable bowel syndrome 232
Jaw pain 236
Kidney disease 238
Kidney stones 240
Knee pain 242
Lung cancer 244
Macular degeneration 246
Menstrual problems 248
Migraines 252
Mouth ulcers 254
Neck pain 256
Obesity 260
Osteoporosis 264
Ovarian cancer 270
Peripheral vascular disease 272
Premenstrual syndrome 274
Prostate cancer 276

Psoriasis 280
Rosacea 282
Sexually transmissible infections 284
Shingles 286
Sinusitis and sinus infections 288
Skin cancer 290
Snoring 292
Stomach bugs 296
Stomach cancer 300
Stomach ulcers 302
Stroke 304
Thrush 308
Tinea 310
Tinnitus 312
Urinary tract infections 314
Varicose veins 316

Recipes for good health

Eat well to live longer 320
Breakfast 322
Salads 324
Soups 332
Chicken 335
Meat 339
Fish and seafood 344
Meatless mains 350
Sides 360
Baked goods 364
Desserts 369

Index 378

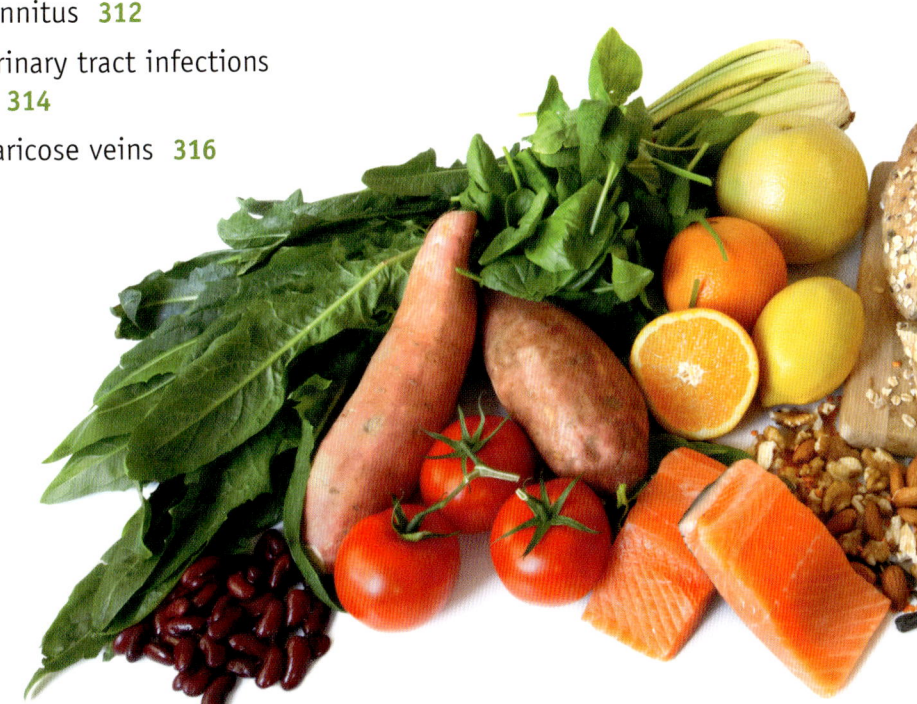

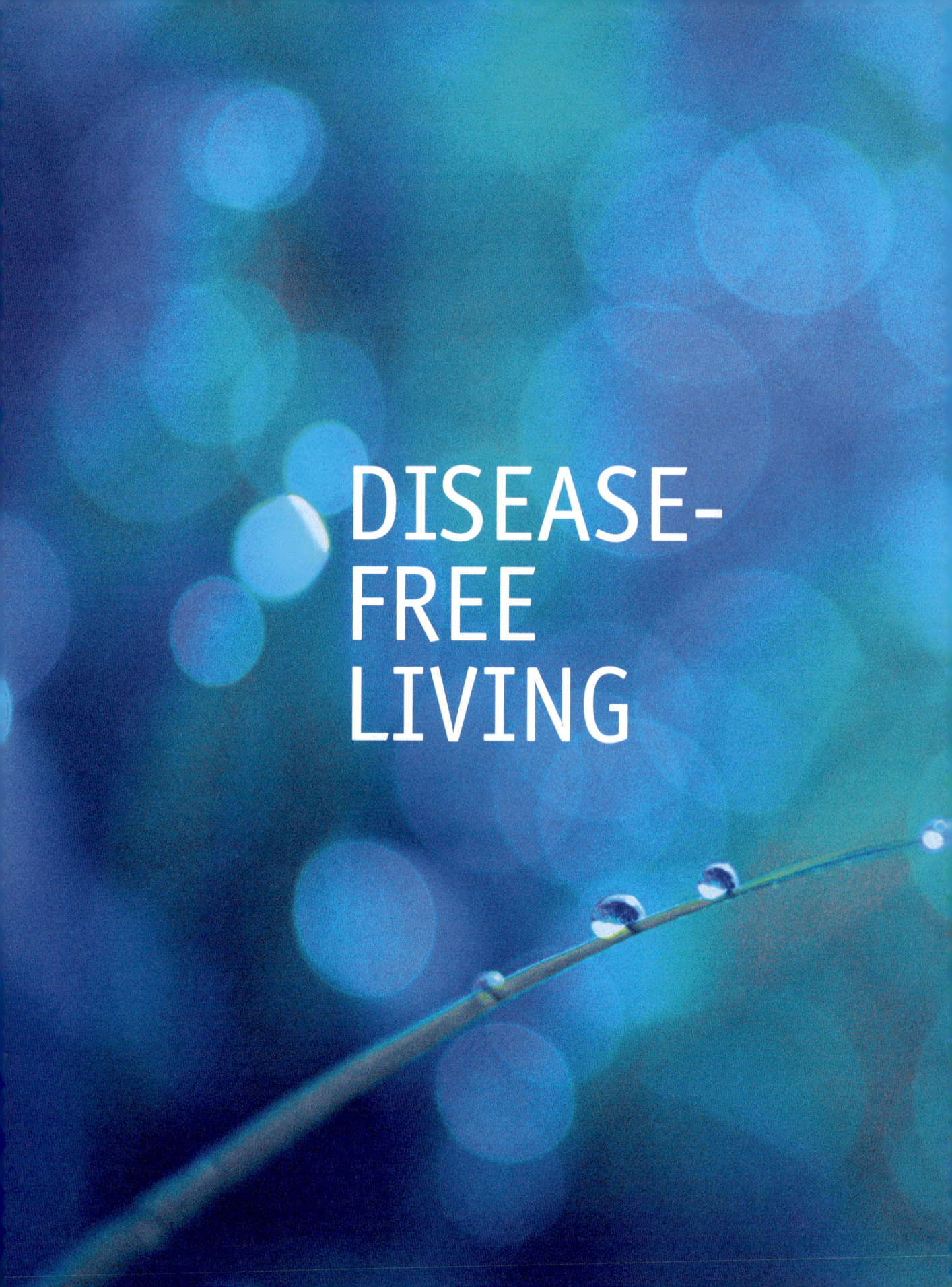
DISEASE-FREE LIVING

Whoever said 'life is short' didn't realise just how long you can live—and how well—when you're free of illness. Fortunately, the good life is also a healthy one.

Healthy choices for a longer life

What if you were told that it's well within your grasp to live an extra decade? We're not talking about 10 years of wheeling around an oxygen cylinder, withering away in a nursing home or even using multiple prescription medications to keep you going, but about *really* living. Travelling or learning another language, pursuing a new hobby (one that keeps you young) or extending your career. Playing with your great-grandchildren or fulfilling other dreams. If you stay disease free, it's not just possible—it's likely.

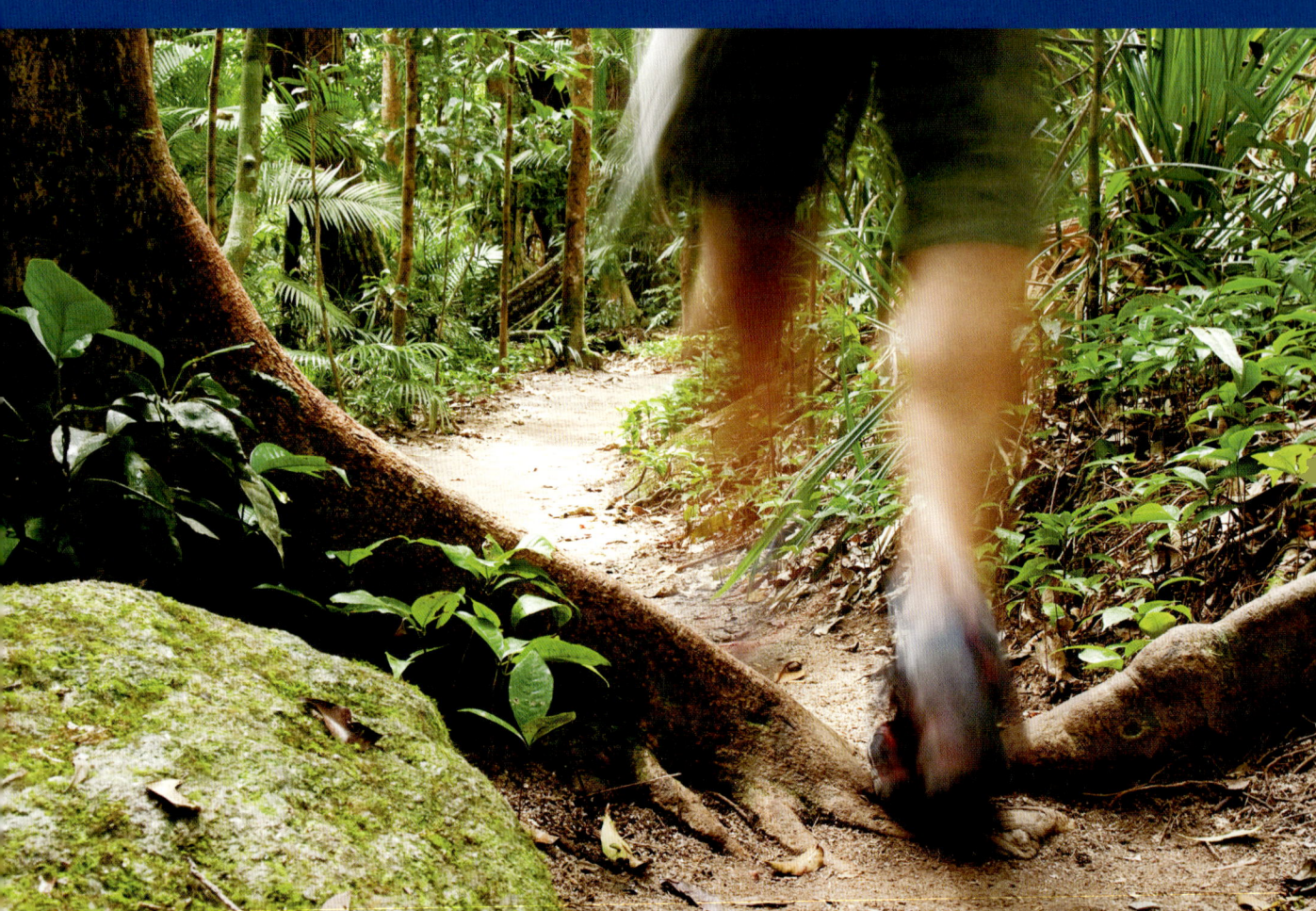

You hold the power

About half of all adults live with one or more chronic conditions, but the diseases people face today are almost entirely preventable. In creating this book, more than 100 doctors specialising in preventive medicine were surveyed by Reader's Digest in the US, and asked a raft of questions relating to chronic diseases and how to avoid them. More than half the doctors in this Disease Prevention Survey said that at least 60 per cent of cases of chronic disease could be avoided.

The upshot of this is that the power you hold to prevent disease and live a long healthy life is nothing short of amazing. One 2008 US study of more than 2000 men found that those who met four simple criteria—they didn't smoke, weren't overweight, exercised regularly and consumed alcohol in moderation, if at all—lived an average of 10 years longer than men who didn't fit at least one of these descriptions—and 10 years of good health at that. More than two-thirds of the men who lived to 90 rated their late-life health as either excellent or very good. And, based on this knowledge, it's reasonable to surmise that the men who lived longer were also happier; you'll find out more about the connection between health and emotional wellbeing later on.

The men in the study didn't do anything outrageous to protect themselves from disease, and you don't have to either, regardless of whether you're male or female. In fact, doing just one thing—getting half an hour of exercise on most days—could dramatically turn your health around and strengthen your resistance to disease. (The experts we polled told us that if you do only one thing for your health, besides quitting smoking, that should be it.) Is living longer and sidestepping crippling conditions like heart disease and diabetes worth a small investment in your time? That's up to you, of course, but it's very hard to see how it isn't.

You may already be taking positive steps to help prevent disease. Do you take an aspirin daily, with your doctor's approval? Did you get a flu shot this year? Have you scheduled your next Pap smear? Study after study confirms that each of these steps saves lives. In 'Key steps to disease prevention', starting on page 60, you'll learn which of these steps rated highest in the survey. All of the steps outlined in that chapter can be seen as a simple 'action guide' for living a healthier life. But first, a few highlights of the survey and our own research.

Your life, your health

Our understanding of what causes chronic disease has radically changed over the past decade. Even as researchers discover more and more links between genetic abnormalities and certain health conditions, it's clearer than ever that the underlying causes of most chronic diseases are lifestyle factors we can control.

For some of us, the initial response to that statement is: 'How can I help or prevent heart disease or diabetes when I have a strong family history?' 'What if I come from a long line of

Say goodbye to disease

The doctors we polled listed the following eight diseases as those that can be virtually eliminated with the right lifestyle measures.

- Chronic obstructive pulmonary disease
- Type 2 diabetes
- Emphysema
- Heart disease
- High blood pressure
- Lung cancer
- Obesity
- Stroke

people who had cancer, heart disease or diabetes?' 'What good is eating salads and exercising like mad going to do if I was dealt a lousy hand of genes at birth?'

These are fair questions, but the science is indisputable: genes may increase your risk for certain conditions, but lifestyle choices have a far greater impact on your health and longevity. Imagine the factors that determine your life span depicted in a pie chart. Studies of identical twins, who share identical genes, suggest that DNA dictates only 25 to 33 per cent of how long you live, or one-quarter to one-third of the pie. The rest? That depends on how you live.

Unfortunately, or fortunately, depending on how you look at it, the way we live—what we eat, the amount of stress we're under, what we do or don't do with our leisure time—is the reason so many of us gather health issues as we age.

The 'new' causes of disease

In the Disease Prevention Survey (see page 11), the number-one cause of chronic disease wasn't bad genes; it wasn't even high cholesterol. It was something many people assume is relatively harmless: high blood pressure, which is why it's often called the silent killer. Fortunately, it's a condition that most doctors listed as one that many people could avoid developing in the first place. If you have untreated high blood pressure, now is the time to deal with it.

Also ranked above genes and high cholesterol in the Disease Prevention Survey was something you might find more or less right under your nose: intra-abdominal fat, the kind of fat that lies deep within the belly, padding internal organs and contributing to everything from diabetes to heart attack. If you have a large waistline, you probably have this type of fat (see page 24 for more in-depth details).

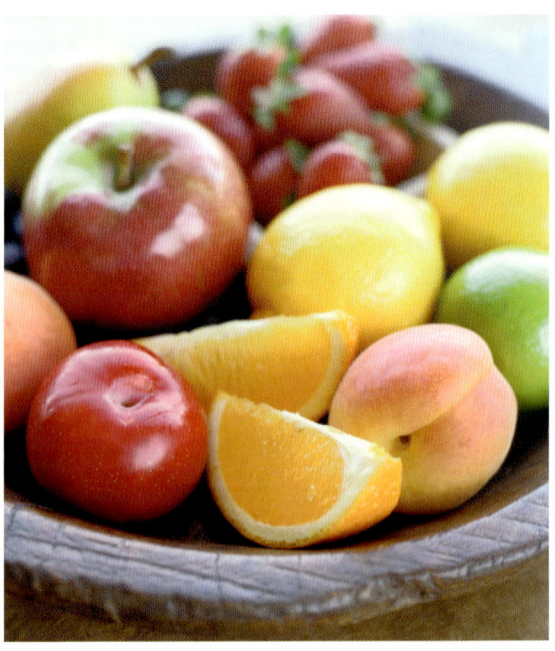

If you're overweight, there's a pretty good chance you have another high-ranking disease risk: insulin resistance, in which the body no longer effectively uses the hormone insulin to transport blood sugar into muscle cells. The most likely explanation for the current wave of insulin resistance is our sedentary lifestyle habits and the foods that many of us tend to favour, including potatoes, white rice, white bread and sugary processed foods—all of which raise blood sugar quickly, and essentially begin to wear out the insulin response. It's a major leap down the path to diabetes, but it's also turning out to contribute to heart attack, stroke and poor circulation.

All three of these root causes—high blood pressure, intra-abdominal fat and insulin resistance—are linked to chronic heart disease, the leading cause of death in the developed world. But they have something else in common: their solutions. If all of us lost weight, exercised more often and ate more fruit and vegetables, all three conditions would be drastically reduced in a relatively short amount of time.

The 'new' keys to health

Although the basic messages about good health haven't changed, we found a new health message in the survey, one that has nothing to do with food or exercise and everything to do with the people we share (or don't share) our lives with.

The experts who answered our survey made it clear that having positive relationships was intimately connected to health. In the survey, 79 per cent of the doctors polled said that being socially isolated was to the 'utmost detriment' of or 'extremely detrimental' to health. And they rated having 'happy interactions with friends and family' above 'cutting most saturated fat from your diet' as prevention strategies.

One reason why family and friends may be so important is because they help combat stress and depression. And many doctors mentioned stress as a contributing factor in major disease. They ranked it as even more dangerous than being 15 kg overweight. It's not surprising that more than half the doctors advocated meditation or other stress-relief techniques as extremely beneficial to health. It's also interesting that depression was ranked significantly higher than high cholesterol as a condition with the greatest potential for causing chronic disease.

Simply put, what happens in your mind and heart (the figurative one this time) affects your body in profound ways. Chronic stress lowers the immune system's ability to function effectively—even making vaccines less effective. It raises levels of stress hormones, such as cortisol, and while high cortisol levels can keep you up at night, they can also raise blood pressure, contribute to high blood sugar and increase intra-abdominal fat.

There's also the more obvious effect that stress, depression and loneliness has on us every day. As one doctor put it, 'Mental stress and conflict, etc., drive the majority of bad physical habits and practices'—in other words, getting too little sleep, being too sedentary and eating too many kilojoules, especially in the form of junk food.

Chronic stress also raises the risk of depression, and if you're depressed the chances are you're not going to exercise or eat well. Depression often goes hand in hand with a whole litany of diseases, from heart disease to cancer, and doctors aren't always sure which causes which.

Surprising advice from the prevention experts

Staying healthy is not all about eating a suitable volume of fruit and vegetables, although that obviously helps. In the Disease Prevention Survey, the following advice convinced us that health really does originate from a life well lived.

'Believe in something good.'

'Focus on a higher sense of purpose.'

'Develop your unique potential.'

'Eat less, exercise more and have fun.'

'Love the ones you're with (spouse, children, extended family, neighbours, colleagues).'

'Achieve balance in your life.'

'Exercise every day, eat a well-balanced diet, maintain meaningful social interactions and relationships, and choose work that is important to you.'

'Find meaning in your life.'

'Get 8 hours or more of sleep a day.'

'Manage stress and enjoy your friends.'

'Stay positive and have a family doctor who helps you to prevent disease and improve health.'

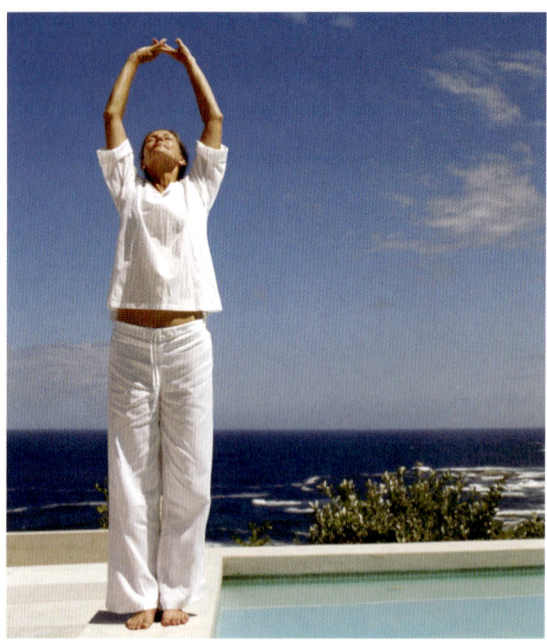

But they do know that having depression and a serious illness tends to make the symptoms of that illness considerably worse.

Considering the known dangers of stress and depression, it's little surprise that many doctors in the survey advocated relaxation techniques such as meditation and happy daily interactions with others. It's important to find something meaningful or fulfilling to do in life, or to believe in a higher sense of purpose to both take our minds off our worries and to provide inspiration for daily life. Many doctors know that it can be just as important as taking regular medication.

It can be difficult to know the answer to the question of whether you are connected to others in a meaningful way, so ask yourself: 'Do I have people I can turn to?', 'Do I get up every day with a sense of optimism or purpose?' or 'Do I dread my to-do list or feel nothing much at all because, in truth, I lost the sense of what was possible many years ago?'. It's never too late to get interested in something new or to reach out and make personal connections with others.

Getting yourself to act

People who exercise and eat well tend to live a long time, often surviving others by up to a decade or more. So why don't more of us get moving? Because it can be hard to get started if exercise has never been a regular habit. Chances are that choosing just one healthy habit to adopt, or one bad habit to quit, will make you feel good both physically and emotionally—good enough to want to choose another. On pages 18–19, the quiz will help you identify your current habits.

It also helps to stop and think of the trouble you'll save yourself by preventing a disease rather than waiting until you need treatment.

Remember that prevention is better than cure

When Benjamin Franklin said that 'An ounce of prevention is worth a pound of cure', he was actually cautioning homeowners to protect their properties against fire. But that comment bears an interesting correlation with your health: when you get sick, you place yourself in the hands of the healthcare system, which does save lives, but it also makes some people sicker. Think about the side effects caused by taking multiple prescription medications and the dangers associated with a hospital stay, not to mention the expense and inconvenience of it all.

For many people, taking medication is as much a part of daily routine as brushing their teeth. One South Australian study showed that 47 per cent of the population used at least one prescription medication, and 5 per cent took six or more. However, some medications, such as aspirin and cholesterol-lowering statins, may form part of your disease-prevention plan. But virtually all medications, even seemingly harmless ones, can produce unwanted side effects.

One example is medication for high blood pressure, which affects about a billion people worldwide. Only about one-third of people who take medication for this condition are able to bring their blood pressure into the safe zone. One well-documented reason is that many people stop taking medication. Some can't afford the cost, while others can't tolerate the side effects, which can include dry cough, swollen extremities, erectile dysfunction, headache, dizziness, fatigue, nausea and vomiting, among others. One study found that nearly 70 per cent of people taking calcium channel blockers developed unpleasant side effects.

A 2008 analysis concluded that there was little proof that widely used antidepressants such as fluoxetine (Prozac) and paroxetine (Aropax) offer any benefit to people with moderate depression. And another recent study showed that the widely prescribed cholesterol-lowering medication ezetimibe (Ezetrol) may not keep arteries clear of heart-stopping plaque.

Meanwhile, regular exercise, a happy personal life and a healthy, balanced diet appear to help prevent both depression and high cholesterol in many people.

It's been said that a hospital is no place for sick people, and it's true. In 2007, an estimated 0.2 per cent of all deaths in Australia were caused by complications of medical or surgical care, including medications. And in one study from a Victorian hospital, one in 14 patients suffered an 'adverse event' during their hospital stay.

In the US, between 5 and 10 per cent of hospital patients acquire one or more infections during their stay, and the risk of hospital-acquired infection is rising rapidly. Simple urinary tract infections are the most common variety, but hospitals the world over are increasingly plagued by 'super-bugs' such as MRSA (methicillin-resistant *Staphylococcus aureus*), the staph infection immune to standard antibiotics. It can cause pneumonia and other life-threatening infections.

All this news could make even the most die-hard armchair sportsman skip the takeaway and eat a bowl of porridge, walk briskly for an extra

Then and now

Available statistics from a century ago show us that people were most likely to die from an infectious disease. But improved hygiene and sanitation later prevented many premature deaths from diseases such as tuberculosis. Today, the diseases that kill us are largely caused by the way we live.

TOP CAUSES OF DEATH IN THE US IN 1900	TOP CAUSES OF DEATH IN AUSTRALIA TODAY
1. Pneumonia/influenza	1. Heart disease
2. Tuberculosis	2. Stroke
3. Diarrhoea, enteritis and ulceration of the intestines	3. Lung cancer
4. Diseases of the heart	4. Dementia and Alzheimer's disease
5. Intracranial lesions of vascular origin (caused by stroke)	5. Chronic lower respiratory diseases (such as chronic bronchitis and emphysema)
6. Nephritis (inflammation of the kidney)	6. Colon and rectal cancer
7. Accidents	7. Diabetes
8. Cancer and other malignant tumours	8. Blood and lymph cancer, including leukaemia
9. Senility	9. Heart failure
10. Diphtheria	10. Kidney disease

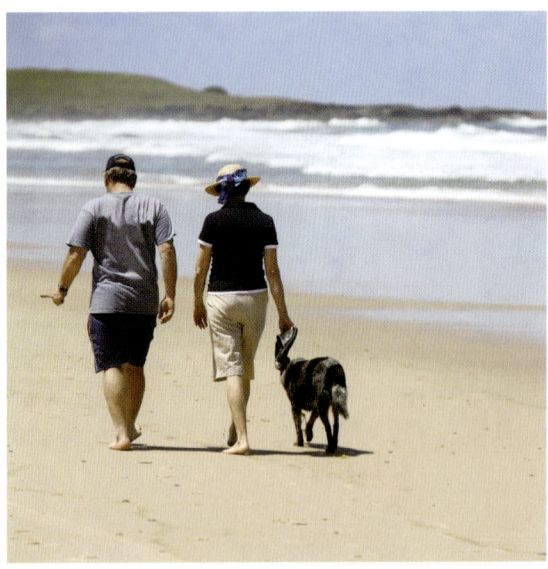

10 minutes, and take other steps to avoid the healthcare system—not to mention a traumatic event such as heart attack or stroke.

Decide to be healthy

That's the sum of it: good health is a goal you can either reach for or ignore. Only you can decide for yourself whether or not your health is a priority. If you don't make any effort to eat well, exercise or control stress, you've decided that it's not, even if you don't think about it that way. But it's never too late to change your mind.

When asked about other significant causes of chronic disease, one doctor wrote, 'Foolish behaviour, even when the patient knows better', which accounts for many cases of poor health. Most of us have an idea of what it takes to stay healthy; we just don't always bother to do it.

The solution for changing old, bad habits isn't always immediately obvious. One solution, suggested by a doctor polled for the survey, was to 'Rely on your inner strength to change your ways'. And the source of that strength will be different for everyone. Perhaps your children or grandchildren make you want to live a longer, healthier life. Maybe you can use the 'you can do it' attitude that made you a success in your career to help transform your lifestyle. Or think of a friend or relative who has struggled with the difficulties of an ongoing illness or condition. You may know first-hand the toll that being sick takes on your mental health, your will to live and your bank balance, and that may be motivation enough to make a few changes in your life. Consider the health problems your parents experienced, and perhaps even died from, and promise yourself that you will try to avoid the same fate. Your health, to a large extent, is up to you, although it's also true that some diseases are unpreventable in some people.

The bulk of this book is geared towards helping you reduce your risk for conditions you're particularly worried about or may be susceptible to. Following our advice in 'Key steps to disease prevention' starting on page 60 will go a long way towards making you less disease prone, but for even more detailed risk-reduction strategies from specific conditions that concern you, turn to the entry outlining that disease or major symptom in Part two.

Working with your doctor

Prevention sometimes gets neglected in doctors' surgeries, so it's up to you to take charge.

In general, healthcare systems are focused on the care and cure of diseases after they have manifested themselves—care that is sometimes delivered too late. There is far too little emphasis on preventing diseases in the first place, and our survey doctors loudly echoed that sentiment.

Studies show that many doctors fail to give even the most obvious prevention advice, such as telling overweight patients to lose weight or encouraging patients who smoke to quit. The fact is, doctors are paid to treat sick people—and that's what they're mainly trained for. Even if they wanted to give prevention advice—and many do—with consultations shorter than the time it takes to hard boil an egg, there just isn't time. According to a 2003 study published in the *American Journal of Public Health*, primary care doctors would need almost 8 hours every day to provide patients with the appropriate counselling, screening and immunisations that are recommended for the highest standard of medical care. Short of cloning themselves, that would also leave doctors insufficient time to take care of patients who are already sick. So it's partially up to you to ask questions and pay attention to prevention.

It's a two-way street, according to Laurel Yates, a doctor and lead author of the study involving men that was mentioned earlier (see page 11). She advocates that, although doctors should know about and practise preventive medicine, you as the patient must also play a part in knowing the importance of prevention, and make sure it's on the agenda.

Whenever you walk into your doctor's surgery, have a list of questions or problems to discuss, with the pressing preventive issues at the top. Raise your concerns at the beginning; never wait until the end of an appointment to start asking questions. Busy doctors can quickly become frustrated with people who say 'By the way, Doctor', with one foot out the door.

If you're already coping with a chronic condition, your doctor may need to spend most or all of a surgery visit discussing medications and other treatments. If you run out of time and don't get to talk about exercise, diet or other protective steps you could be taking, schedule another appointment to discuss this solely.

Make that time discussing these issues an essential element of your medical consultations.

Prevention is not a luxury, and rates of most chronic diseases are rising fast and could produce a healthcare crisis in the not-too-distant future. We're already acutely aware of waiting lists.

Remember, though, prevention is mainly about the things you do outside your doctor's surgery—what you make for dinner, how much time you spend being active in a positive way, whether you're an angry or a happy person. And it's up to you to take charge. As one doctor from the Disease Prevention Survey put it, 'Don't simply wait for health professionals to correct your health problems after they become obvious', because there is no one who can prevent disease and debilitating major symptoms better in people than they can themselves.

So it turns out the old cliché is true: an ounce of prevention is, indeed, worth a pound of cure. If your goal is to stay healthy through the years—and to have lots more of them—then the time to start getting your health on track is now.

Vaccines for adults

No matter how much you exercise and watch what you eat, any plan for disease-proofing your body needs a shot or two in the arm—literally, in some cases. The most obvious form of defence against disease you can seek in a doctor's surgery is a flu shot. In addition to the chills, aches and other miserable symptoms brought on by influenza, the condition can lead to life-threatening complications such as pneumonia. A flu shot cuts your risk by up to 90 per cent. If you haven't discussed vaccinations with your doctor before now, don't assume that you're up to date. You may also be eligible for one of several newer vaccines that guard against conditions such as pneumococcal disease, cervical cancer and shingles.

Quiz: is your health on track?

It's tempting to blame many health issues on genetic predisposition, but in most cases it's the way we live our day-to-day lives that ultimately determines what happens to our bodies—and whether or not we develop health problems that can deplete our energy and general zest for living.

The Reader's Digest Disease Prevention Survey polled more than 100 specialist doctors and, among other questions, asked them how beneficial or harmful they believed certain habits to be. Take this quiz to find out how they would rate your current health profile. If your lifestyle needs modifying to improve your odds of living disease-free, make sure you read 'Key steps to disease prevention', starting on page 60, to find out how you can do that.

Bad health habits

For each bad habit you have, note down the allotted number of crosses in the far right column.

Regularly eat foods containing trans fat (hydrogenated oil)	X X X
Regularly eat packaged goods, canned soups, chips and other processed foods high in sodium	X X X X
Add salt to food at most meals	X X X
Eat out (or have takeaway) more than three times a week	X X X X
Regularly drink more than two standard glasses of alcohol on any one day of the week	X X X
Eat white bread or white rice at most meals	X X X
Have a sweet dessert after dinner on most nights	X X X
Smoke regularly	X X X X X
Smoke a few occasional cigarettes	X X X X
Don't have regular contact with others	X X X X X
Live with frequent and uncontrolled stress	X X X X
Are more than 15 kg overweight	X X X X
Get less than 7 hours of sleep a night	X X X

Good health habits

For each healthy habit you can claim, note down the number of allotted ticks in the far right column.

■ Regularly eat seven serves of fruit and vegetables daily	✓ ✓ ✓ ✓ ✓
■ Have two or more serves of skim milk or low-fat yogurt daily	✓ ✓ ✓
■ Have no more than two standard drinks of alcohol on any day	✓ ✓ ✓
■ Get 20 to 30 minutes of moderate aerobic exercise on most days	✓ ✓ ✓ ✓ ✓
■ Do strength training two or three times a week	✓ ✓ ✓ ✓
■ Meditate or practise another stress-relief technique regularly	✓ ✓ ✓ ✓
■ Always wash your hands after using the bathroom and before cooking	✓ ✓ ✓ ✓ ✓
■ Brush your teeth and floss regularly	✓ ✓ ✓ ✓
■ Get an annual flu shot	✓ ✓ ✓ ✓
■ Have your blood pressure checked regularly	✓ ✓ ✓ ✓
■ Have your cholesterol levels checked regularly	✓ ✓ ✓

Your final score

Add up your bad and good health habits, then subtract the total number of bad habits from the total good habits to get your final score, then see below to interpret the results.

Over 20: Excellent Congratulations! You're living a life that will help to keep you disease-free.

14 to 20: Good Your lifestyle is reasonably healthy. Look for at least one more good habit to adopt and at least one bad habit to lose.

8 to 13: Average You're not doing badly, but there's still room for improvement. Look for a few more good habits to adopt and a few bad ones to lose.

0 to 7: Worrying You're getting by with a lifestyle that is healthy in part, but there's still room for improvement. Look back to see where you missed out on ticks and collected too many crosses.

-1 to -7: Dangerous It's time to take your health more seriously, before you're dealing with treating disease rather than preventing it. Some unhealthy habits are probably dragging down your score; look back to see where you can improve it.

-8 or lower: Very dangerous You're not looking to improve your health, and are clinging to some harmful habits. Start by making just one positive change at a time. Every step counts.

What causes disease?

The Disease Prevention Survey results revealed what over 100 specialist doctors believed caused disease at the most basic level. Here the top six culprits are revealed and the way that they cause serious disease is explained. And in the tables following, the most common symptoms that people often experience are outlined, along with which ones should *never* be ignored, and how to act accordingly.

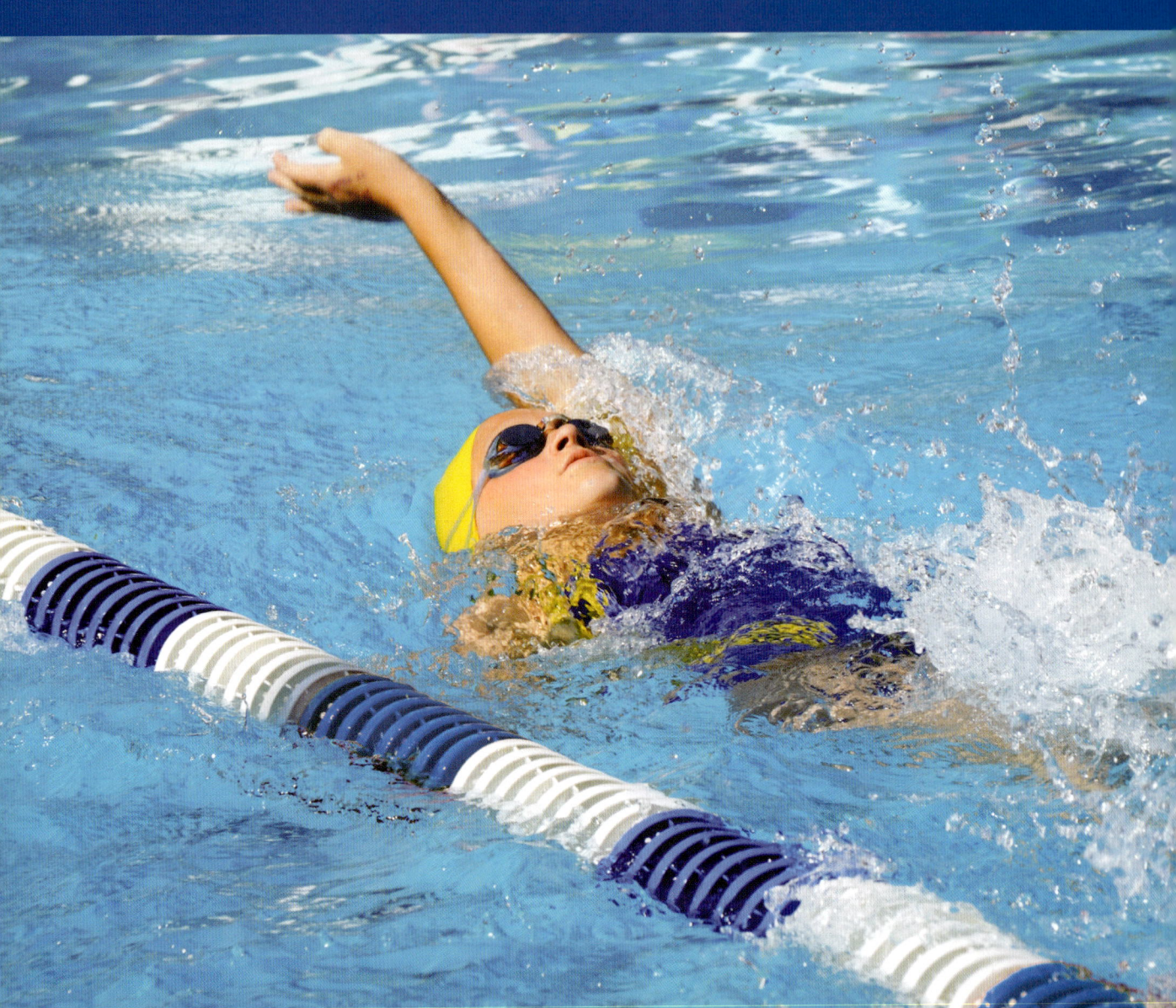

The inside story

As far as the human body goes, for every effect there is a cause. And for every symptom you experience there is a pathological process going on within your body, or in the brain, that can be studied. Not all of these processes are fully understood, especially ones involving the brain, but for the most common major diseases we have a clear idea of the overall picture, and of what happens to the organs and cells involved.

In this chapter, the top six pathological processes leading to chronic disease are looked at in detail so that you can get a better idea of what's going on inside your body. These processes are caused, to a large extent, by our lifestyle choices and they, in turn, lead to disease. One of the most significant of these processes is high blood pressure, which often results in heart attack and stroke, among many other problems.

Intra-abdominal fat is linked to diabetes and colon cancer; depression increases the risk of heart disease and cancer; insulin resistance contributes to a variety of cardiovascular and other disorders; and a bad cholesterol ratio can spell disaster for arteries and blood circulation. And inflammation is a process that can increase your risk for a host of chronic conditions, including Alzheimer's disease.

We look at what causes these pathological processes, describe what happens inside your body and explain why they can be so damaging to your health. We also give you practical prevention strategies from top medical experts so that you can start making positive changes to reduce your risk of developing these disease-causing problems in the first place, and improving, or even reversing, their negative effects if one or more of them is already active in your body.

If you need another reason to get active and eat a healthy diet, remember that it's not only your major organs that are affected, it's also your brain and its ability to function normally. Changing bad habits will improve physical health and also preserve your memory and mental clarity.

Jogging, swimming and other forms of aerobic exercise—essential to any disease-prevention plan—appear to protect the brain, too. One study of nearly 19,000 women found that the most active participants were the least likely to show signs of memory loss or clouded thinking. Studying, reading and other mental challenges are also linked to a lower risk of dementia. And the same is true of coping with emotional stress.

The tables starting on page 34 describe symptoms you should never ignore, explain the most probable causes underlying those symptoms and advise when to seek medical help. But, as always, if you're ever in doubt see your doctor.

Emergency phone numbers

	AUSTRALIA	**NEW ZEALAND**	**SOUTH AFRICA**
Ambulance	Dial 000	Dial 111	Dial 10177
International emergency number for GSM mobile networks	112	112	112
Poisons information	131 126	0800 764 766	Call your nearest Poison and Drug Information Centre

Disease-free living

CAUSE 1

High blood pressure

What is it?

Blood pressure is the force of blood against the walls of your arteries. If your arteries are healthy, they expand and contract easily with every heartbeat, keeping pressure low. But if blood vessels grow stiff, they don't expand as easily and blood pressure rises, just as a wide, lazy river becomes a raging torrent when channelled into a narrow valley. (Stiff blood vessels are both a cause and an effect of high blood pressure.) Pre-hypertension begins at a reading of 120/80 mmHg; hypertension (high blood pressure) begins at 140/90 mmHg.

High blood pressure makes the layer of muscle inside blood vessel walls grow thicker. This narrows the arteries, raising the risk that a blood clot will completely block an artery and cause a heart attack or stroke.

LDL CHOLESTEROL

WHITE BLOOD CELL

PLAQUE BUILDUP

Fast-moving blood damages the delicate layer of cells that line artery walls. Damaged artery walls are magnets for white blood cells and LDL cholesterol, which accumulate and form heart-threatening plaque.

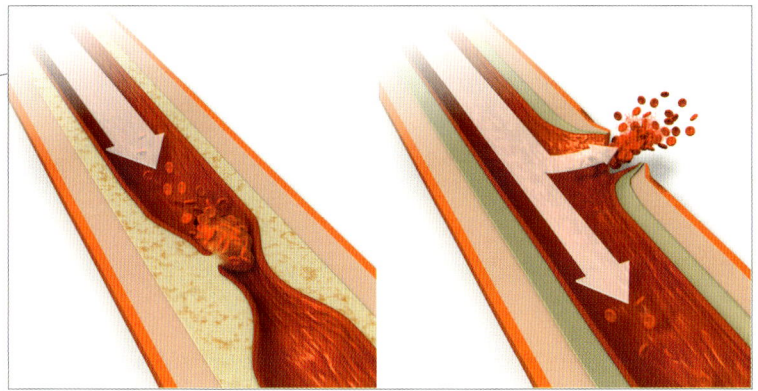

High blood pressure can make blood vessels in your brain grow narrow and weak, raising your risk of two kinds of stroke. A blood clot can block blood flow, causing an ischaemic stroke (at left), or an artery may rupture, causing a haemorrhagic stroke (at right).

As arteries narrow, the heart works harder and the left ventricle grows bigger. But a bigger heart can't expand fully or fill completely with blood, so it becomes less efficient at pumping, raising your risk of a heart attack, sudden cardiac death and congestive heart failure.

What causes it?

Family history, advancing age, diabetes, being male and being indigenous all increase risk. So do smoking, being overweight, stress, lack of exercise, eating foods high in salt and saturated fat, and skimping on fruit and vegetables and dairy products. Many of these risk factors contribute to high blood pressure in part by reducing production of nitric oxide, a chemical that makes blood vessels flexible.

Why is it dangerous?

It makes artery walls thicker, narrower, stiffer and weaker, which means less blood, oxygen and nutrients get to your organs. And blood clots are more likely to get stuck in narrowed arteries, which can trigger a heart attack, a stroke or peripheral vascular disease. Blood vessel damage can also raise your risk of dementia, kidney failure, vision problems and even blindness.

TOP PREVENTION STRATEGIES

▸ **STOP SMOKING** if you haven't already.

▸ **EXERCISE** to lower blood pressure and lose weight.

▸ **SKIP** high-sodium processed foods and avoid adding salt to food.

▸ **EAT MORE** fruit, vegetables, low-fat dairy products and foods high in potassium.

CAUSE 2

Intra-abdominal fat

What is it?

Fat packed deep within the abdomen, in and around your internal organs. Women with waistline measurements of over 88 cm and men with measurements over 102 cm are likely to have it. (For people of Asian descent, risk rises with measurements over 80 cm for women and 95 cm for men.) A large waist measurement is dangerous even if your body weight is within the healthy range for your height. To measure your waist, wrap a tape measure snugly around your midsection at about belly-button height.

A high-kilojoule diet, lack of regular physical exercise and chronic stress all conspire to prompt your body to store dangerous fat around the liver, pancreas and other internal organs.

Intra-abdominal fat pumps free fatty acids and inflammatory compounds into the portal vein—the 'superhighway' delivering blood from your lower abdomen to the liver, pancreas and other internal organs.

What causes it?

Too many fatty foods, being sedentary and too much of all those other activities that keep you sitting down, such as working in front of a computer and driving. In other words, a diet high in kilojoules and a life devoid of exercise. Chronic stress plays a role, too, especially for women, since the stress hormone cortisol directs your body to store more fat in your abdomen.

An influx of free fatty acids causes your liver to produce more 'bad' LDL cholesterol, less 'good' HDL cholesterol, more blood sugar and less adiponectin, a hormone that regulates the use of blood sugar and keeps appetite in check. The result is that your risk of heart disease and diabetes rises.

What causes disease?

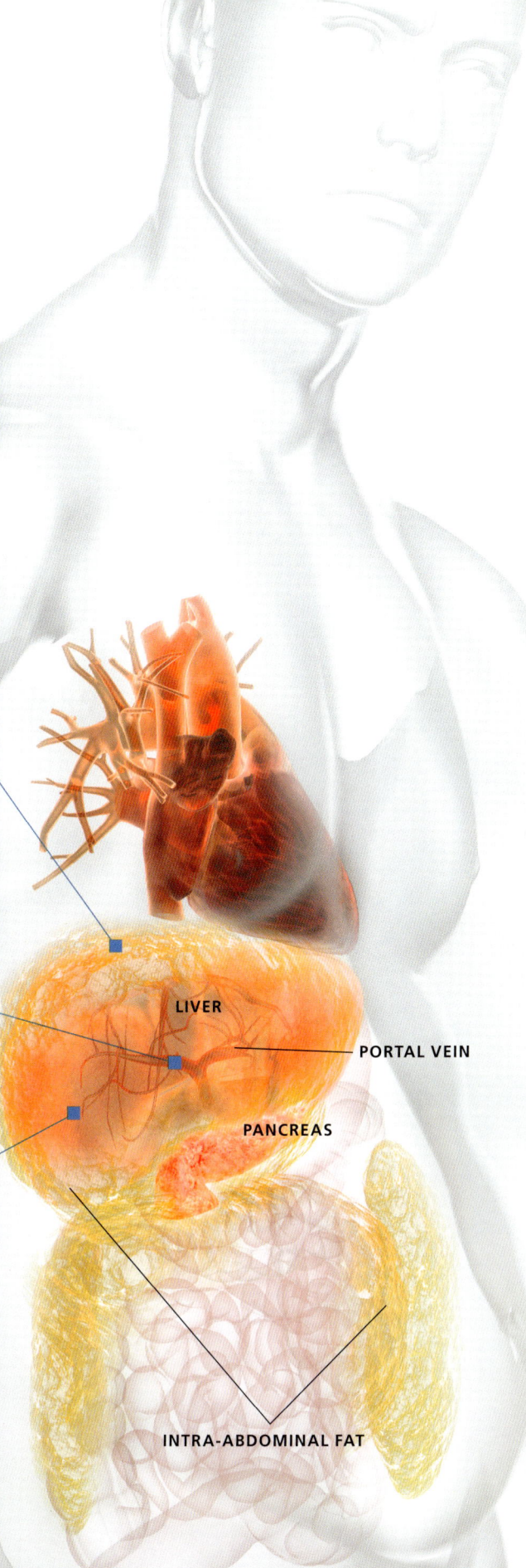

LIVER
PORTAL VEIN
PANCREAS
INTRA-ABDOMINAL FAT

Why is it dangerous?

Unlike the relatively harmless fat on your buttocks, hips, thighs and even just under the skin at your waist, intra-abdominal fat churns out substances that raise your risk of diabetes, high blood pressure, heart attack, stroke, colon cancer and even memory problems. These include inflammatory compounds that make blood stickier as well as free fatty acids that prompt your liver to produce more blood sugar and LDL ('bad') cholesterol.

The inflammatory compounds secreted by fat cells encourage the growth of plaque inside artery walls, boost blood pressure and make blood more likely to clot—all of which is a recipe for a heart attack. They also make cells resistant to insulin, which in turn contributes to diseases such as Alzheimer's and cancer.

TOP PREVENTION STRATEGIES

- **EAT MORE** fruit, vegetables and whole grains, and less saturated fat.
- **EXERCISE** to lower pressure and lose weight.
- **FIND TIME** to relax every day.
- **CORRECT** persistent snoring caused by obstructive sleep apnoea.

CAUSE 3

Depression

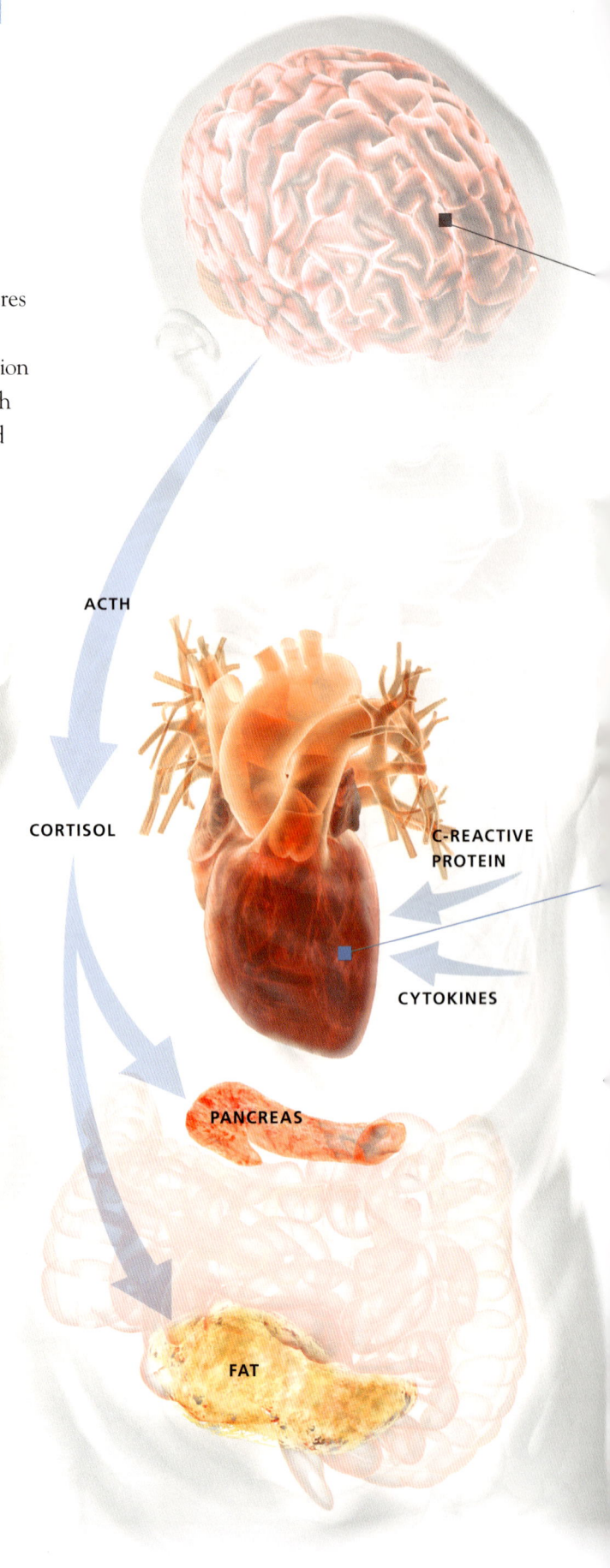

What is it?

More than a passing bad mood, depression interferes with your life, relationships, sense of yourself and health. It ranges from dysthymia—low-level depression that can last for years—to major depression, which can make working, performing daily activities and relating to your spouse, family and friends nearly impossible. Another type is seasonal affective disorder, which occurs only during certain times of the year (usually winter).

Depression releases a hormone called ACTH that increases levels of the stress hormone cortisol in the body. Extra cortisol may be the reason people with depression have higher rates of diabetes, because it reduces production of insulin in the pancreas, allowing blood sugar to rise. Cortisol also prompts the body to store more abdominal fat, which is a risk factor for many chronic diseases.

What causes it?

Often a combination of genetics, chronic stress and difficult life experiences. Levels of the neurotransmitters serotonin, dopamine and noradrenaline, which brain cells use to communicate with each other, may be out of balance. And areas of the brain that regulate mood, thought, sleep, appetite and behaviour may function abnormally.

What causes disease? 27

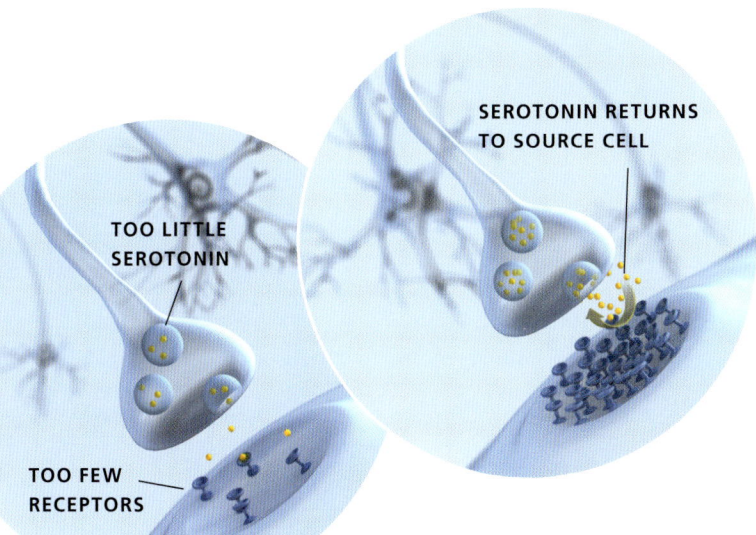

TOO LITTLE SEROTONIN

TOO FEW RECEPTORS

SEROTONIN RETURNS TO SOURCE CELL

If you are depressed, you may have abnormally low levels of the brain chemical serotonin. The brain may not produce enough serotonin, brain cells may not have enough receptors to receive it or it may bounce back instead of being delivered from cell to cell.

People with depression may have higher levels of C-reactive protein, an inflammatory compound linked with increased heart attack risk. Depression also increases the release of other inflammatory compounds, called cytokines, that fuel the growth of heart-threatening plaque in artery walls.

Why is it dangerous?

Serious depression may lead to suicide. Outside of this risk, depression often coexists with diabetes, heart disease, stroke, cancer and other major health conditions, making symptoms of these illnesses more severe and more difficult to manage. The combination can be fatal: people with diabetes and depression face a higher risk of dying from heart disease. According to new evidence, depression may even help trigger diabetes, heart disease and osteoporosis by raising levels of inflammation and stress hormones.

Depression raises the risk of osteoporosis and bone fractures. Research suggests that the mood disorder triggers production of the hormone noradrenaline in bones, which reduces the body's ability to maintain healthy bone density.

TOP PREVENTION STRATEGIES

- **SEEK** professional help as early as possible.
- **EXERCISE** regularly; studies show it can help prevent or lift depression.
- **RELIEVE STRESS** every day in whatever way works best for you.
- **CULTIVATE** a positive attitude.
- **CONNECT** with family and friends for social support whenever you can.

CAUSE 4: Insulin resistance

What is it?

When you eat, some of the food is turned into blood sugar (glucose), the body's main source of fuel. The pancreas responds by secreting the hormone insulin, which triggers cells throughout the body to allow sugar to enter. But when cells are insulin-resistant, they turn partially 'deaf' to insulin's signals. The pancreas turns up the volume by churning out more and more insulin.

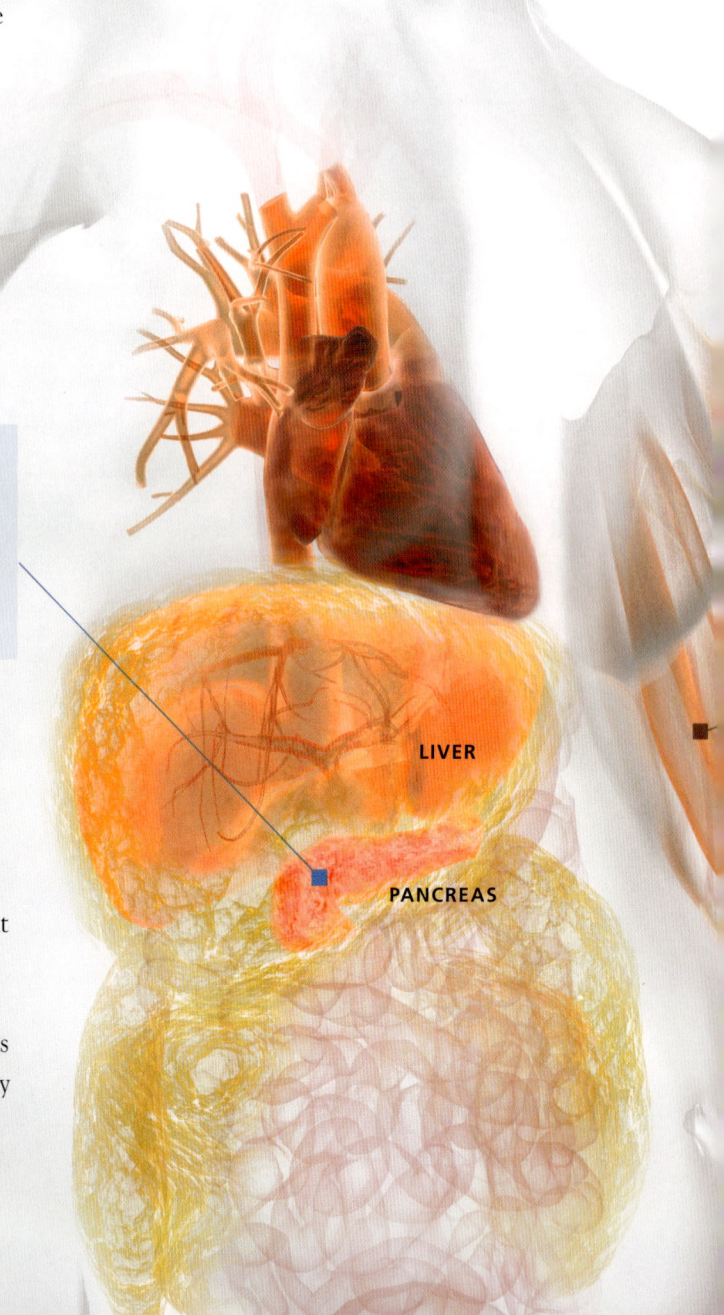

After a meal or snack, the pancreas secretes insulin to help sugar enter cells. The insulin finds its way to various cells in the body, especially muscle cells, which burn sugar for energy.

LIVER

PANCREAS

What causes it?

Scientists aren't exactly sure, but genetics, advancing age, lack of exercise and excess weight (especially intra-abdominal fat) play key roles. Diets high in saturated fat and simple carbohydrates also contribute, as do chronic infections (such as gum disease), which release inflammatory chemicals that interfere with chemical signals from insulin.

Why is it dangerous?

High insulin levels can damage blood vessels and trigger the liver to produce more heart-threatening triglycerides and LDL ('bad') cholesterol and less HDL ('good') cholesterol. They also increase the risk of blood clots and prompt the body to retain more sodium, raising blood pressure. Excess insulin may even spur the growth of some cancers and contribute to Alzheimer's disease. If your pancreas can't keep pace with your body's need for extra insulin, blood sugar levels may begin to rise after years or even decades of insulin resistance, resulting in diabetes.

Insulin binds to receptors on the cell, which triggers a series of chemical signals that allow molecules of sugar to be transported into the cell.

INSULIN

SUGAR (GLUCOSE)

DAMAGED INSULIN RECEPTOR

NORMAL INSULIN RECEPTOR

FATTY ACIDS

The result is the cell can't easily absorb the sugar, and the pancreas has to churn out extra insulin. Eventually, blood sugar levels may begin to rise.

In insulin resistance, some insulin receptors are damaged, so the signals don't get through. Signals may also get scrambled if a cell is packed with too many fatty acids (thanks to genetics and/or excess abdominal fat). Inflammatory chemicals released by belly fat and by chronic infections can also interfere with the signals.

TOP PREVENTION STRATEGIES

- **EXERCISE** on most days; exercise increases sensitivity to insulin.
- **CUT** kilojoules and reduce the amount of saturated fat in your diet.
- **LOSE** just 5 to 7 per cent of your body weight.
- **EAT MORE** fruit, vegetables and whole grains instead of refined grains and highly processed or sugary foods.

Disease-free living

CAUSE 5
Bad cholesterol ratio

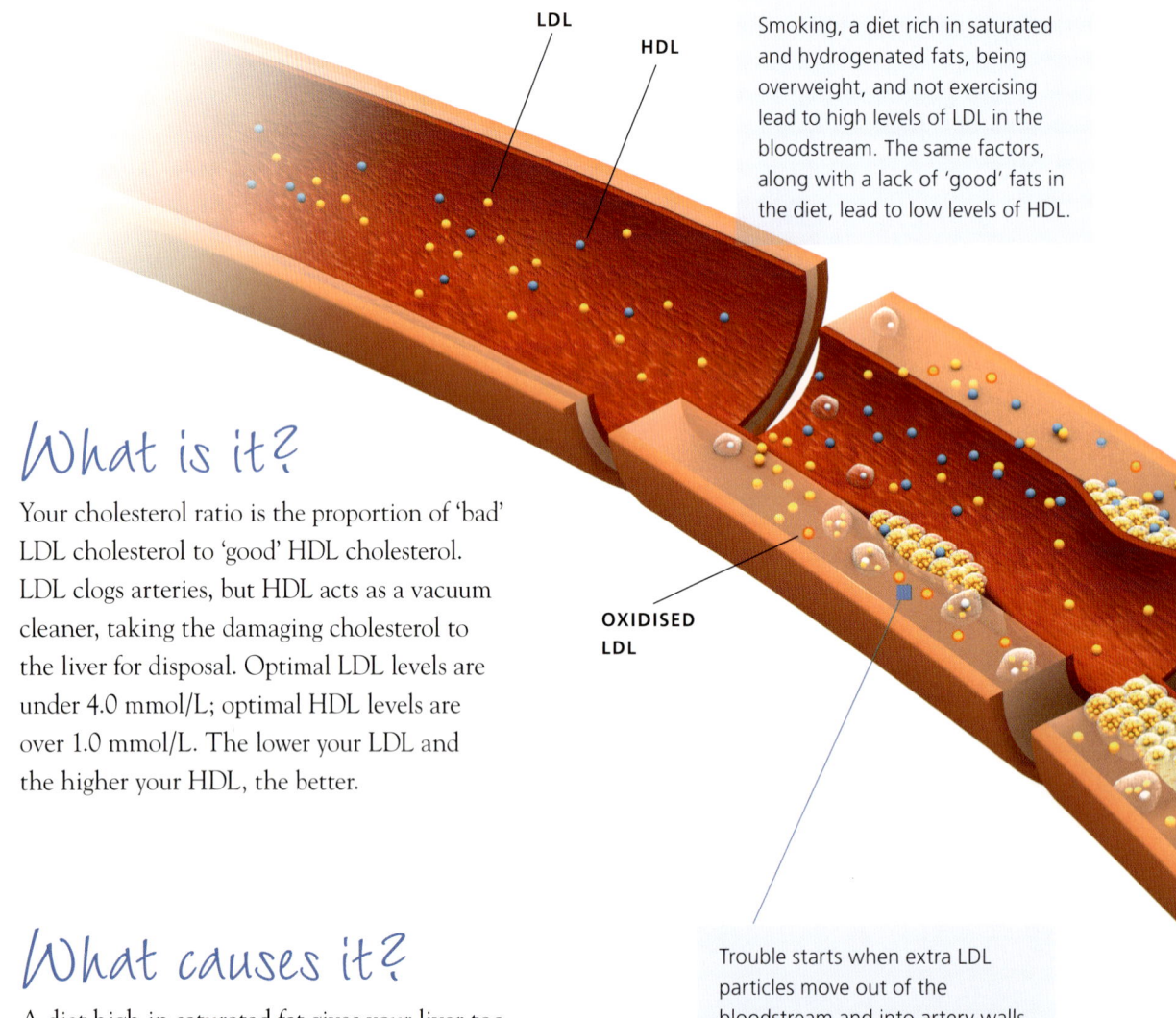

LDL
HDL
OXIDISED LDL

Smoking, a diet rich in saturated and hydrogenated fats, being overweight, and not exercising lead to high levels of LDL in the bloodstream. The same factors, along with a lack of 'good' fats in the diet, lead to low levels of HDL.

Trouble starts when extra LDL particles move out of the bloodstream and into artery walls. There they can be damaged by a process called oxidation, making them targets for white blood cells, which rush to the rescue.

What is it?

Your cholesterol ratio is the proportion of 'bad' LDL cholesterol to 'good' HDL cholesterol. LDL clogs arteries, but HDL acts as a vacuum cleaner, taking the damaging cholesterol to the liver for disposal. Optimal LDL levels are under 4.0 mmol/L; optimal HDL levels are over 1.0 mmol/L. The lower your LDL and the higher your HDL, the better.

What causes it?

A diet high in saturated fat gives your liver too much of the raw material it needs for producing LDL and reduces its ability to remove excess LDL from the bloodstream. Eating hydrogenated fats, smoking, being overweight and a lack of exercise can also raise LDL and depress HDL. Skimping on monounsaturated fats (in olive oil, nuts and avocados) and soluble fibre (in oats, barley, legumes and pears) also makes an impact on your ratio.

What causes disease?

HDL is your bloodstream's clean-up crew, removing LDL from circulation and returning it to the liver for elimination or re-use. HDL can even extract cholesterol from plaque in artery walls. But if levels are low, the LDL wins.

LIVER

PLAQUE

BLOOD CLOT

WHITE BLOOD CELL

Why is it dangerous?

LDL normally moves through artery walls and into cells, where it's put to good use. But excess LDL gets 'stuck' in artery walls, beginning the formation of artery-narrowing plaque. HDL can clean up this LDL, but if levels are low, it can't get the job done, putting you at risk for a heart attack or stroke.

The combination of LDL and white blood cells in artery walls eventually leads to the buildup of dangerous plaque. Eventually plaque can burst, leading to the formation of blood clots that can stop the flow of blood to your heart or brain.

TOP PREVENTION STRATEGIES

- **STOP SMOKING** if you haven't already.
- **EAT LESS** saturated fat and hydrogenated oils (giving rise to trans fats).
- **EAT MORE** soluble fibre (from oats, barley and legumes) and good fats (from fish, nuts and olive or canola oil).
- **DO MORE** brisk walking.
- **ENJOY** alcohol in moderation.

CAUSE 6
Inflammation

What is it?

Inflammation is a side effect of the immune system at work. When you have an injury or infection, immune system cells and chemicals rush to the site to kill germs and repair damaged tissue. You can see inflammation in action when the skin around a cut becomes red and swollen. Short bouts are beneficial, but when the body is constantly barraged by inflammation—due to ongoing low-grade infections or 'injuries' from smoking and other irritants—it ceases to help and starts to harm.

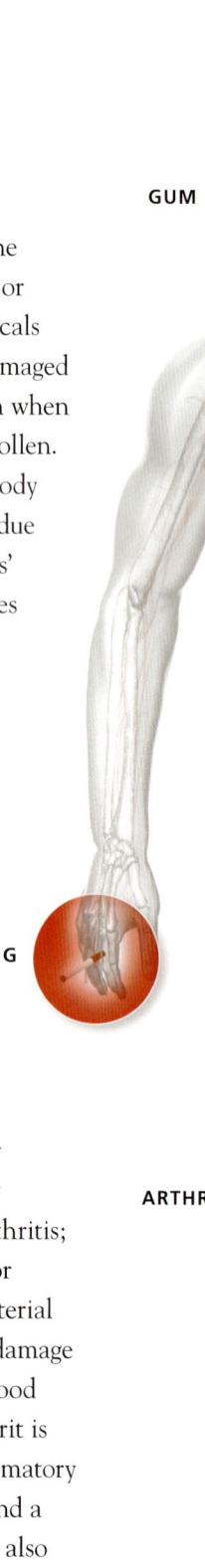

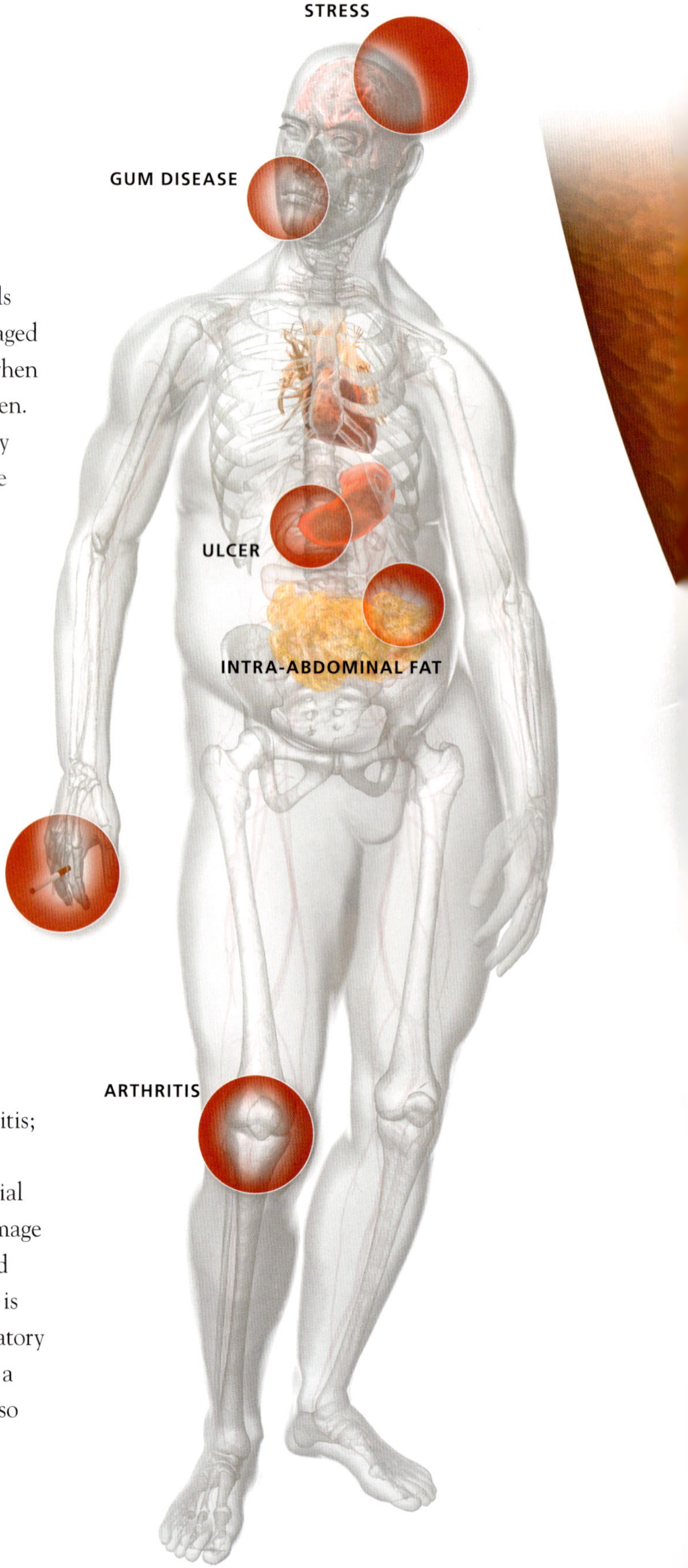

STRESS

GUM DISEASE

ULCER

INTRA-ABDOMINAL FAT

SMOKING

ARTHRITIS

What causes it?

Chronic inflammation can be triggered by allergens, toxins and radiation, but also by medical conditions such as rheumatoid arthritis; infections such as untreated gum disease or stomach ulcers, which are caused by a bacterial infection; or microscopic injuries such as damage to artery walls caused by smoking, high blood pressure or high cholesterol. Another culprit is intra-abdominal fat, which secretes inflammatory chemicals. Stress, anger, lack of exercise and a diet full of fast food and hydrogenated fats also increase inflammation.

What causes disease? 33

In your blood, levels of inflammatory chemicals called cytokines rise in response to smoking, bacteria, intra-abdominal fat and other stressors to the body. Cytokines alert the body that something is wrong and set off a chain of events that causes inflammation.

Why is it dangerous?

It accelerates the growth of plaque in artery walls and then makes that plaque less stable and more likely to burst open and block an artery. Chronic inflammation also contributes to insulin resistance and raises your risk of a whole host of chronic diseases, including diabetes, Alzheimer's disease, lung disease, osteoporosis and even cancer.

WHITE BLOOD CELL

INFLAMMATION

PLAQUE

BLOOD CLOT

TISSUE FACTOR

LDL

FATTY STREAK

OXIDISED LDL

White blood cells release more cytokines that eat away at the protective cap covering the plaque. Eventually, the plaque may burst open and spill its contents into the bloodstream. A distress signal sent by white blood cells, called tissue factor, triggers a clotting response. If a blood clot blocks the artery, a heart attack or stroke can result.

White blood cells rush to the site of the infection or injury—such as artery walls damaged by oxidised cholesterol (LDL) particles. When LDL burrows into artery walls, the immune cells engulf them in order to dispose of them. But if there's too much LDL, the white blood cells become overstuffed, collect in the artery wall and form plaque that narrows the artery.

TOP PREVENTION STRATEGIES

- ▶ **STOP SMOKING** as it inflames artery walls.
- ▶ **EAT MORE** fatty fish, fruit and vegetables, and less fried food and hydrogenated oils.
- ▶ **SLEEP** at least 7 or 8 hours a night.
- ▶ **EXERCISE** moderately.
- ▶ **TREAT** any existing infections, such as gum disease or *Helicobacter pylori*.

Symptoms you should never ignore

Thankfully, the vast majority of illness turns out to be harmless. However, some symptoms should never be ignored or overlooked because they may signal the onset of serious illness, and early diagnosis and treatment can be vital. In the following tables you'll find common symptoms that may be the first sign that a dangerous condition is brewing, what the underlying problem might be and what steps to take. A timely phone call or visit to your family doctor—or, where we have indicated, a call to the ambulance service or a trip to your local emergency department—can either help put your mind at rest or steer you to the treatment you need (for a table of emergency numbers, see page 21). Of course, you should always consult your doctor whenever a symptom is worrying you, regardless of whether or not it is listed in this section.

If you need to go to hospital, take all your regular medications with you, or a list of what you normally take, including over-the-counter preparations and herbs, vitamin supplements, or any other alternative treatments.

Abdominal pain

DESCRIPTION	POSSIBLE CAUSES	RESPONSE
A burning sensation just below the breastbone, particularly after a large meal	Heartburn (reflux)	Take over-the-counter antacids and avoid large greasy meals. If pain persists for several weeks, see your doctor.
Pain around and below your navel accompanied by gas	Constipation or flatulence	Take an over-the-counter laxative or anti-gas medication. If pain persists for more than two weeks, see your doctor.
Sudden pain around your navel; may be accompanied by nausea, fever, vomiting, loss of appetite, pressure to have a bowel movement or stiffening of the abdominal muscles	Appendicitis	Go to the hospital. Appendicitis must be treated quickly or the appendix will rupture and leak infected fluid into other parts of the abdomen. Stiffening of abdominal muscles is a sign that infection is starting to spread.
Sudden pain in the right side of your abdomen that may radiate to other parts of your abdomen or back	Gallstones or gall bladder inflammation	If pain persists or worsens after eating greasy foods, see your doctor.
Sudden pain below your navel that radiates to either side of your navel	A colon disorder, a urinary tract infection or pelvic inflammatory disease	If pain continues to worsen, call your doctor, who may order diagnostic tests or advise you to go to the emergency department.

DESCRIPTION	POSSIBLE CAUSES	RESPONSE
Sudden sharp pain near your lower ribs that radiates down your groin	Kidney stones or, if accompanied by fever, a kidney or bladder infection	Increase your water intake and call your doctor. Most kidney stones eventually pass on their own, although in rare cases surgery is necessary. If you also have a fever, call your doctor.
Sudden pain and tenderness in your lower left abdomen may be accompanied by fever, nausea or vomiting	Crohn's disease, ulcerative colitis or diverticulitis	See your doctor, who may recommend a colonoscopy. Long-term treatment may be required.
Sudden pain accompanied by bloody diarrhoea, blood in the stool or vomiting blood	A blockage in the bowel, a perforated appendix or bleeding from the bowel	These are symptoms of internal bleeding; go straight to the nearest hospital.
Mild pain or discomfort that comes on slowly and continues or recurs for weeks or months, sometimes accompanied by diarrhoea, constipation, bloating or flatulence	A chronic ailment such as lactose intolerance, irritable bowel syndrome, ulcers, food intolerance, Crohn's disease, ulcerative colitis or coeliac disease	See your doctor, who may refer you to a gastroenterologist for follow-up.
Sudden abdominal pain in an older person especially one who smokes or has high blood pressure; may be accompanied by lightheadedness	Abdominal aortic aneurysm	The widening of the aorta can cause fatal bleeding. Go to the emergency department immediately.

Back pain

DESCRIPTION	POSSIBLE CAUSES	RESPONSE
Back pain if accompanied by fever, chills, immune suppression or recent bacterial infection, back surgery, epidural/spinal anaesthesia or injecting drug use	Serious infection	Call your doctor or, after hours, go to the emergency department.
Back pain that is worse at night or when lying down or accompanied by weight loss, sensory changes, leg weakness, bladder or bowel dysfunction, or a history of cancer	Cancer	Call your doctor; if there are sensory changes, leg weakness or bladder or bowel dysfunction, go to the emergency department immediately, as urgent treatment may be necessary to restore function.
Back pain if accompanied by osteoporosis	Fracture	Call your doctor.

Black or bloody stools

DESCRIPTION	POSSIBLE CAUSES	RESPONSE
Black or tarry stools; may be accompanied by a burning in the stomach and oesophagus	An ulcer in the upper gastrointestinal tract	Go to the emergency department, where you may be admitted for an endoscopy for visual inspection and to take tissue samples for biopsy.
Maroon or black stools with no other worrying symptoms	Consuming black licorice, blueberries, lead, iron pills, tomatoes or spinach	Stop eating the suspicious food to see if stool colour returns to normal. If not, call your doctor. If you've ingested lead or iron, call the Poisons Information Centre or a hospital.
Maroon or bright red stools accompanied by pain and pressure while moving your bowels	Anal fissures (small tears around the anus) or haemorrhoids (swollen blood vessels near the rectum, which can rupture)	Over-the-counter haemorrhoid creams, ointments or pads can bring relief; surgery may be necessary for persistent haemorrhoids. If bleeding continues, see your doctor.
Maroon or bright red stools accompanied by discomfort in the lower abdomen and other GI symptoms, such as gas, constipation, diarrhoea or pain	A serious condition such as ulcerative colitis, Crohn's disease, diverticular disease, a tumour or benign or cancerous polyps	See your doctor, who will refer you to a gastroenterologist for follow-up and treatment.

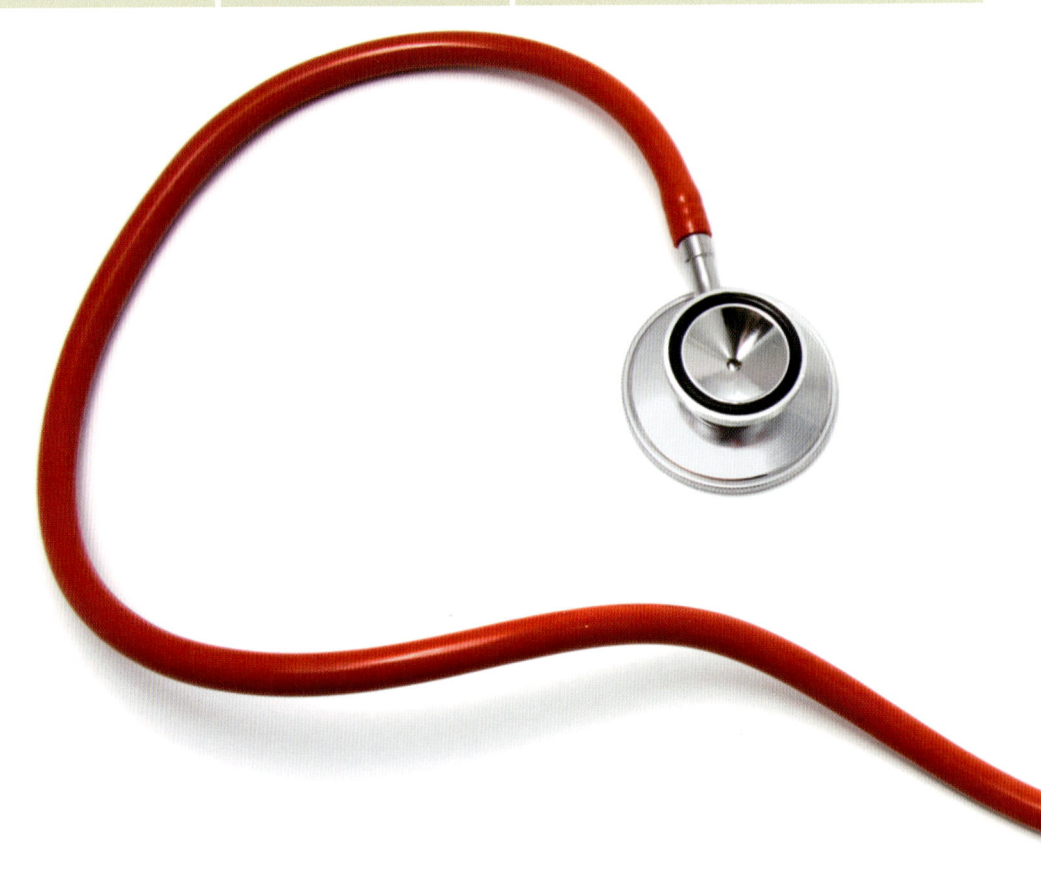

Blood in the urine

DESCRIPTION	POSSIBLE CAUSES	RESPONSE
Blood in the urine after starting a new medication	A side effect of medications such as aspirin, some antibiotics, blood thinners and cancer drugs	Talk with your doctor about whether a different medication should be substituted. Side effects sometimes disappear after a few days or weeks of taking a new medication.
Pink, red or brownish urine accompanied by pain, burning during urination, a frequent strong urge to urinate or foul-smelling urine	A bladder infection	See your doctor, who will order diagnostic urinalysis. Treatment is usually an oral antibiotic.
Blood in the urine, usually accompanied by fever and back pain	A kidney infection	See your doctor. An antibiotic is prescribed when a bacterial infection in the bladder moves to the kidneys.
Blood in the urine accompanied by severe pain	Kidney stones	See your doctor, who will order a CT scan, ultrasound or abdominal X-ray. Many kidney stones pass on their own. If they don't pass, they may need to be surgically removed or shattered with shock waves.
In men, blood in the urine accompanied by difficulty urinating or a strong need to urinate often	Prostate enlargement	See your doctor, who will order diagnostic ultrasound or other imaging tests. Treatment includes medication or laser therapy to destroy excess prostate tissue.
Unexplained blood in the urine with no other symptoms	Bladder cancer, kidney cancer or a genetic kidney disorder	See your doctor, who will order diagnostic ultrasound, CT scans and other imaging tests.

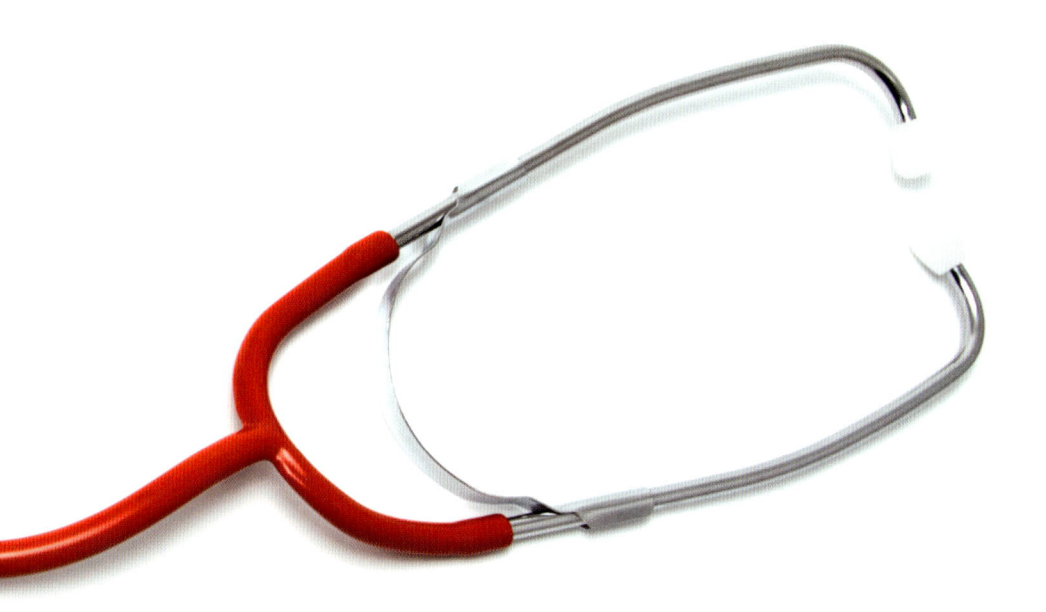

Changes in appetite

DESCRIPTION	POSSIBLE CAUSES	RESPONSE
Decreased appetite accompanied by fatigue, hair loss or decreased tolerance to the cold	Hypothyroidism (underactive thyroid)	See your doctor, who will order a diagnostic blood test. If your thyroid is underactive, treatment is thyroid hormone replacement medication.
Decreased appetite accompanied by other symptoms, including a change in bowel habits, fatigue, nausea or blood in stools, urine or vomit	Cancer	See your doctor, who may order diagnostic tests.
Decreased appetite after starting a new medication	A side effect of medications such as cancer drugs, some antibiotics, narcotic pain relievers and some cough and cold preparations	Talk with your doctor about whether a different medication should be substituted. Side effects sometimes disappear after a few days or weeks of taking a new medication.
Increased appetite accompanied by insomnia, excessive thirst, increased sweating, more frequent bowel movements or hair loss	Hyperthyroidism or other hormone imbalance	See your doctor, who will order diagnostic blood tests. If your thyroid is overactive, prescription medication can slow it down.
Increased appetite accompanied by excessive thirst, fatigue, increased urination or poor wound healing	Diabetes	See your doctor, who will order a test to measure your blood sugar. Early diabetes can often be treated with lifestyle measures.
Increased appetite after starting a new medication	A side effect of medications such as corticosteroids, some antidepressants and some allergy medications	Talk with your doctor about whether a different medication should be substituted. Side effects sometimes disappear after a few days or weeks of taking a medication.

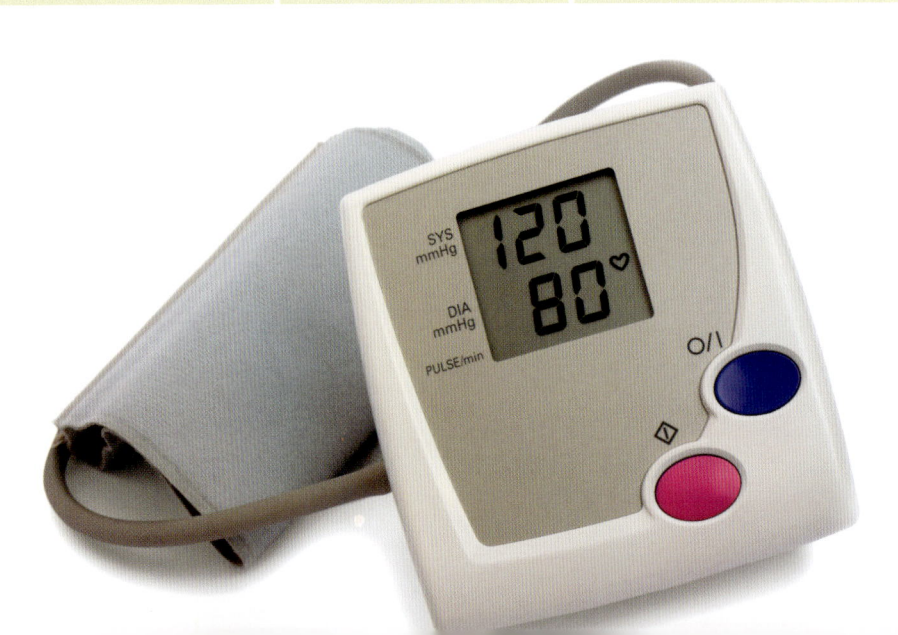

Chest pain

DESCRIPTION	POSSIBLE CAUSES	RESPONSE
Squeezing, tightening pain that usually occurs around the breastbone and may radiate to the arms, jaw, back or teeth and worsens with exertion; may come on suddenly (unstable) or regularly during exertion (stable)	Angina, which occurs when the heart is not getting enough blood or oxygen	Go to the emergency department; unstable angina can be very dangerous. Stable angina usually goes away within a couple of minutes if you stop the exertion that brought it on, but it is still a serious condition that requires medical care.
Pain accompanied by shortness of breath, coughing or wheezing	Asthma or chronic obstructive pulmonary disease (smoker's lung)	If you have an inhaler, use it. If you don't, make an appointment with your doctor. If you can't breathe, go straight to the emergency department.
Sharp pain that worsens when you cough or take a deep breath; may be accompanied by flu-like symptoms; sometimes hurts when you press your hand against your chest	A lung condition such as pneumonia, a blood clot in the lung, a collapsed lung, inflammation of the lung's lining or inflammation of ribcage cartilage	Call your doctor or, if you can't breathe, go straight to the emergency department, where doctors will consider whether you need specific diagnostic tests.
Burning pain accompanied by gastrointestinal symptoms such as indigestion or reflux	An ulcer, pancreatic disease or an inflamed gall bladder	See your doctor, who may recommend diagnostic tests or refer you to a gastroenterologist.
Crushing, squeezing, tightening pressure on your chest that comes on suddenly; may be accompanied by pain that radiates from your chest to your jaw, back, neck, shoulders or arm, particularly your left arm; may also be accompanied by nausea, racing pulse or shortness of breath	Heart attack	Call an ambulance or have someone drive you to the hospital immediately. If your doctor has prescribed nitroglycerin to have on hand, take the suggested dose. After you have called an ambulance, chew a regular aspirin (300 mg) or three low-dose aspirin (100 mg each) straight away.
Pain accompanied by anxiety, racing pulse or shortness of breath	Panic attack	Breathe deeply and try to relax. If symptoms persist, call your doctor. Panic attack symptoms can mimic those of more serious conditions such as heart attack. If it's your first panic attack, call your doctor or go to the emergency department to exclude a more serious condition.

Chronic cough

DESCRIPTION	POSSIBLE CAUSES	RESPONSE
A cough accompanied by postnasal drip, repeated throat clearing, nasal discharge or excessive phlegm	Allergies or a sinus infection	See your doctor, who may prescribe allergy medication or refer you to an allergist for diagnosis and treatment. If you have a sinus infection, your doctor may prescribe an antibiotic.
A night-time cough that brings up no mucus and may end with wheezing or a rattling sound	Asthma	See your doctor, who may prescribe a broncho-dilator, inhaled corticosteroid or other medication to control asthma.
A cough after starting to take an ACE inhibitor	A drug side effect; ACE inhibitors cause dry cough in 5 to 10 per cent of patients	Talk with your doctor about whether another medication should be substituted.
A dry cough accompanied by shortness of breath	Chronic obstructive pulmonary disease, a condition that includes chronic bronchitis and emphysema and is almost always caused by smoking	See your doctor, who may do a test to measure lung capacity and order a chest X-ray. There is no cure, but symptoms can be treated and further lung damage prevented.
A cough accompanied by bouts of heartburn that occur more than twice a week	Gastro-oesophageal reflux disease (GERD), a condition involving chronic heartburn	See your doctor, who will prescribe antacids and medications that inhibit stomach acid production and may recommend gastroscopy to assess damage to the oesophagus.
A cough that worsens over time and may be accompanied by fatigue, chest pain, coughing up blood, hoarseness or shortness of breath	Lung cancer	See your doctor, who will order diagnostic tests such as a chest X-ray, CT scan, MRI scan and blood tests.

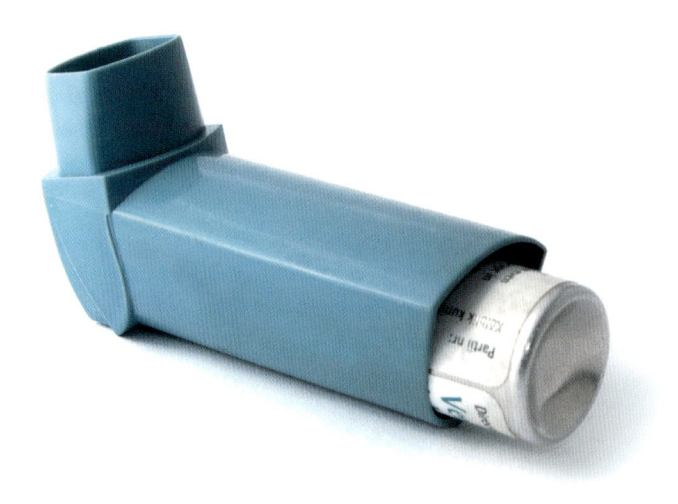

Confusion and memory loss

DESCRIPTION	POSSIBLE CAUSES	RESPONSE
Sudden confusion; may be accompanied by blurred vision, slurred speech, sudden numbness on one side of the body or sudden severe headache	Stroke or transient ischaemic attack (TIA)	Go to the hospital immediately. Prompt treatment can save your life, lessen damage to your brain and reduce your risk of permanent disability.
Sudden confusion or memory loss after an accident	Head injury or concussion	Go to the hospital immediately.
In the elderly, memory loss or confusion that begins gradually but doesn't worsen quickly or interfere with everyday life	Normal age-related memory loss	Keep your mind active with crossword puzzles and other mental challenges. Use a detailed date book, always put keys and other items in the same place and repeat a person's name to yourself several times when you meet.
In the elderly, memory loss or confusion that begins gradually, starts to worsen quickly and interferes with the functions of everyday life	Alzheimer's disease, a neurodegenerative disorder, or a brain tumour	Consult with your doctor, who will determine whether testing is needed.
Confusion that comes on gradually after a period of vomiting, diarrhoea or significant exposure to heat or sunlight	Dehydration	Rehydrate by sipping water frequently. If dehydration is caused by vomiting or diarrhoea, choose nondairy beverages or an over-the-counter electrolyte solution. Call your doctor if you can't keep liquids down or confusion persists.
Memory loss or confusion after starting a new medication	A side effect of medications such as narcotic pain relievers and benzodiazepines	Talk with your doctor about whether a different medication should be substituted. Side effects sometimes disappear after a few days or weeks of taking a medication.
Confusion that comes on quite suddenly; may be accompanied by hunger or lightheadedness	Low blood sugar	Have a sweet snack or drink.

Constipation

DESCRIPTION	POSSIBLE CAUSES	RESPONSE
Occasional constipation may be accompanied by bloating, a feeling of fullness and the need to strain to have a bowel movement	Poor diet (low in fibre and fluids and high in fat), not enough exercise or too much alcohol or caffeine	Symptoms usually clear up once you resume a healthy diet with plenty of fibre and fluids. Natural fibre supplements can also ease symptoms; always drink plenty of water if you take them.
Constipation after starting a new medication	A side effect of medications such as painkillers, antacids that contain aluminium and calcium, calcium channel blockers, drugs for Parkinson's disease, antispasmodics, antidepressants, iron supplements, diuretics, and anticonvulsants	Talk with your doctor about whether a different medication should be substituted. Side effects sometimes disappear after a few days or weeks of taking a medication.
Constipation that occurs regularly and is accompanied by abdominal pain and bloating; may occur during periods of stress	Irritable bowel syndrome	See your doctor, who may prescribe medication, fibre supplements, physical activity or stress reduction techniques, such as meditation, to help reduce symptoms.
Constipation during or after pregnancy, travel or other lifestyle changes	A temporary reaction to change	Symptoms should clear up on their own.
Constipation accompanied by bloating, gas or pain	A disease or condition of the colon or rectum, such as diverticular disease, tumours or scar tissue in the intestines	See your doctor, who may order diagnostic tests.
Constipation accompanied by excessive thirst, increased urination, fatigue, depression, weight gain or headache	A metabolic or endocrine disorder such as diabetes, hypothyroidism (underactive thyroid) or hypercalcaemia (too much calcium in the blood)	See your doctor, who will order diagnostic tests.

Diarrhoea

DESCRIPTION	POSSIBLE CAUSES	RESPONSE
Diarrhoea that comes on suddenly for no apparent reason; may be accompanied by fever, vomiting, cramping or headache	A viral infection (stomach flu)	Symptoms usually clear up on their own within a few days. During that time, stay well hydrated. Drink nondairy, decaffeinated fluids or an over-the-counter electrolyte solution throughout the day.
Diarrhoea after eating certain foods, such as milk or eggs	Food allergy or intolerance	Eliminate the trigger food from your diet and talk with your doctor about whether to have allergy tests.
Diarrhoea starting 2 to 6 hours after a meal	A bacterial infection caused by spoiled, undercooked or contaminated food; most cases of food poisoning are due to common bacteria such as staphylococcus or *E. coli*	Symptoms usually clear up on their own within 12 to 48 hours. Avoid solid food until your stools return to normal. Call your doctor if symptoms last more than two or three days or if you're unable to stay hydrated; you may need intravenous fluids. If you ate contaminated mushrooms or shellfish, go straight to the emergency department.
Diarrhoea while travelling overseas	An infection caused by contaminated water; most often due to common bacteria and sometimes parasites	Symptoms usually clear up on their own in one to two days. If they persist or are accompanied by other symptoms such as persistent vomiting and headache, see a doctor, who may prescribe an antibiotic or anti-parasitic medication.
Diarrhoea while taking medications	A side effect of medications such as antibiotics, diuretics, laxatives containing magnesium, or cancer drugs	Talk with your doctor about whether a different medication should be substituted. If you're taking an antibiotic, eat yogurt with active cultures to replenish the 'good' bacteria in your gut.
Diarrhoea that lasts more than four weeks	A chronic condition such as lactose intolerance, Crohn's disease, ulcerative colitis, irritable bowel syndrome or coeliac disease (intolerance to gluten—a protein found in wheat, rye and barley)	See your doctor, who may refer you to a gastroenterologist and/or dietitian.

Dizziness

DESCRIPTION	POSSIBLE CAUSES	RESPONSE
Dizziness accompanied by dry mouth, thirst, dark urine and decreased urination	Dehydration	Rehydrate with noncaffeinated drinks or an over-the-counter electrolyte solution. Call your doctor if you can't keep liquids down and dizziness persists.
Dizziness accompanied by ear pain, reduced ability to hear and fever	An ear infection	See your doctor, but understand that most ear infections clear up on their own within a few days. Use an over-the-counter pain reliever or a heating pad to reduce pain.
Dizziness accompanied by blurred vision, slurred speech, sudden numbness on one side of the body or sudden severe headache	Stroke or transient ischaemic attack (TIA)	Go to the hospital immediately. Prompt treatment can save your life and reduce your risk of permanent disability.
Sudden severe dizziness accompanied by chest pain, racing pulse, shortness of breath, sweating or pain	Heart attack	Call an ambulance. If your doctor has prescribed nitroglycerin to have on hand, take the suggested dose. After you call an ambulance, chew a regular aspirin (300 mg) or three low-dose aspirin (100 mg each) straight away.
Sudden severe dizziness accompanied by chest pain, shortness of breath, racing pulse or fainting	Heart arrhythmia (irregular heartbeat)	An unusually fast or slow heartbeat is usually harmless, but the symptoms of arrhythmia are so similar to those of heart attack that only a trained medical professional can tell them apart. If you've never had them before, call an ambulance.
Dizziness triggered by standing up or moving suddenly	Positional vertigo (an inner ear disorder)	Sit or lie still until the dizziness passes. Avoid moving quickly.
Dizziness after starting a new medication	A side effect of various medications, especially those for diabetes, high blood pressure, depression and anxiety	Talk with your doctor about whether a different medication should be substituted. Side effects sometimes disappear after a few days or weeks of taking a medication.
Dizziness accompanied by anxiety, racing pulse or shortness of breath	Panic attack	Breathe deeply and try to relax. If symptoms persist, call your doctor. Frequent panic attacks can be treated with therapy, medication and relaxation techniques such as meditation. If it is your first panic attack, go to the emergency department to exclude a more serious condition.

Excessive thirst

DESCRIPTION	POSSIBLE CAUSES	RESPONSE
Thirst accompanied by chest pain, increased or decreased urination, appetite loss, nausea, vomiting, swelling or numbness in the hands or feet, muscle cramps, trouble concentrating, shortness of breath, or dizziness	Heart, liver or kidney failure	Call your doctor immediately. A thorough physical examination can determine the existence and extent of these conditions.
Thirst, possibly accompanied by insomnia, unexplained weight loss, increased sweating, more frequent bowel movements or hair loss	Hyperthyroidism or other hormone imbalance	See your doctor, who will order a diagnostic blood test. If your thyroid is overactive, prescription medication can slow it down.
Thirst after starting a new medication	A side effect of medications such as diuretics, anti-histamines, some anti-depressants, cancer drugs and steroids	Talk with your doctor about whether to continue the medication, but don't stop it without medical permission. Check the package inserts or call your pharmacist for advice on whether to, or how much to, increase your fluid intake.
Thirst possibly accompanied by increased urination, unexplained weight loss, increased hunger or blurred vision	Hyperglycaemia (high blood sugar) or diabetes	See your doctor, who will order a test to measure your blood sugar levels.
A strong desire to drink with no other physical symptoms	Psychogenic polydipsia, a mental disorder	See your doctor, who may refer you to a mental health professional.
Thirst accompanied by excessive urination	Diabetes insipidus, a rare disorder caused by a deficiency of antidiuretic hormone or the inability of the kidney to respond to it	See your doctor, who will order diagnostic blood tests.

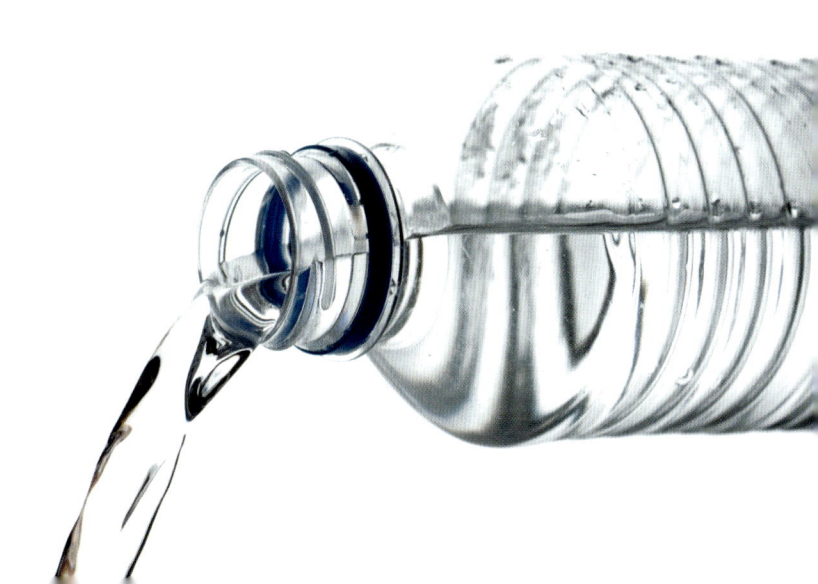

Fatigue

DESCRIPTION	POSSIBLE CAUSES	RESPONSE
Sudden fatigue accompanied by viral symptoms	An illness such as a cold or the flu	Rest while your body fights off the virus.
Fatigue accompanied by loss of interest in favourite activities, unintentional weight gain or loss, irritability, feelings of hopelessness, or trouble concentrating	Depression or anxiety	Seek support from friends and family and see your doctor, who may refer you to a mental health professional. Long-term depression or anxiety, common in older people, can be treated with therapy, medication or both.
Fatigue while taking medication	A side effect of drugs such as beta-blockers, antihistamines, anti-anxiety medications, cough and cold remedies, and some antidepressants	Ask your doctor or pharmacist if fatigue is a common side effect of any of the medications you take. If the answer is yes, talk with your doctor about whether a different medication should be substituted.
Fatigue lasting more than two weeks	A problem such as infection, allergies, a sleep disorder such as apnoea, anaemia, heart disease, diabetes, kidney disease or liver disease	See your doctor, who will order diagnostic tests and may refer you to a specialist.
Fatigue accompanied by unexplained weight gain, dry skin, hair loss, change in sleep patterns, constipation or depression	Hypothyroidism (underactive thyroid)	See your doctor, who will order a diagnostic blood test. If your thyroid is underactive, treatment is thyroid hormone replacement medication.
Severe, persistent, unexplained fatigue accompanied by muscle aches or difficulty concentrating	Chronic fatigue syndrome	See your doctor, who will rule out other possible causes. There is no cure, but symptoms can be controlled. Make sure your doctor has experience in treating CFS.

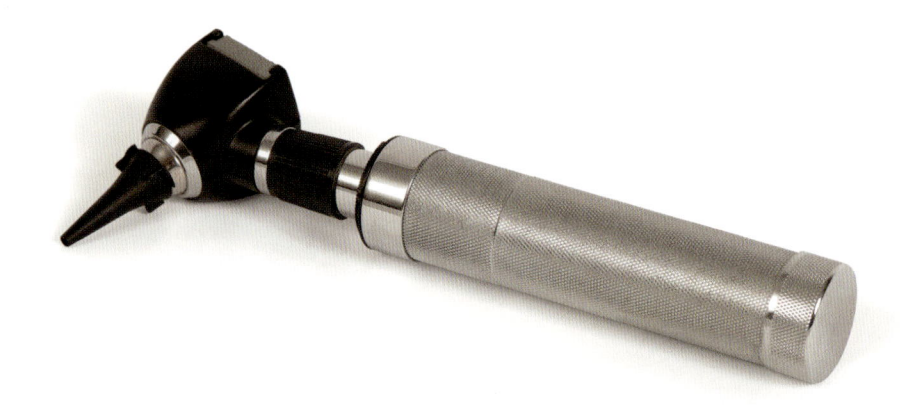

Fever

DESCRIPTION	POSSIBLE CAUSES	RESPONSE
A small increase in body temperature (0.5 to 1°C) with no other symptoms	Exercise, heat, heavy clothing, intense emotion	Normal body temperature is about 37°C. In adults and children over the age of six, a variation of 1.5 degrees is normal. To reduce your temperature, turn on airconditioning, loosen clothing, drink fluids or bathe in lukewarm water.
A rapid, dramatic increase in body temperature after exposure to heat, sun or intense exercise; may be accompanied by rapid pulse, nausea and disorientation	Heatstroke or heat exhaustion	Move to a cool place then spray yourself with and drink cool water. If symptoms are extreme (temperature of 39°C or higher), call an ambulance. Heat exhaustion is less serious; heatstroke is a medical emergency.
A moderate fever (38.5 to 39.5°C); may be accompanied by nasal discharge, sore throat, cough, earache, vomiting or diarrhoea	A viral or bacterial infection such as a cold, the flu, strep throat, an ear infection, bronchitis or a urinary tract infection	Paracetamol or ibuprofen can reduce the fever. If your fever is above 39°C or lasts for more than three days, call your doctor. If you have a bacterial infection, your doctor may prescribe an antibiotic. Stay hydrated with water or an electrolyte solution.
A high fever (39.5°C or higher); may be accompanied by confusion, a stiff neck, difficulty breathing, hallucinations or convulsions	A viral or bacterial infection, or pneumonia, meningitis, a kidney infection, mononucleosis or other serious condition	Go to the emergency department, especially if the patient seems lethargic or unresponsive. Paracetamol or ibuprofen can reduce the fever, as can bathing in lukewarm water. Stay hydrated by drinking water or an over-the-counter electrolyte solution.
Fever after starting a new medication	A side effect of medications such as some antibiotics, antihistamines, barbiturates, anti-seizure and hypertension medications	Talk with your doctor about whether a different drug should be substituted. Side effects sometimes disappear after a few days or weeks of taking a medication.
A mild fever that occurs after a vaccination	A side effect of some routine immunisations, such as diphtheria, tetanus and pneumonia	Fever usually subsides in a day or two; take ibuprofen or paracetamol to reduce discomfort.
A fever that occurs with other unexplained symptoms, such as weight loss, muscle or joint aches, or stomach pain, and may come and go	A wide variety of conditions and diseases, such as cancer, ulcerative colitis, Crohn's disease, lupus, HIV/AIDS, rheumatoid arthritis and autoimmune disorders	See your doctor, who may order diagnostic tests.

Headache

DESCRIPTION	POSSIBLE CAUSES	RESPONSE
Dull pain in the head, neck or shoulders that comes on gradually; may feel like a vice around your forehead, temples or back of your head and neck	Tension headache; can be triggered by stress, fatigue, anger or depression, or can have no known trigger	Take aspirin, ibuprofen or paracetamol.
Pain after physical exertion such as running, sexual intercourse, coughing or bowel movements	Exertion headache; related to cluster headaches, migraines or, rarely, to aneurysms, tumours or malformed blood vessels	Pain usually goes away in less than an hour. It can be treated with aspirin or medications for migraines or cluster headaches. If headaches persist, see your doctor.
Throbbing pain that comes on several days after consuming a large amount of caffeine	Caffeine withdrawal	Reduce or eliminate caffeine intake.
Throbbing pain, usually on one side of the head, often accompanied by nausea and sensitivity to light and sound; occasionally accompanied by flashing lights, blind spots or tingling in the arm or face prior to head pain	Migraine; occurs more commonly in women and can be triggered by menstruation, ovulation or menopause	Migraines typically last from 4 hours to three days. Take aspirin immediately or a prescription migraine medication if you have one, and lie down in a darkened room. If you have more than two migraines a month, see your doctor, who may recommend preventive medication. If this is your first migraine, do not take any medication and call your doctor immediately.
Sudden sharp, severe pain on one side of the head, sometimes around the eye; may be accompanied by excessive sweating, tearing and nasal congestion	Cluster headache; 90 per cent of sufferers are men	Headaches may last anywhere from a few minutes to several hours but are likely to recur later that day. See your doctor, who may prescribe medication to treat them. There are also preventive medicines that help ward off attacks. Avoid alcohol.
Unexplained pain that becomes progressively worse; may be accompanied by blurred vision, confusion or loss of consciousness	Cancer; infection; high blood pressure; a disease or disorder of the brain; disorders of the eyes, ears or nose; blood clots; temporal arteritis; or aneurysms	Go to the hospital, where doctors may order diagnostic tests or consult a specialist.
Sudden severe pain; may be accompanied by numbness on one side of the body, dizziness, blurred vision, headache or confusion	Stroke	Go to the hospital immediately. Prompt treatment can save your life, lessen damage to your brain and reduce your risk of permanent disability.

Lesions and skin rashes

DESCRIPTION	POSSIBLE CAUSES	RESPONSE
Pinpoint rash accompanied by a fever	Meningococcal disease	Go to the emergency department immediately.
Pinpoint rash without a fever	Low platelet count	See your doctor, who will order a blood test.
Mouth ulcers	Medication reaction, low white cell count or viral infection	See your doctor, who may order blood tests.
A mole that changes shape, size or colour, or is bleeding	Melanoma	See your doctor promptly. Early diagnosis can save lives.
Blisters	Chickenpox, shingles, eczema, impetigo, allergic reaction or autoimmune skin disease such as bullous pemphigoid	See your doctor for investigation and treatment.
Unexplained bruises	Bleeding disorder, liver problems, medication side effects	See your doctor promptly. Early diagnosis can save lives.
Skin ulcer that doesn't heal	Skin cancer, circulation problem, infection	See your doctor for investigation and treatment.

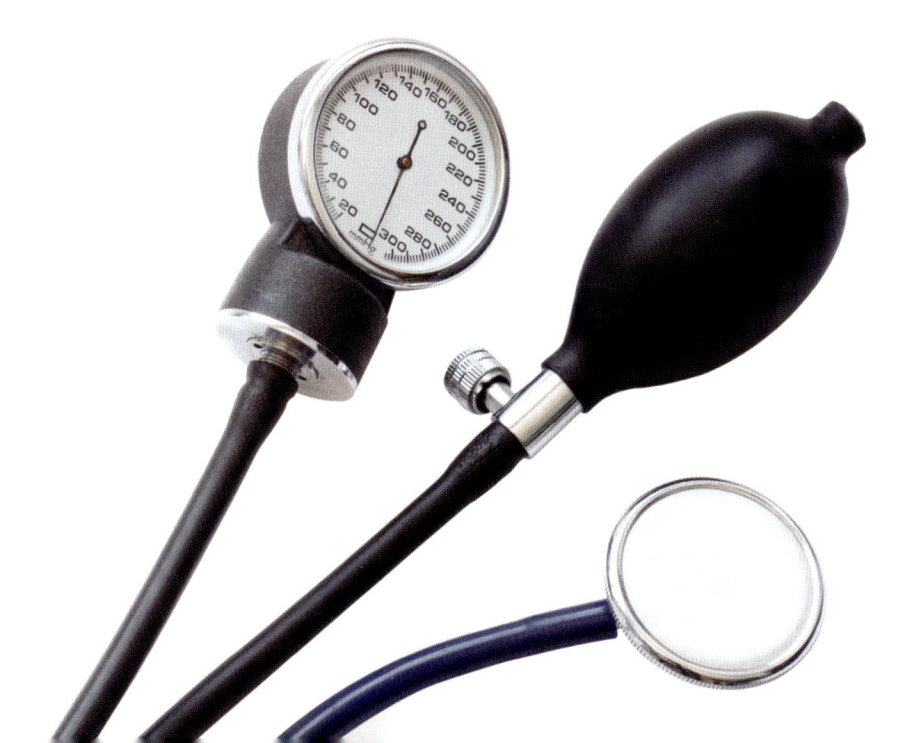

Nausea and vomiting

DESCRIPTION	POSSIBLE CAUSES	RESPONSE
Nausea and vomiting in women in early pregnancy	Morning sickness	See your doctor, who may recommend ginger or vitamin B_6.
Nausea and vomiting after starting a new medication	A side effect of a medication	Talk with your doctor about whether a different drug should be substituted. Side effects sometimes disappear after a few days or weeks of taking a medication.
Nausea or vomiting accompanied by sudden pain in your upper right abdomen that may radiate to other parts of your abdomen or your back	Gallstones or gall bladder inflammation	If pain persists or worsens after eating greasy foods, see your doctor.
Nausea or vomiting starting 2 to 6 hours after a meal	A bacterial infection caused by spoiled, undercooked or contaminated food; most cases of food poisoning are due to common bacteria such as staphylococcus or *E. coli*	Symptoms usually clear up on their own within 12 to 48 hours. Call your doctor if symptoms last more than two or three days or if you're unable to stay hydrated; you may need intravenous fluids. If you ate contaminated mushrooms or shellfish, go to the emergency department.
Nausea or vomiting accompanied by crushing, squeezing, tightening pressure on your chest that comes on suddenly; pain that radiates from your chest to your jaw, back, neck, shoulders or arm, particularly your left arm; racing pulse; or shortness of breath	Heart attack	Call an ambulance or have someone drive you to the hospital immediately. If your doctor has prescribed nitroglycerin to have on hand, take the suggested dose. After you call an ambulance, chew one regular aspirin (300 mg) or three low-dose aspirin (100 mg each) straight away.
Nausea or vomiting after an accident, sports injury or fall	A concussion or brain injury	If symptoms continue to worsen, call your doctor or go straight to the emergency department.
Nausea or vomiting accompanied by black or tarry stools, a burning sensation in the stomach and oesophagus, indigestion, or reflux	An ulcer in the upper gastrointestinal tract or gastro-oesophageal reflux disease (GERD)	See your doctor, who will probably refer you for an endoscopy, in which a scope is inserted through your mouth and into your upper gastrointestinal tract for visual inspection and to take tissue samples for biopsy.
Nausea or vomiting accompanied by other unexplained symptoms, such as fatigue, pain or weight changes	Cancer	See your doctor, who will order diagnostic tests.
Nausea or vomiting after eating certain foods, such as milk or eggs	Food allergy or intolerance	Eliminate the trigger food from your diet and talk with your doctor about whether to have allergy tests.

DESCRIPTION	POSSIBLE CAUSES	RESPONSE
Nausea or vomiting that comes on suddenly; may be accompanied by pain around your navel, fever, loss of appetite or pressure to have a bowel movement	Appendicitis	Go to the hospital. Appendicitis must be treated quickly or the appendix will rupture and leak infected fluid into other parts of the abdomen.
Nausea or vomiting accompanied by excessive thirst, fatigue, increased urination or poor wound healing	Poorly controlled diabetes	See your doctor, who can help you get your diabetes under control.
Nausea or vomiting that comes on gradually and continues or recurs for weeks or months; may be accompanied by pain or discomfort in the abdomen, diarrhoea, constipation, bloating, flatulence, and other gastrointestinal symptoms	A chronic condition such as lactose intolerance, irritable bowel syndrome, ulcers, food allergies, Crohn's disease, ulcerative colitis or coeliac disease	See your doctor, who may refer you to a gastroenterologist.
Nausea and vomiting accompanied by chest pain, excessive thirst, increased or decreased urination, appetite loss, swelling or numbness in the hands or feet, muscle cramps, trouble concentrating, shortness of breath, or dizziness	Heart, liver or kidney failure	Call your doctor immediately. A thorough physical examination can determine the existence and extent of these serious conditions.
Nausea or vomiting accompanied by throbbing headache on one or both sides of the head and sensitivity to light and sound; may be accompanied by flashing lights, blind spots or tingling in the arm or face prior to head pain	A migraine	Migraines typically last from 4 hours to three days. Take an aspirin immediately or a prescription migraine medication if you have one, and lie down in a darkened room. If you have more than two migraines a month, see your doctor, who may recommend preventive medication. If this is your first migraine, do not take aspirin; call your doctor.

Numbness and tingling

DESCRIPTION	POSSIBLE CAUSES	RESPONSE
Numbness and tingling along the arm or down the back of the leg, sometimes after an accident or fall	An injury to a nerve in the neck or back	See your doctor.
Pain in the lower back radiating to the buttock or down the back of the leg that may include numbness in the leg or foot	Sciatica caused by pressure on the spinal nerve from a herniated disc in the back	Avoid activity that hurts, but do exercise, or the muscles around the disc will weaken. Over-the-counter painkillers and physical therapy can also help, as can weight loss if you are overweight.
Numbness or tingling in the hand, wrist and fingers that develops over time, usually due to overuse of the hands for repetitive motion; may be accompanied by loss of feeling in the fingers	Carpal tunnel syndrome	See your doctor. Treatment options include wrist splinting, stretching exercises, nonsteroidal anti-inflammatory drugs, corticosteroids and, in some cases, surgery.
In people with diabetes, numbness and tingling, usually in the feet; may be accompanied by a reduced ability to feel pain, heat or cold; loss of balance; or sharp pains that worsen at night	Diabetic neuropathy	See your doctor. There is no cure, but symptoms can be managed with medication. To prevent progression, keep your blood sugar and blood pressure under control and take your diabetes medication as prescribed.
Numbness or tingling that comes on suddenly and affects one side of the body; may be accompanied by dizziness, blurred vision, headache or confusion	Stroke or transient ischaemic attack (TIA)	Go to the hospital immediately. Prompt treatment can save your life and reduce your risk of permanent disability.
Numbness or tingling that comes on gradually in your fingers, hands and lower extremities; may be accompanied by fatigue or muscle weakness anywhere in the body	Abnormal levels of calcium, potassium, sodium or vitamin B_{12}	See your doctor, who may suggest blood tests and a supplement; be sure to discuss any other supplements you take.

Painful urination

DESCRIPTION	POSSIBLE CAUSES	RESPONSE
A burning sensation during urination; may be accompanied by a frequent need to urinate	A urinary tract infection	See your doctor, who will order diagnostic urinalysis. Treatment is usually an antibiotic.
A burning sensation during urination accompanied by fever over 38.5°C and back pain	A kidney infection	See your doctor. An antibiotic is prescribed when a bacterial infection in the bladder moves to the kidneys.
Itching and burning during urination; may occur after antibiotic treatment	A yeast infection	See your doctor, who may collect a mucus specimen from your vagina to check for the presence of yeast.
Painful urination after starting a new medication	A side effect of medications such as ibuprofen and some antidepressants, osteoporosis drugs, and cancer drugs	Talk with your doctor about whether a different medication should be substituted. Side effects sometimes disappear after a few days or weeks of taking a medication.
Pain or pressure in the bladder area with difficulty emptying the bladder completely	An ovarian cyst pressing against the bladder	See your doctor, who will order tests such as an ultrasound and may biopsy the cyst if cancer is suspected.
Severe pain in the back and side; may be accompanied by a frequent need to urinate, inability to urinate, bloody urine, fever, chills or foul-smelling urine	Kidney stones	See your doctor, who will order a CT scan, ultrasound or abdominal X-ray. Many kidney stones pass on their own. If they don't pass, they may need to be surgically removed or shattered with shock waves.
Painful urination possibly accompanied by sores, blisters, scabs or pustules in the genital area; painful intercourse; and unusual discharge from the vagina or penis	A sexually transmissible infection such as genital herpes, genital warts, syphilis, gonorrhoea or HIV/AIDS	See your doctor; prompt treatment can often prevent more serious symptoms. Avoid intercourse until you've seen your doctor.

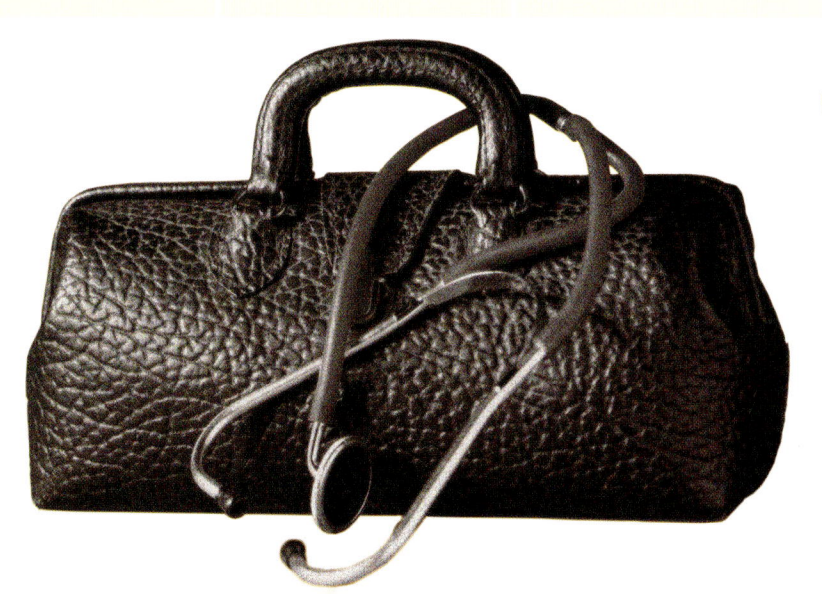

Shortness of breath

DESCRIPTION	POSSIBLE CAUSES	RESPONSE
Sudden shortness of breath accompanied by chest pain or pressure, pain that radiates outward from the chest, or sweating	A heart attack, arrhythmia or a blood clot that travels from the legs to the heart	Call an ambulance.
Sudden shortness of breath after inhaling a piece of food, liquid or other foreign object; may be accompanied by frequent cough, fever, the feeling that something is stuck in your throat or pain when trying to take a deep breath	Airway obstruction or infection (acute pneumonia) caused by aspiration of a foreign object	If the person is choking, slap them between the shoulder blades. Otherwise, go to the emergency department, where a bronchoscope or laryngoscope can be used to remove a foreign object. If infection is present, antibiotics may be prescribed.
Sudden shortness of breath after exposure to an allergen such as nuts, shellfish or eggs; may be accompanied by itching, hives, swelling of the tongue or reddened skin	Anaphylactic shock	Call an ambulance immediately. Use an EpiPen if your doctor has prescribed one.
Sudden shortness of breath after exposure to a known trigger such as dust, pollen or pet dander	Asthma or an environmental allergy	Use an inhaler if you have one; take an antihistamine.
Shortness of breath before, during or after a very stressful or anxiety-provoking experience; may come on suddenly and may be accompanied by sweating, hyperventilation, nausea, chest pain or tightness in your throat	Panic attack	If you are hyperventilating, breathe through pursed lips (as if you were going to blow out a candle) or cover your mouth and one nostril and breathe through the other nostril. If it's your first panic attack, go to the emergency department to exclude a more serious condition. If attacks continue, see your doctor, who may recommend medication or behavioural therapy.
Shortness of breath that comes on gradually, lasts for a week or more and is accompanied by fever or cold or flu symptoms	Bronchitis or pneumonia	See your doctor, who may order an X-ray. Treatment options include antibiotics, antifungal medication and oxygen therapy.
Shortness of breath that comes on gradually and becomes chronic	Asthma, chronic obstructive pulmonary disease, cardiovascular disease, emphysema, tumours, pulmonary hypertension, muscular dystrophy or amyotrophic lateral sclerosis (ALS)	See your doctor, who will order diagnostic tests.

Unintentional weight gain

DESCRIPTION	POSSIBLE CAUSES	RESPONSE
Gradual weight gain with no other symptoms	Decrease in exercise, increased kilojoule intake, or ageing	Eat less and get more exercise. As you age, your energy (kilojoule) needs decrease.
Weight gain accompanied by swelling, chest pain or shortness of breath	Heart or lung disease	See your doctor, who will order diagnostic tests.
Weight gain accompanied by fatigue, hair loss, decreased cold tolerance, constipation or depression	Hypothyroidism (underactive thyroid)	See your doctor, who will order a diagnostic blood test. If your thyroid is underactive, treatment is thyroid hormone replacement medication.
Weight gain after starting a new medication	A side effect of medications such as corticosteroids, lithium and some anti-depressants	Talk with your doctor about whether a different medication should be substituted. Side effects sometimes disappear after a few days or weeks of taking a medication.
In women, gradual weight gain possibly accompanied by irregular or nonexistent periods, excess hair growth, acne or infertility	Polycystic ovary syndrome	See your doctor, who can prescribe medications to help control symptoms.
Weight gain during a period of high stress or anxiety	Anxiety or intense stress	Look for ways to change whatever is causing the stress or anxiety. Relaxation techniques such as meditation, yoga and visualisation may help you cope. Longer-lasting anxiety can be treated with therapy, medication or both.
Weight gain accompanied by sadness, fatigue, loss of interest in enjoyable activities or thoughts of suicide	Depression	See your doctor, who may refer you to a mental health professional for medication, therapy or both.
Weight gain after quitting smoking	Emotional eating and the slowing of metabolism that comes with smoking cessation	Suck on sugarless lollies or chew sugarless gum, snack on raw vegetables, drink plenty of water, and start an exercise regimen.
Weight gain accompanied by excessive thirst, fatigue, increased urination or poor wound healing	Diabetes	See your doctor, who will order a test to measure your blood sugar levels.

Unintentional weight loss

DESCRIPTION	POSSIBLE CAUSES	RESPONSE
Weight loss accompanied by insomnia, unusual thirst, increased sweating, increased bowel movements and hair loss	Hyperthyroidism or other hormone imbalance	See your doctor, who will order a diagnostic blood test. If your thyroid is overactive, prescription medication can slow it down.
Weight loss after starting a new medication	A side effect of medications such as sedatives, SSRI antidepressants and narcotic pain relievers	Talk with your doctor about whether a different medication should be substituted. Side effects sometimes disappear after a few days or weeks of taking a medication.
Weight loss during a period of high stress or anxiety	Anxiety or intense stress	Look for ways to change whatever is causing the stress or anxiety. Relaxation techniques such as meditation, yoga and visualisation may help you cope. Longer-lasting anxiety can be treated with therapy, medication or both.
Weight loss accompanied by feelings of sadness, fatigue, loss of interest in enjoyable activities or thoughts of suicide	Depression	See your doctor, who may recommend medication, therapy or both.
Weight loss accompanied by gastrointestinal complaints such as bloating, gas, constipation or diarrhoea	Coeliac disease, an autoimmune disorder in which the gluten in wheat, rye and barley damages the intestines and decreases the body's ability to absorb nutrients	See your doctor, who will order a diagnostic blood test or gastroscopy. Switching to a gluten-free diet for life is the only treatment.
Weight loss accompanied by intestinal pain and diarrhoea or loose stools	Ulcerative colitis or Crohn's disease, which prevent digestion and absorption of some of the food you eat	See your doctor, who may recommend dietary changes, surgery, or medication that reduces inflammation.
Weight loss accompanied by excessive thirst, fatigue, increased urination or poor wound healing	Diabetes	See your doctor, who will order a test to measure your blood sugar levels.
Weight loss with no other symptoms or accompanied by unexplained gastrointestinal symptoms such as bloating, abdominal pain, bloody urine, bloody stools or nausea	Gastrointestinal cancer	See your doctor, who will order diagnostic tests.

Vaginal bleeding or discharge

DESCRIPTION	POSSIBLE CAUSES	RESPONSE
Fishy-smelling discharge from the vagina; may be accompanied by swelling, redness, itching or burning	Bacterial vaginosis, an inflammation of the vagina caused by bacteria	See your doctor, who will prescribe an oral antibiotic or an antibiotic cream or suppositories; these can clear up the symptoms within a few days.
Yellow or greenish bubbly discharge with a foul odour; may be accompanied by pain during intercourse; symptoms worsen after a menstrual period	Chlamydia, gonorrhoea, trichomoniasis or other sexually transmissible infection	See your doctor, who will prescribe antibiotic injections or tablets. Ask whether your partner should also receive treatment, and avoid intercourse until the infection clears up.
White, cheese-like discharge; may be accompanied by swelling, pain during intercourse and itching; may occur shortly after beginning a course of oral antibiotics	Thrush	See your doctor, who will prescribe an antifungal drug to be administered orally or vaginally.
Bleeding between menstrual periods	Uterine fibroids, or cancer of the uterus, vagina, endometrium or ovaries	See your doctor, who will order diagnostic tests.
Bleeding between menstrual periods, possibly accompanied by excess hair growth, acne or infertility	Polycystic ovary syndrome	See your doctor, who may prescribe medication to help control symptoms.
Bleeding while using an IUD, contraceptive injection or contraceptive implant	These methods of contraception can cause occasional spotting	See your doctor if bleeding continues or becomes heavy.
Bleeding during pregnancy	A miscarriage, ectopic pregnancy or other serious complication	Call your doctor immediately.
Bleeding or discharge; may be accompanied by fever or pain in the pelvic or lower abdominal area	Pelvic inflammatory disease, an inflammation or infection of the ovaries, fallopian tubes or uterus; can be caused by sexually transmissible bacteria or after surgery, including insertion of an IUD	See your doctor. Prompt treatment with antibiotics can prevent damage to your reproductive system that could contribute to infertility, ectopic pregnancy and other reproductive disorders.
Bleeding after intercourse	A sexually transmissible infection, cancer of the cervix or dry vaginal walls caused by lack of oestrogen	See your doctor for testing.

Vision loss

DESCRIPTION	POSSIBLE CAUSES	RESPONSE
Sudden loss of vision that occurs after an accident, sports injury, chemical burn or contact with irritating foreign material	An injury to the retina, cornea or nerves, including corneal abrasion and torn retina	Sudden vision loss is always an emergency. Go to the hospital immediately.
A sudden change in vision accompanied by confusion, slurred speech, sudden numbness on one side of the body or sudden severe headache	Stroke or transient ischaemic attack (TIA)	Go to the hospital immediately. Prompt treatment can save your life and reduce your risk of permanent disability.
A gradual decrease in your ability to focus on nearby objects	Presbyopia, an age-related change that typically begins around the age of 40	Buy reading glasses from a pharmacy or consult an optometrist for bifocals.
Blurred vision, burning, dryness, irritation or a gritty feeling in the eyes; often occurs in women during menopause	Dry eyes	Use over-the-counter or prescription eyedrops. In severe cases, a doctor can insert plugs into the tear ducts to maintain moisture in the eye.
Blurred vision and dry eyes after starting a new medication	A side effect of medications such as diuretics, beta-blockers, antihistamines, sleeping pills and some pain relievers	Talk with your doctor about whether a different medication should be substituted. Side effects sometimes disappear after a few days or weeks of taking a new medication.
In people with diabetes, blurred or spotty vision	Diabetic retinopathy, in which blood vessels in the retina are damaged	See your doctor. Surgery (laser or conventional) can reduce loss of vision.
In older people, blurred, cloudy vision; may be accompanied by faded appearance of colours, glare or halos around lights, poor night vision, or double vision	Cataracts, a condition in which the eye's lens is clouded by clumps of protein	See your doctor. Clouded lenses can be surgically removed and replaced with artificial ones, improving vision in 90 per cent of cases.
Blank spots in your field of vision possibly accompanied by blurred vision, loss of peripheral vision, eye pain, headache and rainbow-coloured halos around lights	Glaucoma, a disease caused by pressure within the eye that damages the optic nerve	See your doctor. Surgery and medication (eyedrops or tablets) can slow glaucoma's progression but can't bring back lost vision.
Blurriness or loss of central vision; may be accompanied by straight lines appearing wavy, difficulty recognising faces and the need for extra light while reading	Age-related macular degeneration, a disease that occurs when the macula—the central part of the eye—breaks down or is damaged	See your doctor. Treatments include laser surgery, photodynamic therapy (medication combined with light therapy) and medications that are injected into the eye as often as every month. Treatment can't restore lost vision but can usually delay further loss.

Wounds that won't heal

DESCRIPTION	POSSIBLE CAUSES	RESPONSE
Cuts or bruises that heal unusually slowly but do not appear infected	Weakened immunity, which can be caused by poor nutrition, vitamin deficiency, steroid medications or cancer treatment	Talk with your doctor about vitamin supplementation or changes in steroid use; follow-up with a dietitian may be useful.
A wound that is swollen, red or hot, or has pus or red lines radiating from it; may be accompanied by fever	Cellulitis (a bacterial infection of the skin) or a foreign object stuck in the wound	See your doctor, who may prescribe an antibiotic. If symptoms are worsening quickly, go to the emergency department. Cellulitis can cause serious infection that can spread.
Poor wound healing accompanied by chest pain, shortness of breath and changes in urinary habits	A disease of the heart, lungs, kidneys or other major organs	See your doctor, who will probably order diagnostic tests.
Poor wound healing accompanied by excessive thirst, increased urination, unexplained weight loss, increased hunger or blurred vision	Undiagnosed or poorly controlled diabetes	See your doctor, who will order a test to measure your blood sugar levels. If you have diabetes that is poorly controlled, you may need to switch from a family doctor to an endocrinologist.
In people with diabetes, poor wound healing in the feet; may be accompanied by a reduced ability to feel pain, heat or cold; loss of balance; or sharp pains that worsen at night	Diabetic neuropathy	See your doctor. There is no cure, but symptoms can be managed with medication. To prevent progression, keep your blood sugar and blood pressure under control and take your diabetes medication as prescribed.
Sores on the legs or feet that won't heal accompanied by cold feet, leg or foot pain or numbness, or changes in the toenails or amount of hair on the legs or feet	Peripheral arterial disease, a restriction of blood flow in the arteries of the leg caused by accumulation of arterial plaque	See your doctor. Circulation can be improved with exercise, quitting smoking and a heart-healthy diet; in some cases, medication or surgery is needed.
A sore in the mouth or on the lip or skin that doesn't heal; may be accompanied by other symptoms, such as unexplained weight loss	Oral cancer or skin cancer	See your doctor, who may order diagnostic tests.

Key steps to disease prevention

When preventive medicine specialists were polled about what really helps to prevent disease, their answers were surprising, and challenged us to look at health in new ways. Exercising, eating more fruit and vegetables, and quitting smoking are still important, as is getting necessary screening tests, but while you're having your cholesterol levels measured, you may want to measure your level of happiness, too. That's right—a happy, stress-free life driven by a higher purpose emerged as the real picture of healthy living.

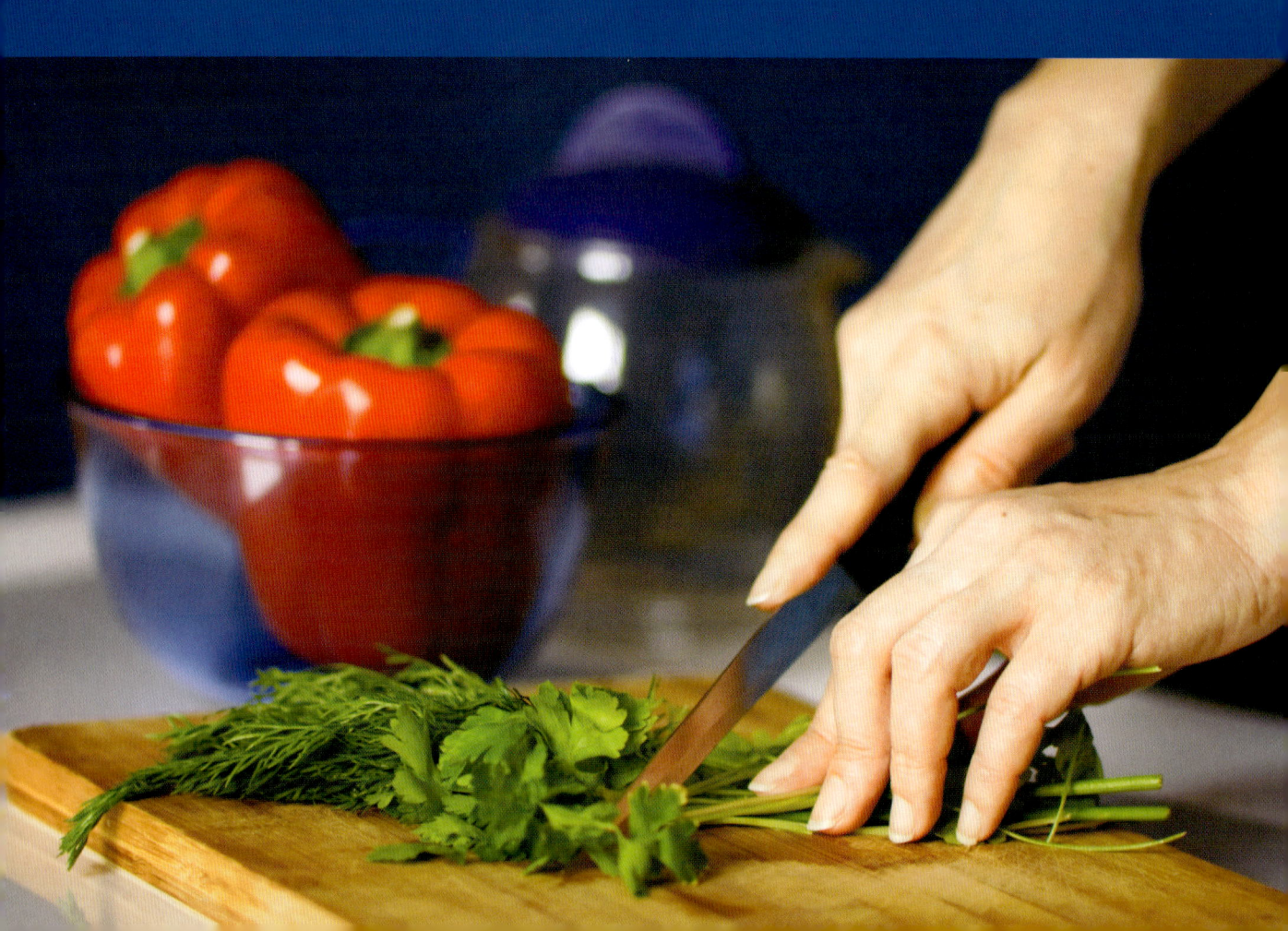

Getting organised

Now that you've read about the main causes of disease and completed the quiz on pages 18–19, it's time to take a closer look at the key steps that are going to put your health back on track—and keep it on track. By following the steps outlined in this chapter you'll lower your risk for a collection of major diseases, from cardiovascular disease and stroke to Type 2 diabetes and lung cancer, and ensure that health issues are not going to become an obstacle to your enjoyment of life. Even if your quiz score was good, there's still room for improvement. But if your score was lower than it should be, then you'll want to make sure you start incorporating all of the steps outlined on the following pages, to reap the maximum health benefits.

All 12 key steps are important lifestyle measures that most of us can manage, but the top three—quitting smoking, getting 30 minutes of light exercise on most days, eating at least seven serves of fruit and vegetables daily—can drastically reduce your risk for disease. And of those, giving up smoking rated highest in our Disease Prevention Survey.

It's really no surprise that quitting smoking rates as the first and most important key step, but for some people it is one of the most challenging things they'll ever do. To help you quit, we have outlined five easy ways to make breaking the habit a successful enterprise. For other people, making time for regular physical activity is what's hardest to achieve—even if they don't smoke and enjoy a diet rich in fresh produce. Everyone needs to get moving to burn kilojoules in order to maintain a healthy weight and to prevent obesity and the complications arising from it. The underlying message is that each of the key steps works in combination with the others.

Getting started usually happens once you get organised, but how do you do that? Make a list of the key steps that aren't already part of your everyday life, then read through each of those steps, noting down what the advice on offer is. For example, if you've tried to quit smoking a number of times, using only willpower, and failed, talk to your GP about the possibility of taking medication to help you succeed this time. By approaching lifestyle changes in an organised way, you'll increase your chances of sticking with them in the long run.

What is risk?

Risk is the chance that something might happen in a set time frame. In health terms, that chance can be high (catching at least one cold each winter) or low (getting pancreatic cancer).

For some conditions, you may be able to affect personal risk. For example, the average Australian's chance of developing melanoma is about 5 per cent (1 in 20), but you can reduce that risk by avoiding excessive sun exposure, and by so doing your risk will drop to about 1 per cent (1 in 100). This can be described as an 'absolute risk reduction' of four percentage points. Alternately, the same scenario can be described in terms of a 'relative risk reduction' of 80 per cent, because you are now 80 per cent less likely to get a melanoma than you would have been. Obviously, the relative risk reduction figure sounds more dramatic than the absolute risk figure.

Throughout this book relative risk reduction is used, partly because this is easier for researchers to calculate, but also in the hope that the larger numbers will motivate you to act on the advice of our experts in order to see a significant improvement in your overall health outcomes.

Step 1
Quit smoking

If you smoke, nothing else you do will offer anywhere close to the health benefits you'll get from quitting. It's no surprise that when our panel of preventive medicine experts ranked the habits they considered most detrimental to well-being, 99 per cent put smoking first on the list, ahead of other threats such as being significantly overweight or not getting enough sleep.

It's not news that cigarettes (as well as cigars and pipes) are lethal. Around the world, tobacco kills 5.4 million people annually thanks to lung cancer, breast cancer, heart attack, stroke, diabetes, progressive lung diseases and hundreds of other health problems it triggers or makes worse. And we now know why it's so difficult to quit: in terms of addictive power, experts put nicotine in the same class as heroin and cocaine. So if you've tried to quit smoking before and it hasn't worked, don't worry—and don't give up. It can take as many as five or more attempts. And you don't have to go it alone; in fact, the latest research shows that using several strategies to help you quit, such as nicotine replacement and support from your doctor, can double or even triple your chances of succeeding.

Quitting gives your health an immediate boost. Within 8 hours, levels of toxic carbon monoxide gas in your bloodstream drop to normal. Within a day, your heart attack risk begins to drop. Over your first smoke-free year, your circulation will improve, your senses of taste and smell will sharpen, and you'll have fewer lung infections, cough less and have less sinus congestion. After just a year, your odds of developing heart disease drop by half. And the payoffs mount with each smoke-free year: after four years, your chance of having a heart attack falls to that of someone who has never smoked. After 10 years, your lung cancer risk drops to nearly that of a nonsmoker, and your odds for cancers of the mouth, throat, oesophagus, bladder and kidney decrease significantly, too. To help yourself quit successfully, try these strategies.

Line up help *before* your quit date After you smoke that last cigarette, a relapse can occur very quickly. Within two days, half of all people light up again; by the end of the first week, two-thirds are back to smoking. Help at the right moment can be crucial, and it's easy to get. Before your quit date, set up a visit with your doctor, a cognitive behavioural therapist or a smoking-cessation support group for your first smoke-free week. Or plan to call a telephone quitline. All of these resources can offer custom-tailored help to cope with specific challenges, such as what to do if you've always had a cigarette after dinner (schedule an activity for that time—mow the lawn or take an evening walk with a friend), or smoked when life threw a few challenges your way. In one US study, 43 per cent of people who used a telephone quitline were still smoke free after nine months compared to just 5 per cent who didn't. In Australia, you can call 131 848; in New Zealand, call 0800 778 778; and in South Africa, call 011 720 3145.

Consider a behavioural therapy program or support group When researchers at Oxford University in the UK reviewed 55 smoking-cessation studies, they found that people who joined therapy groups doubled their odds of succeeding, compared to those who tried to kick the habit by themselves.

Use the correct nicotine-replacement dose Chewing gum, patches, lozenges, sprays and inhalers containing nicotine can all be helpful. They all release nicotine very slowly into the bloodstream, easing symptoms of withdrawal without all the other toxins in cigarette smoke.

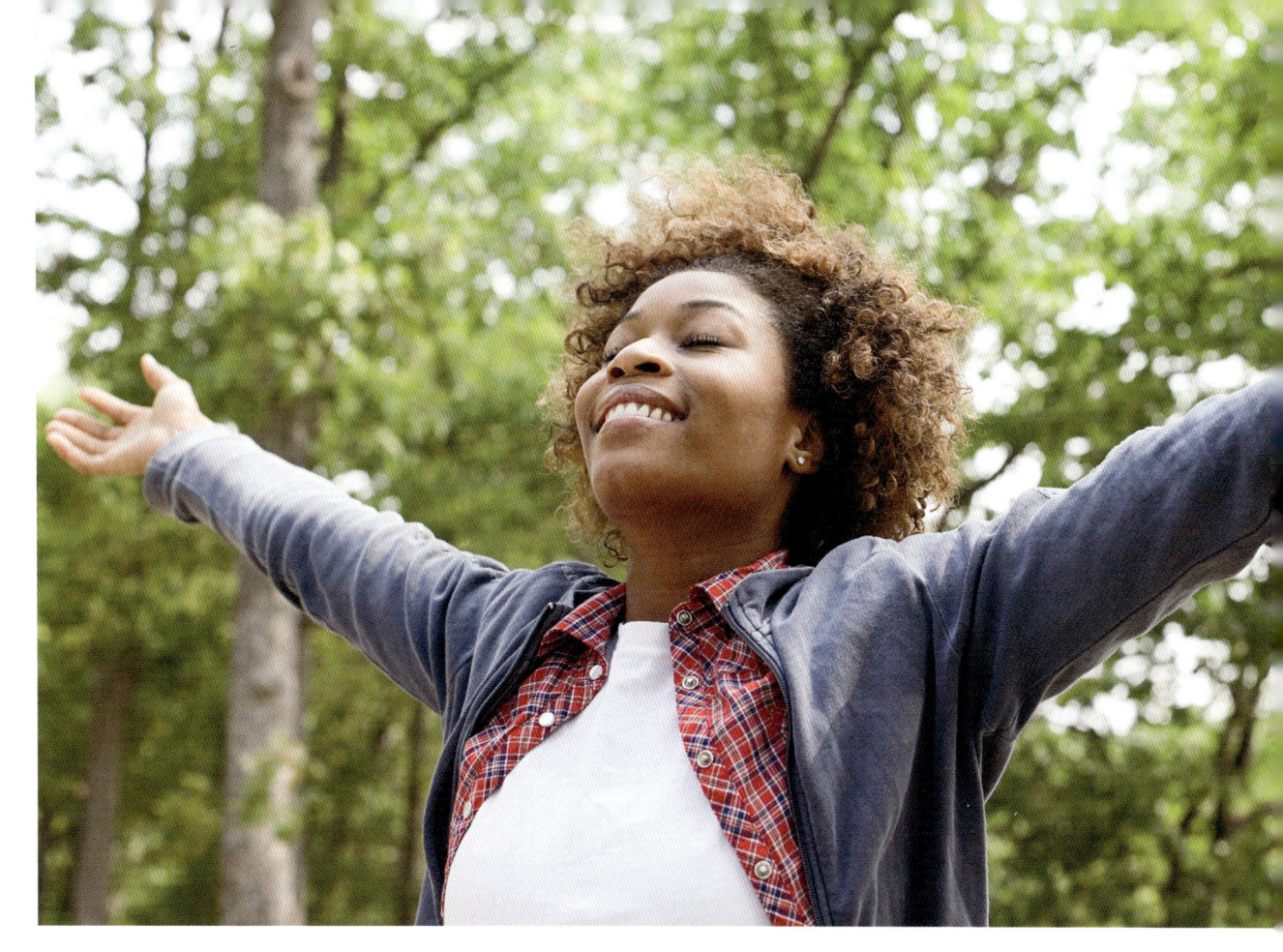

Studies find that the patch increases quit rates by about 7 per cent compared to a placebo, the gum and inhaler by about 8 per cent, and the nasal spray by 12 to 16 per cent. But make sure you're getting enough. If you smoke more than 10 cigarettes a day, for example, choose a higher-dose (usually 21-mg) patch. And if you have your first cigarette within half an hour of waking up in the morning, start the day with a 4-mg lozenge rather than a 2-mg dose.

If you still have cravings, using a patch plus a faster-acting product such as gum, lozenges or a spray or inhaler can further boost your chances of succeeding, according to experts.

Use medications to help you There's a choice of two prescription medications to help you quit smoking: bupropion (Zyban) and varenicline (Champix). They are not addictive and work by decreasing cravings, although doctors are not sure how they do this, but both medications significantly increase your chances of quitting and staying smoke free. Varenicline is taken for at least 12 weeks and the commonest side effect is nausea (it can't be used by pregnant women, but they can use nicotine-replacement therapy). Bupropion is taken for at least seven weeks and the commonest side effect is headache. It is not suitable for anyone who has had a seizure (fit) or is at risk of seizures. Before prescribing either medication, your doctor will need to know your full health history and your regular medications.

Schedule exercise Exercising three times a week may work even better than a behavioural therapy program. In one study, nearly 20 per cent of people who exercised were still smoke free after a year compared to 11 per cent of the therapy group; they also gained less weight. Of course, counselling plus exercise is an even better idea.

Step 2
Get 30 minutes of light exercise on most days

In the short amount of time it takes to watch many TV programs, you could cut your risk of diabetes by 34 per cent, of stroke by 20 per cent, of a hip fracture by 41 per cent and of dying over the next few years by half—and at the same time sharpen your thinking skills, reduce your waistline and improve your general sense of wellbeing.

How? By exercising regularly. The Disease Prevention Survey panel of experts ranked exercise high on their list of health-enhancing 'moves'. And it couldn't be easier: just half an hour of light activity (a walk, a swim, working in the garden) on most days of the week is enough to reap dramatic, body-wide benefits. Even if you have limited mobility, you can still be active.

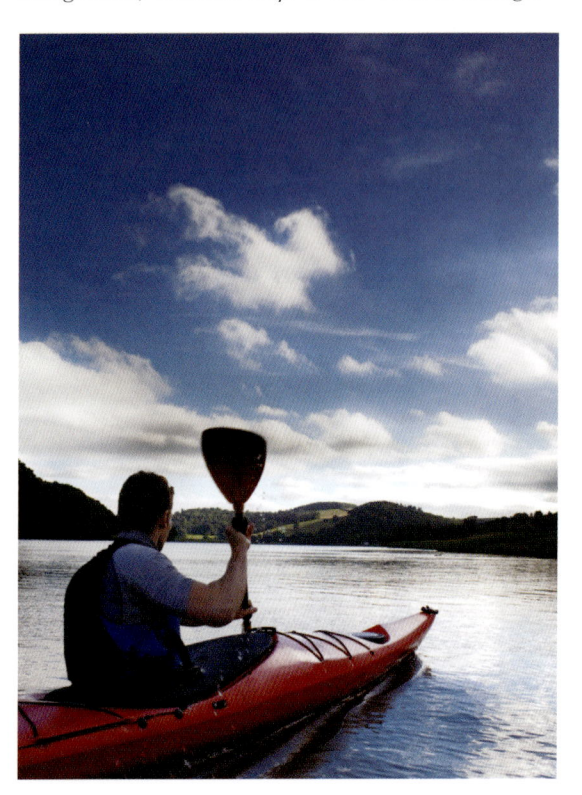

However, the real question about exercise and health isn't whether it works, because most of us have heard that lecture at least 1000 times before. Rather, it's why don't most of us do it?

The honest answer is that many of us have trouble getting off the couch and out the door, possibly because we're scared of exercise, but more probably because inertia takes over when we become accustomed to sitting on the couch and not exercising. And sometimes sitting around all day can make you feel tired, so the impetus to exercise isn't there. Sound familiar?

If you've been putting it off until you feel like exercising, forget it. Waiting for the perfect wave of enthusiasm to get you on your feet just doesn't work. Instead, make a commitment to do just 10 minutes of exercise on a certain schedule. Regular exercisers say that simply getting out there—whether you feel motivated or not—creates the energy that gets you moving and buoys your mood. Just tell yourself you'll walk for 10 short minutes, then once you get started, 10 minutes will soon become 20 minutes and eventually 30 minutes.

Walking or cycling is a great way to start
It's also important to engage in physical activities that strengthen your muscles and build bones, such as working with hand weights or elastic exercise bands, doing moves like sit-ups and push-ups, using the strength machines at the gym, or even working hard in the garden. You begin losing muscle mass in your thirties, and as a result your body burns fewer kilojoules every day—making it tougher to maintain a healthy weight. Some strength training can reverse this trend and give you the strength for everyday activities, such as carrying heavy grocery bags, as well as for dancing, bowling and keeping up with

younger children. It's well worth investing a little time and energy in learning how to do the right strength-training moves for your age and fitness level by buying a few sessions with a personal trainer or taking a class at your local gym.

Your best exercise accessory is a mind-set that helps you find a routine that works for you. Try adjusting your attitude with these ideas.

Anything is better than nothing If you don't have time for a 30-minute walk or a 45-minute gym workout, then use the 5, 10 or 15 minutes you do have. Numerous health studies show that three 10-minute walks burn off kilojoules just as effectively as one 30-minute walk and may be even better at things such as keeping blood pressure lower and healthier all day. Dancing, playing energetically with children, walking rather than driving and taking the stairs instead of the lift can all boost cardiovascular health just as well as a formal work-out.

Willpower is not the answer If you're like most people, willpower alone won't get you up every day for that 7 am walk, or pull you away from the day's work for those sit-ups. Instead, set an exercise 'date'—a regular walking or jogging time with a friend, a class at the gym or even an appointment with your personal trainer, then write it in pen on your calendar.

It should be enjoyable It's no wonder many people think they dislike exercise—how much fun is it to sit in the living room pedalling an exercise bike that's going nowhere? If you're a competitive person, consider taking up squash or tennis. Or if you're social, try to schedule walks with different friends or join a spin or water aerobics class. If you're a nature lover, map out some beautiful places to explore near your home. Or simply plan to work in the garden more often and in a more directed fashion. Exercise isn't just a means to an end; it's part of your life, so it shouldn't feel like a drag.

Opportunities are everywhere That carpark at the back of the supermarket, the stairs next to the escalator, the dog with a leash in his mouth, the young child longing for an outing to the playground—these are all golden opportunities to fit more old-fashioned kilojoule-burning movement into your day. Fifty years ago, we burned about 2950 more kilojoules per day than we do today, not by running marathons but through a host of daily activities that we've since engineered out of our lives, from walking to the bus stop to washing the dishes. It's up to you to create a new trend.

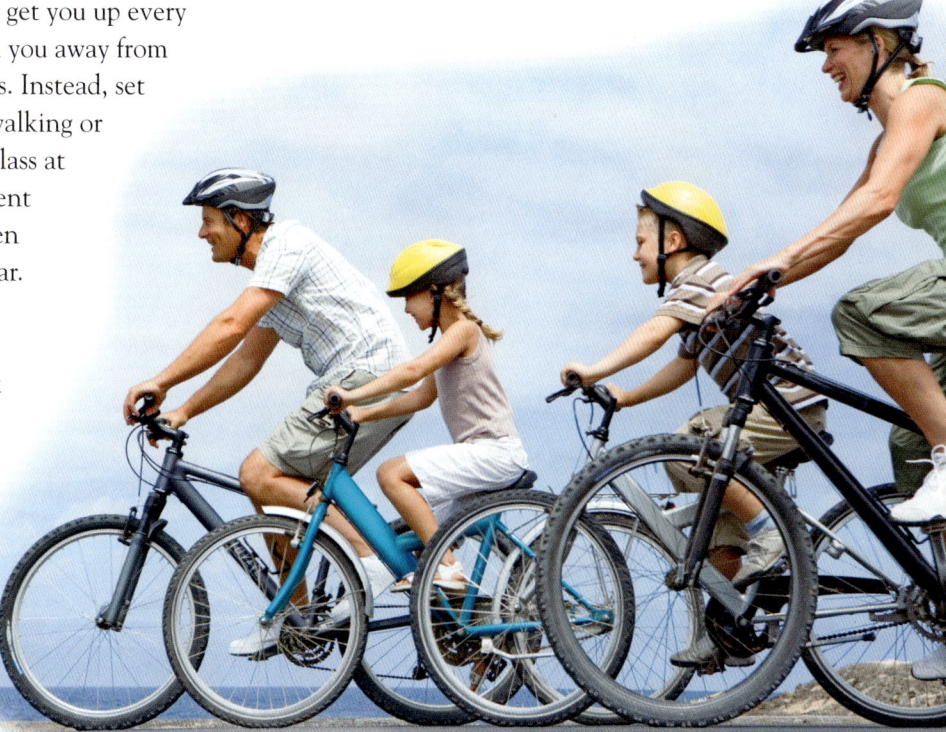

Step 3
Eat at least seven serves of fruit and vegetables daily

If everyone followed the simple advice of our health experts by eating at least seven serves of fruit and vegetables a day, the results would be nothing short of miraculous—there would be emptier hospitals, shorter lines at the pharmacy and far fewer of the major diseases that disable and kill millions each year around the world.

The fact is, we are designed to eat these foods in volume every day. Our bodies are meant to be flooded on a daily basis by those miraculous, health-giving chemicals called anti-oxidants, which protect cells from damage. And we need them now more than ever. Modern life triggers the production of more free radicals in our bodies than previously—thanks in large part to fried foods (and simply overeating), more air pollution and the fact that we're living longer, along with permanent environmental damage such as the thinning atmosphere, which could also be a significant contributing factor.

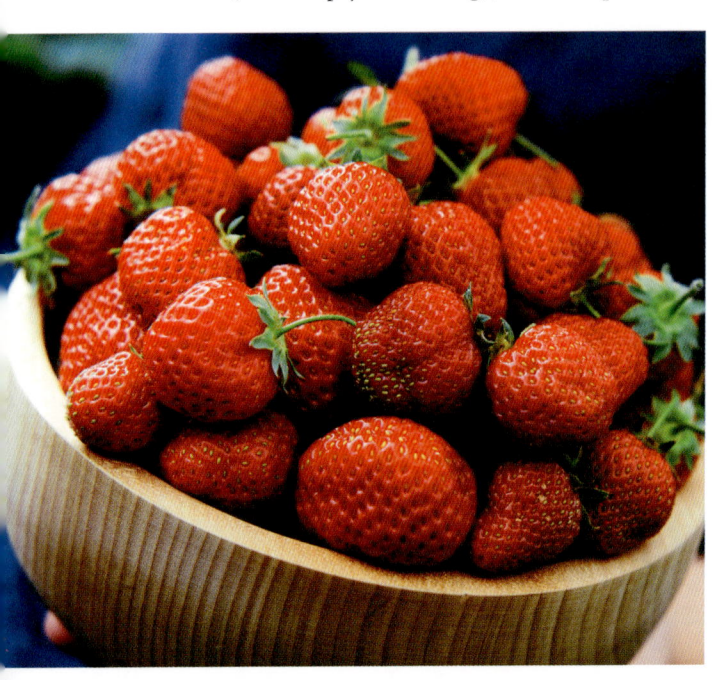

Free radicals are atoms or groups of atoms with an odd number of electrons. They form naturally when we digest food, convert blood sugar into energy or are exposed to sunlight or pollution. Free radicals destroy cell walls or, even worse, DNA itself. The result is an increased cancer risk, cholesterol that's more likely to burrow into artery walls, and damaged cartilage that isn't able to cushion joints properly. Your body uses the anti-oxidants in fruit and vegetables to neutralise these free radicals before they can do harm to cells. If you shortchange yourself by not getting enough of them in your diet, then you're essentially allowing rogue elements to take over your body and wreak havoc.

Fruit is simple to eat and it can transform a meal. Think about grapes in chicken salad or the burst of sharp sweetness a few strawberries add to cereal. With a little creativity, vegetables can be just as delicious—ripe red tomatoes dressed with basil, roasted zucchini or kumara (orange sweet potatoes) with just a pinch of cinnamon or nutmeg.

Putting fresh, healthy food on your plate doesn't have to take longer than picking up fast-food or tossing a frozen meal into the microwave, and it's more than worth it for health gain. And thanks to the convenience of prewashed and precut fresh vegetables that are now available in most supermarkets, you'll be surprised at how easy it can be to put a meal together quickly. Try these strategies to reach your daily target.

Assign specific servings to each meal For example, you might always have a small glass of freshly squeezed orange juice plus a handful of berries or a slice of melon at breakfast, start lunch with a salad (three serves of vegetables),

Key steps to disease prevention

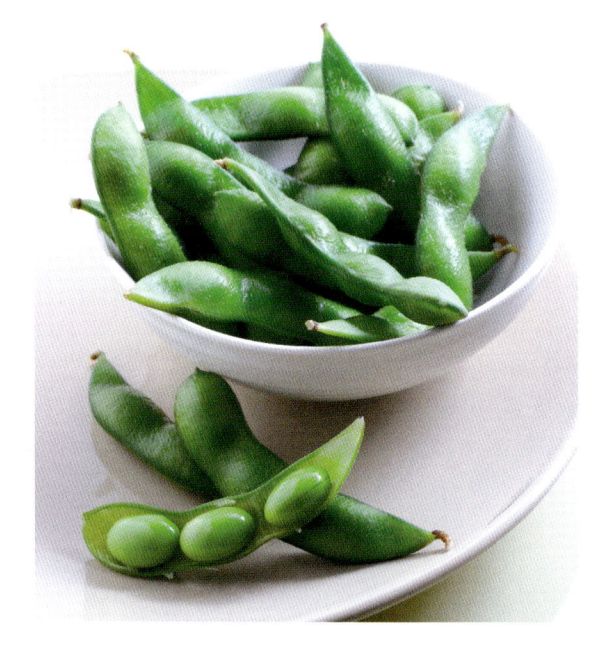

have fruit as a snack and serve another two to three serves of vegetables with dinner. That's more than seven serves right there.

Aim to always have two colours of fruit or vegetables on your plate Start breakfast with a spinach and capsicum omelette, have carrots and black beans (legumes count as vegetables) on your salad at lunch, top pasta with tomatoes and steamed broccoli at dinner, and snack on berries and melon in yogurt. It's an automatic two serves per meal and fills your body with a variety of anti-oxidants and other beneficial phytochemicals essential for good health.

Double each vegetable portion you'd normally eat This is a good approach if you're already eating several serves a day.

Load up on ready-to-use produce Try cans of fruit in natural juice (not syrup), frozen plain (no sauce) vegetables, frozen berries and presliced, pretrimmed vegetables. And look for prewashed spinach, rocket and other salad leaf mixes.

Keep salads interesting Plain green salads can be boring, but varied toppings will fix that. Try roasted sesame seeds, canned artichoke hearts, a few olives, roasted beetroot, capsicums, chillies or even a few raspberries or orange segments.

New reasons to eat less

Big portions and high-fat, high-kilojoule, processed foods are the number-one enemies of good health. Excess weight puts you at higher risk for heart disease and diabetes. But a growing body of research links obesity to an increased risk of most types of cancer, too. Not surprisingly, cutting back on overeating is a top priority in reducing your risk for these diseases and many others.

Eating too much not only packs on visible kilos, it also crowds internal organs with fat that fuels the development of major disease processes. But extra kilojoules are dangerous for a second reason: digestion creates destructive particles called free radicals that play a role in a host of health problems, from joint pain to cancer. More food, more digestion, more free radicals. Eating just enough is a challenge in today's world, but it can be done. Here's how:

- **Dole out single serves** Don't serve platters of food or sit near an open bag of snacks.

- **Eat at home** Women who eat out five times a week or more consume 1260 kilojoules more each day than those who don't.

- **Bulk up your meals with extra vegetables** These add fibre, water and volume to your meal—three factors that make you feel fuller while you're eating hundreds fewer kilojoules. Researchers say this strategy also stretches the stomach wall, activating 'fullness receptors'.

- **Eat only until you're 80 per cent full** This ancient Japanese custom gives your mind time to register what you've eaten. Leave the table when you still have room for a little more instead of finishing everything that's there. Within 20 minutes, you'll feel satisfied.

Step 4
Get recommended screening tests

Left to their own devices, some invisible health problems turn into big ones. A slightly raised blood sugar level becomes full-blown diabetes; pre-hypertension becomes high blood pressure; suspicious-looking cells become cancer. Your best defence is to catch these and other silent health issues early on, when they can most easily be reversed and even cured.

There's no doubt that a healthy lifestyle is the best way to prevent most major medical nightmares from developing in the first place, but trouble can still arise in the healthiest of bodies. That's why our preventive medicine specialists ranked getting recommended screening tests highly on their list of 'prescriptions' for staying disease free. Unfortunately, many of us skip these important, easy-to-get tests. Laziness, lack of time, fear of finding out that something's wrong or the mistaken conviction that you really don't need the screenings because you're feeling fit and healthy can cause you to not get tested—and then seriously regret it later on.

See the table on the page opposite for a list of common screening tests and when to get them. (The guidelines suggested are set out for Australians and New Zealanders; South Africans should ask their doctor about timing guidelines.)

Get screened during a regular visit to the doctor If you're already scheduling an appointment for a sore throat, sinus infection, earache or other minor problem, ask if you can get simple screening tests such as cholesterol, mammography, blood pressure and blood sugar at the same time, rather than making a separate appointment for an annual physical.

Hate going to the doctor? Go with your spouse or a friend to increase your odds of getting the screenings you need by seeing your family doctor together for things such as a Pap smear, cholesterol and blood pressure testing, and colon cancer screenings. You can also offer to be each other's support team when it's time for specialised checks for breast and prostate cancer.

Speak up about your family history Make sure your doctor knows about any relevant family history. If a close relative has had a stroke or heart attack or was diagnosed with cancer or diabetes, it's important to let the doctor know.

Mention depression Doctors should screen for depression, but they don't always. If you're constantly overwhelmed by feelings of sadness or hopelessness, let your doctor know. There are treatment options that may help.

Ask about vaccinations Aside from a yearly flu vaccine, you should get a one time-only shingles vaccine if you've never had chickenpox, and a one-time-only pneumonia vaccine if you're aged 65 or older (50 or older if you're an indigenous Australian or New Zealander).

Keep track Don't wait for your doctor to tell you it's time to check your cholesterol again. Keep a record of the tests and vaccinations you've had and when in a small notebook or wherever you record birthdays and appointments.

The screening tests you need

	TEST	WHEN TO GET IT
Women	Mammogram	Between 40 and 50, ask your doctor if you need to have this test, especially if you have a family history. Otherwise, get tested every two years from 50 to 70.
	Pap smear	Every two years if your last Pap smear was normal. Your doctor will advise you about the correct timing if your last smear showed any abnormalities.
Men	Prostate specific antigen (PSA test)	Every year from the age of 50 (45 if you have a family history of the disease). However, this is a controversial recommendation so talk to your doctor about the pros and cons of having the test.
	Digital rectal exam	Every year from the age of 50 (45 if you have a family history of the disease). However, this is a controversial recommendation, so talk to your doctor about the pros and cons of having the test.
Everyone	Dental examination and cleaning	Every six months.
	Blood pressure reading	Every two years when you're younger and every year when you're older (over 50); every six months if you have risk factors for cardiovascular disease.
	Cholesterol test	Every two years after the age of 45 if you have any risk factors for cardiovascular disease; every year if you also have a chronic disease.
	Fasting plasma blood sugar test	Every three years.
	Skin cancer check	Every year, or every three months if you have a higher than normal risk.
	Eye exam, hearing test and falls risk	Every year for older people.
	Faecal occult blood test (for bowel cancer)	Every two years from the age of 50; after 75, discuss this with your doctor. People at high risk may need more frequent testing from a younger age.
	Kidney health check	Every five years; every year if you have risk factors such as high blood pressure.
	Weight	Every two years; more often if you have diabetes, cardiovascular disease, gout, liver or gall bladder disease, or are an indigenous person.

Step 5
Get at least 7 to 8 hours sleep a night

Blame it on insomnia, our infatuation with caffeine, shift work or pay TV and the Internet; whatever the cause, we've become sleep-deprived. And we're paying the price with higher rates of obesity, diabetes, depression, anxiety and some forms of cancer—all partly due to a lack of sleep.

Researchers are beginning to suspect that sleep deprivation exerts its far-reaching effects on the body by disrupting levels of key hormones and proteins. These include the appetite-regulating hormones ghrelin and leptin, which is why lack of sleep contributes to weight gain; stress hormones, such as cortisol, that raise blood sugar and blood pressure (a reason lack of sleep makes diabetes worse); and proteins involved in chronic inflammation, a condition in which the immune system remains on high alert, raising the risk of heart disease, stroke, cancer and diabetes. Lack of sleep also seems to reduce levels of melatonin, which is a hormone that may help to protect our bodies against cancer.

If you have insomnia or you're a heavy snorer and often wake up exhausted, turn to 'Insomnia' and 'Snoring', on pages 228 and 292, respectively. More often than not, many of us are our own worst enemies when it comes to getting enough sleep. If that's you, put these three simple strategies to work in order to get 7 to 8 hours of deep, refreshing sleep every night.

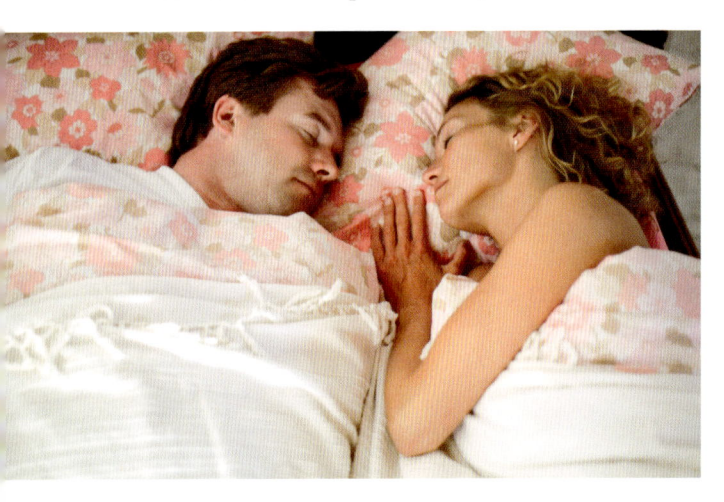

Pick your perfect bedtime, then stick with it for two weeks Count back 8 hours from the time you have to get up in the morning. This is your new, not-negotiable lights-out time. Subtract another half an hour: this is your new 'get into bed' time. Subtract another half an hour to find the time when you should start relaxing, getting your mind and body ready for sleep before turning in. Here's an example: if you have to be up at 6:30 am, you'll need to start relaxing by 9:30 pm, get into bed by 10 pm and turn out the lights by 10:30 pm.

Turn off all electronics Half an hour before you get into bed, turn off the TV, computer, mobile phone and personal digital assistant. Politely tell anyone who calls on your home phone that you'll talk to them tomorrow (or better yet, screen your calls and return non-urgent messages in the morning). Lock up the house, have a shower or bath and climb into clean, comfortable pyjamas. Brush your teeth, comb your hair, do a few minutes of gentle stretching or deep breathing, then read a few pages of your book. And skip snacks during this winding-down time: too often we turn to food to fuel a burst of late-night energy.

When it's time, turn out the lights If you've trained yourself to fight back fatigue and keep on going, you may be tempted to stay up just a little later. But make a habit of simply turning out the lights when it's time to sleep. It will soon become a habit in itself and you'll feel much better for it.

Step 6

Consider taking a low-dose aspirin every day

Taking a low-dose aspirin daily only applies if your doctor has recently confirmed that it's appropriate for you to do so.

Aspirin can protect against two of the biggest killers: heart disease and stroke. Taking one a day can cut your risk of having a heart attack by as much as 23 per cent and a stroke by 15 per cent. New research suggests it may even cut the odds for the most common form of breast cancer by 16 per cent. Yet fewer than half of the people who could benefit from this inexpensive health 'insurance policy' take this potent medication.

Aspirin guards your heart by making platelets, the special clotting cells in your bloodstream, less sticky. This means they're less likely to form a clot that can then travel to your heart, causing a heart attack, or to your brain, causing a stroke. And aspirin's anticancer benefits are probably due to its anti-inflammatory effects (chronic inflammation plays a significant role in the development of cancer).

It sounds very convincing, but don't start taking aspirin every day without medical consideration. In some people, long-term use can provoke serious digestive upset and excessive bleeding, including bleeding in the brain. Doctors usually recommend daily aspirin therapy only to people with risk factors for heart attack and stroke, such as smoking, high cholesterol, diabetes or a family or personal history of either condition. If you're already taking an aspirin daily, drink alcohol in moderation (no more than one drink a day for women or men), because the combination of aspirin and excessive intake of alcohol can cause damage to your liver.

The rules for taking aspirin

If you take aspirin daily or are thinking about it, these essential tips can help to keep you safe.

- **Tell your doctor if you bleed easily** due to a clotting disorder or have asthma, stomach ulcers or heart failure, all conditions that may prevent you from taking a daily low-dose aspirin.

- **Take the dose your doctor recommends** Some studies have found benefit from as little as 75 mg a day (less than the 100 mg in low-dose aspirin), but some doctors prefer to prescribe half a regular-strength, 300-mg tablet, daily.

- **Ibuprofen interferes with aspirin's anti-clotting ability, reducing its effectiveness** If you need a single dose of ibuprofen for pain, take it 2 hours after taking aspirin. If you use ibuprofen regularly, talk to your doctor about ways of getting the most from both drugs.

- **Tell your surgeon and dentist** If you need a surgical procedure or dental work, inform your doctor about your aspirin use ahead of time to avoid problems like excessive bleeding.

- **Before you begin taking aspirin on a daily basis,** tell your doctor if you take another blood-thinning drug, such as warfarin (Coumadin), or any herbs and supplements, especially vitamin E, St John's wort or ginkgo biloba. All can interact with aspirin and thin the blood too much.

Step 7
Know your blood pressure reading

Simply knowing what your blood pressure is could cut your risk for heart attack, stroke, kidney failure or blindness. If you don't know what your reading is, you may not know whether you're developing high blood pressure, the disease that nearly every doctor in the survey said has the greatest potential for causing chronic disease. And if you don't know your blood pressure is creeping up over the years, you can't take steps to bring it back down, leaving the door open for years or even decades of damage to occur.

You can't feel high blood pressure, but it wreaks havoc on your cardiovascular system—thickening heart muscle, promoting the growth of plaque in artery walls, rupturing blood vessels in your brain, tearing vessels in your eyes, weakening your kidneys and even raising your risk of dementia. You should have your blood pressure checked every year, but some doctors don't do that, so ask to have it done and record the results.

Until just a few years ago, doctors thought you were in the clear if your blood pressure was below 140/90 mmHg. Now we know the risk of heart disease and stroke begins to rise when blood pressure is as low as 115/75 mmHg. Being in the 'pre-hypertensive' range—with a reading between 120/80 and 140/90 mmHg—raises your risk of dying from heart disease by 58 per cent, making this 'little' problem more deadly than smoking.

More than one in four adults have what's called pre-hypertension. Even if your pressure is normal now, consider that 90 per cent of us will develop high blood pressure after the age of fifty-five. And don't depend on your doctor to catch rising blood pressure early, when it's easiest to fix. According to studies, some doctors opt to 'wait and see' what develops when their patients' pressures start creeping up. So it's up to you to keep tabs on your own blood pressure and to take action if it starts rising, even if your reading is still within the healthy range.

Live a healthy blood-pressure lifestyle At breakfast, lunch and dinner, you can choose the power foods that fight hypertension. One top eating strategy is to follow the DASH diet, which is packed with fruit and vegetables, whole grains, and several serves of low-fat dairy foods, every day. Keep sodium low, too. Quitting smoking, treating obstructive sleep apnoea and getting regular exercise can all make big dents in raised blood pressure.

Ask about medication If lifestyle changes alone don't lower your blood pressure, medication can help. Forward-thinking doctors are beginning to prescribe blood pressure-lowering medications even to people in the pre-hypertensive category if they have other risk factors for heart disease or kidney problems, such as diabetes or kidney disease.

What the numbers mean

115/75 mmHg or lower: Ideal

Below 120/80 mmHg: Healthy

120–139/80–89 mmHg: Pre-hypertensive

140/90 mmHg: High blood pressure

Step 8
Stay connected with family and friends

A growing body of scientific research is proving that positive, happy relationships literally change the biochemistry of your brain for the better, while loneliness raises your risk of problems such as high blood pressure, depression and even an early death. In fact, an overwhelming 79 per cent of the doctors polled in the Disease Prevention Survey said that social isolation is extremely detrimental to health. Good times with friends and family, on the other hand, pump up feelings of joy, boost immunity, lower your risk of heart trouble and can even extend your life.

Experts are beginning to realise that we're hardwired for personal connection. Back in prehistoric times, being alone was perilous— no one was around to help fend off marauding wolves or forage for roots and berries if you were sick. And although today we're remarkably self-sufficient, our ancient responses haven't really changed. When you're alone for too long (and the definition of 'too long' is different for each of us), levels of the stress hormone cortisol rise, increasing your odds of heart disease, high blood pressure, depression, confusion and sleep problems. One US study even found that our brains register social isolation in the same way that they register physical pain, which is quite alarming.

Here are some easy ways that you can improve your health by staying connected socially.

Reach out Stop waiting for the perfect moment. Plenty of people you know are shy and would love it if you called with an invitation to a movie or to come over to enjoy dinner together. Thinking that you need an elaborate plan, a perfectly clean house or a new haircut before you can make a date only postpones happiness.

Have physical contact more often Sit closer to your spouse or partner. Hold hands more often— and while you're at it, make love more often. Studies show that these physical connections buffer stress and even cut heart attack risk. If you need more touch in your life and don't have a life partner, don't forget about hugging the younger people in your life, along with our furry, four-legged friends. Plenty of research shows that animals can have profound health benefits, including reducing levels of stress hormones and calming high blood pressure. Having regular, gentle touch is very important for happiness in our everyday lives.

Expand your network Old friends know us best, but relying on a small group of companions could be a setup for loneliness. Invest in your future health by reaching out to a new person this week. An easy way to begin is to strike up a conversation with someone you might see often in your neighbourhood, at your gym, at work or somewhere else. Then go a step further and ask if they'd like to join you for a cup of coffee or a walk during your lunch hour or on a weekend.

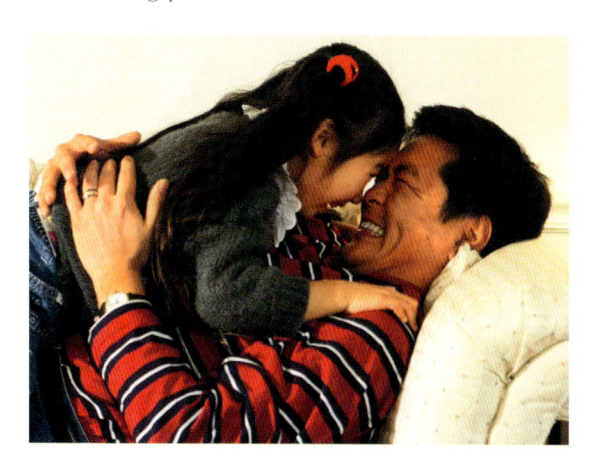

Step 9
Cut back on saturated fat

Steering clear of fast-food drive-throughs and the fatty meats, butter and full-fat milk and cheeses at the supermarket could lower your LDL ('bad') cholesterol by an impressive 10 per cent. And this medication-free drop in bad cholesterol could, in turn, cut your risk of having a heart attack by 20 per cent. Not a bad return on a smart food investment, which is why cutting back on saturated fat when you're ready to make some healthy dietary modifications is highly recommended.

These days, experts say that getting LDL lower than ever (below 3.5 mmol/L for most people and as low as 2.5 mmol/L if you have diabetes or have had a heart attack or stroke) is essential. The best way to do it is to cut back on saturated fat, the body's raw material for manufacturing LDL.

Your goal is to keep saturated fat at less than 7 per cent of the kilojoules you eat. That's less than 16 g worth if you eat about 8000 kilojoules a day, or less than 19 g if you eat 10,000 kilojoules. You can see that there's no room for butter, at 7 g of saturated fat per tablespoon; heavy cream, at about 3.5 g per tablespoon; or full-fat cheddar cheese, at 6 g per 30 g (about one slice). Here's how to minimise intake of saturated fat:

Buy low-fat or skim milk and dairy products
Choosing skim over full-fat milk will save you about 4 g of saturated fat per cup, and having low-fat cheese will save the same amount per slice. If you don't like low-fat cheese, try soft cheeses, such as goat's cheese, which are naturally a little lower in saturated fat than hard cheeses. Or choose a strong-flavoured cheese such as Romano and use less of it in dishes.

Replace butter with something healthier
If you like margarine, choose a brand that doesn't contain hydrogenated oils, which are as bad for your heart as saturated fat is. Even better, try dipping your bread in olive oil, or use avocado as a spread instead of butter or margarine (but don't use too much as it's also a source of fat, even though it's healthy fat).

Opt for lean beef Whenever possible, avoid beef mince and choose cuts of meat such as eye fillet or those that have been trimmed and have very little visible fat (marbling). And avoid fatty underbelly cuts such as rib eye, spareribs and brisket. A 90-g (small) piece of grilled top sirloin has about 1.5 g of saturated fat. If you do cook with beef mince, opt for the leanest grade. A 90-g beef patty made from 80 per cent lean mince has approximately 8 g of fat, one made from 90 per cent lean mince has about 4 g and extra-lean beef mince (95 per cent lean) will cut the saturated fat to around 2 g per serve.

The Australian Dietary Guidelines suggest no more than three to four 65–100-g serves of lean red meat per week. Most cancer experts agree that higher intakes can raise your cancer risk.

Eat skinless chicken and turkey Well-trimmed pork tenderloin or pork chops, skinless chicken, and turkey are all good lean meat choices. But avoid processed meats such as salami and ham.

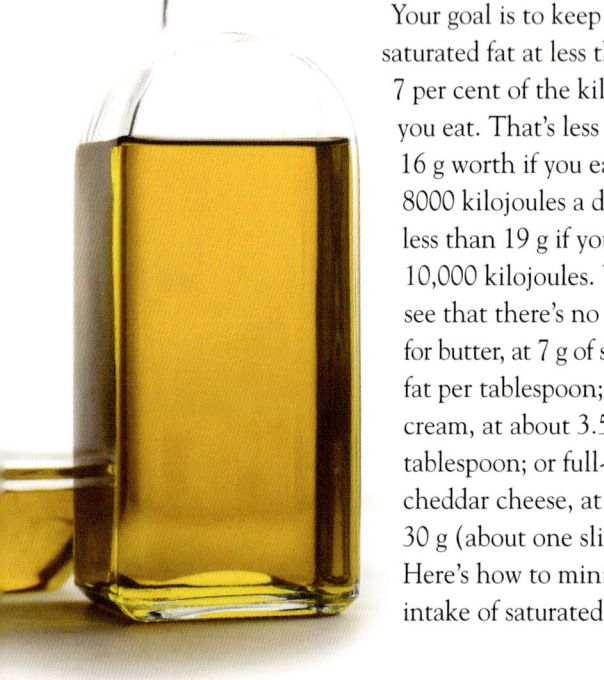

Key steps to disease prevention 75

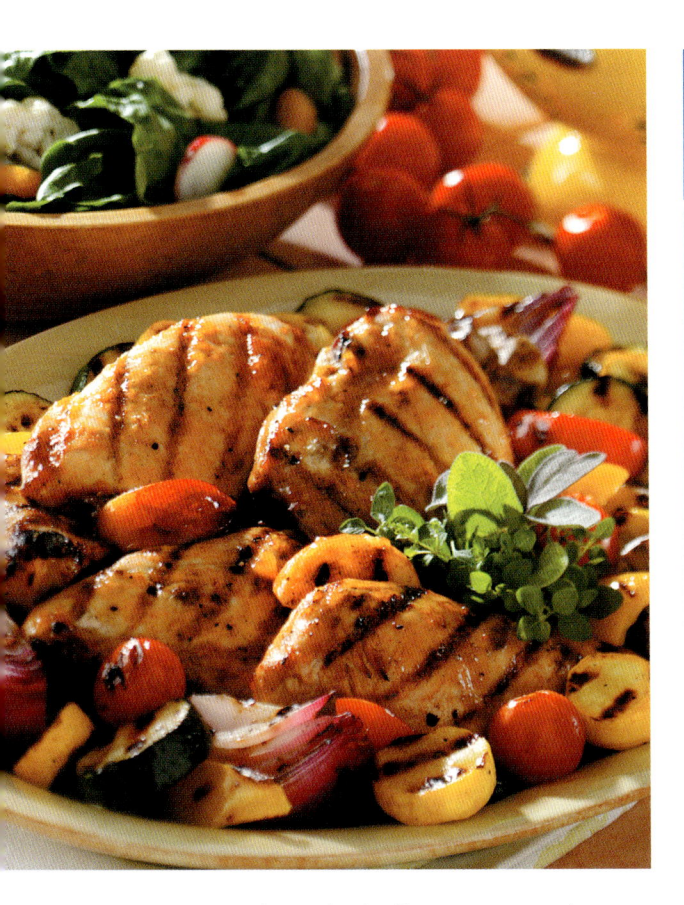

Steer clear of tropical oils Coconut, palm and palm kernel oil are rich in saturated fat, and appear in some commercial baked goods such as biscuits and plain crackers. Some food manufacturers are using these oils at the same time they remove trans fats (partially hydrogenated vegetable oils linked to higher risk of heart disease). So if the label says 'no trans fats', check the ingredients list for tropical oils and look at the nutrition panel to see what the overall saturated fat content is.

Swap bad fat for good Try a fish burger instead of a beef burger. Instead of butter, use olive oil. Fish and olive (and canola) oil offer substantial heart benefits. And instead of snacking on chips or doughnuts, have a small handful of walnuts or almonds, which actually lower cholesterol.

Can carbohydrates keep you disease free?

Many people are cutting down on their carbohydrate intake to keep their weight in check. Is that a smart idea? That depends.

Most experts agree that carbohydrates in the form of sugary drinks, shop-bought baked goods such as muffins, packaged snacks and lollies make blood sugar and blood fats (such as triglycerides) soar, raising your risk for Type 2 diabetes, heart disease and even some cancers.

Instead, stock up on 'smart carbs'—whole grains such as oats, barley, wholegrain bread and brown rice, as well as fruit and vegetables, and legumes—and you'll fortify your body with very powerful disease-fighting compounds. The following strategies can help you replace refined carbohydrates with more healthy alternatives.

- **Look for breads and cereals with the word 'whole' in the first ingredient**

- **Minimise your intake of 'white' foods**
  White potatoes, white pasta and white rice make blood sugar soar; in comparison, wholegrain side dishes such as barley, quinoa and burghul keep it lower and steadier.

- **Have legumes for dinner a few nights a week** Rinse canned beans, peas or lentils to reduce excess sodium. Then add them to soups, salads, casseroles or pasta dishes, or enjoy them with your favourite seasonings as a side dish.

- **Drink unsweetened herbal tea or water**
  Besides containing hundreds of empty kilojoules, soft drink (even one can a day) has been linked with a higher risk of diabetes, heart disease and obesity, so skip the sugary drinks.

Step 10
Reduce chronic stress

Our bodies are reasonably adept at dealing with short-term stress. If you swerve to avoid a car accident, a burst of adrenaline occurs before your mind has time to fully process what happened. But living with chronic stress is another story altogether, one with surprising health implications. It increases levels of cortisol and other stress hormones and leaves them set on 'high' for days, weeks, months and sometimes even years on end. The result is often tension headaches, insomnia, disrupted digestion, the list goes on. Researchers are finding links between this kind of stress and higher blood sugar levels, dangerous intra-abdominal fat and possibly even a higher risk of certain cancers. So it's no wonder that living with uncontrolled stress is potentially more destructive than major disease triggers such as being 15 kg overweight or eating too many processed foods on a regular basis.

All of us have stress in our lives, whether it's the result of a dramatic event such as divorce or a major illness, or the low-level frustrations that come with a busy job, a tense home life, financial worries or regrets about the roads not taken in life. Bandaid recommendations such as a bubble bath, a hot cup of tea or a good cry are all very nice, but it's more important to get to the bottom of your stress. The best place to start is by being completely open and honest with yourself about what's bothering you, before looking for solutions.

Admit to yourself what's really stressing you
Whatever it is, it deserves your attention and respect. Once you bring it out into the open, you can start dealing with it rather than letting it eat away at you on the inside. Don't downplay the issues that are gnawing away at you, even if they seem commonplace. When US researchers at Pace University quizzed people over the age of

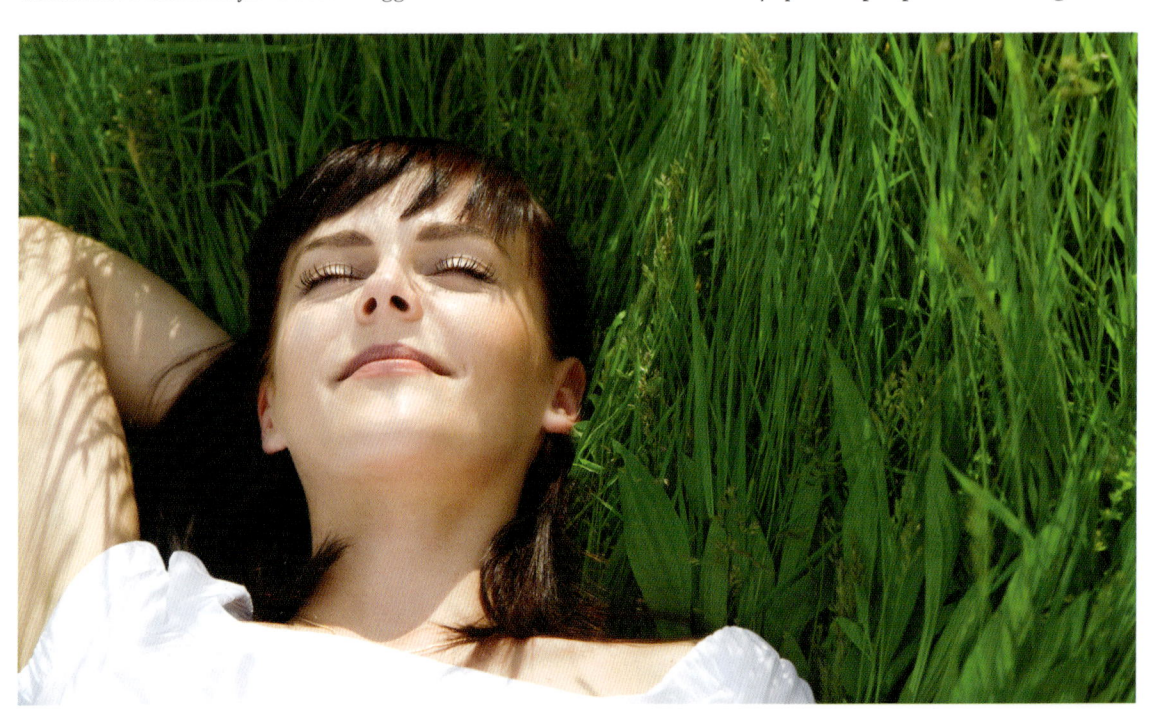

50 about the biggest sources of stress in their lives, a decreasing circle of friends, slowing down physically, diminishing time left to spend with children and grandchildren, regret over earlier life choices, physical pain, memory problems, and the headache of growing red tape (filling out health insurance and income tax forms, for example) were issues that showed up on the list. Once you've identified the things that are really stressing you, write them down, leaving room beside each one to note whether it's something you can't really change and need to accept (such as a milestone birthday coming up) or something you do have some control over. If it's the latter, allow yourself some time to think, then list a few concrete steps you can take to start addressing it. Introducing even one small improvement into your life can make you feel remarkably better by finally giving you a sense of control.

Ask for help where you need it It's human nature: people are often unwilling to ask for help. Or they assume there's nowhere to turn, when often there are resources available. Financial planners, marriage counsellors, life coaches, your doctor or a trusted adviser from your spiritual congregation, if you have one, are good resources that can help you address specific problems in your life. And friends, relatives, neighbours or even acquaintances are usually willing to help out with small tasks if you have the courage to reach out. It's just as likely that they could use your help in return, too.

Build, or rebuild, a social network Loss is a theme that occurred again and again when the Pace University researchers asked people about larger stressors. Their advice was to rebuild a web of caring connections through community groups, volunteering and church groups or other religious organisations. Don't depend on a small, close-knit circle of friends—now is the time to branch out. Scientific journals are now supplying evidence that having friends around changes the biochemistry of your brain—by pumping up feelings of joy and wellbeing that bolster immunity, for example, while being lonely puts you at increased risk for an earlier death, high blood pressure, depression and even accidents at home and on the road.

Learn and practise relaxing Most of us aren't very aware of our bodies. If our muscles are tensed or our breathing is faster and shallower than it should be, we don't manage to notice, let alone make the connection to stress. A good solution is to find a relaxation technique you like and use it every day, regardless of how you feel that day. You can try formal meditation and mindfulness-based stress reduction (locate a class nearest you at **www.umassmed.edu/cfm/mbsr**), yoga and breathing exercises (inhale slowly for four counts, pause for one to two counts, exhale for seven to eight counts, pause for one to two counts, and inhale again). The health benefits of relaxation include better weight control, lower blood sugar, stronger immunity, less depression, an easing of chronic pain and even faster recovery from the serious skin condition psoriasis.

Step 11
Seek treatment for depression

Depression isn't a bad mood. It's a common, serious illness that puts your health in danger—the Disease Prevention Survey's medical experts ranked it as more dangerous than having high cholesterol. It's linked with a higher risk of diabetes, heart disease and a host of other serious health conditions. Having depression plus diabetes and heart disease (a common combination) is a deadly triple threat that increases your risk of early death by as much as 30 per cent.

It's not clear why depression accompanies so many serious health problems. Some experts are beginning to suspect that stress hormones and changes in the nervous system play important roles. What is clear, though, is that fighting depression is imperative for good health.

The trouble is often a case of people not getting the help they need. Thanks to archaic beliefs that this illness is a sign of weakness (or something you can 'tough out' on your own), and to doctors who fail to recognise or treat depression, millions of people plod along on their own. If that sounds like your situation, call your doctor today and make an appointment specifically to talk about this issue and to get help.

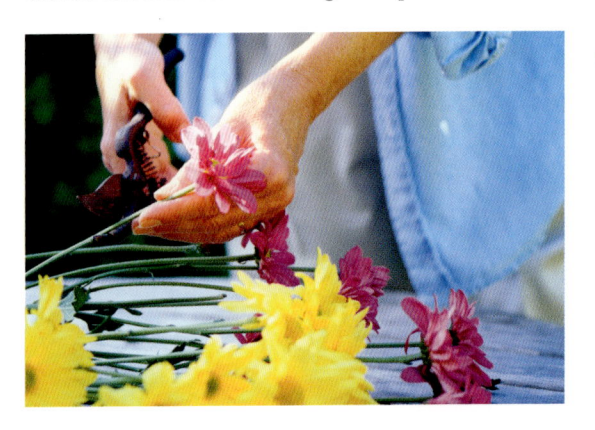

We know that one of the hardest things about depression is trying to believe that you can feel better, but that belief should be your goal—and your doctor's. Mental health experts now say that feeling a bit better isn't enough. You can, and should, feel as good as you felt before the depression began. However you choose to get there, call on the following three courageous qualities (and expect them of your doctor, too) on your journey towards feeling happier again.

Be patient Nearly 70 per cent of the 3700 people in a recent landmark study of depression treatments eventually felt that they had found success. Just 37 per cent got there with the first treatment (an antidepressant) they tried. The rest needed as many as four different therapies before finding the right one for them. What worked? For some, it was one antidepressant. For others, it was a combination of two drugs. For still others, cognitive therapy was the turning point. The point is that you won't know what works for you until you try—and keep trying until you hit on the right combination.

Have high expectations of treatment Expect to feel significantly better. If you have lingering down times after giving a therapy a good try (usually 8 to 12 weeks), talk to your doctor about what else he or she can do to help you.

Be persistent Plenty of people stop taking antidepressants or going to therapy as soon as they begin to feel better, but many relapse. The reason is that a single episode of depression can last for 9 to 12 months. Stopping treatment early leaves you vulnerable, so stick with the one that's making your life better. If you think you're ready to go it alone, talk with your doctor about the best way to taper off a medication and how to create your own relapse-prevention plan.

Step 12
Focus on a higher sense of purpose

Have you ever noticed that people with a deep love or passion for something outside themselves—helping others, nature, music, art or perhaps their religion—complain less about themselves, their health and their lives and seem to manage better when bad things happen? Quite possibly they are more joyful, more thankful or feel more at peace with the world around them, and, luckily, those feelings ultimately pay off in the form of better health. The benefits are so strong, in fact, that the doctors who participated in the Disease Prevention Survey ranked meditating or embracing a higher sense of purpose, such as when praying, as more important to disease prevention than consuming more omega-3 fatty acids or eating less sugar in our daily diets. The problem is that we're not accustomed to hearing this sort of advice from medical experts, but it's heartening because many people have known this fact intuitively for a long time.

It is amazing how many of our survey doctors answered along the following lines when they were asked what actions were important for maintaining health and preventing disease. One doctor advised that people should 'believe in something good; practise being a loving person'. Another recommended that we 'love the ones you're with (spouse, children, extended family, congregation, neighbours, colleagues, community members)'. A third wrote: 'Volunteer in the community to improve the life of others less fortunate than yourself'. A fourth put it this way: 'Strive to achieve something bigger than yourself'.

Meditation is a very effective way to quiet the noise of everyday life and concentrate on the big picture with focus and a renewed clarity.

Studies show that faith, a strong core belief system and the support of a friendly community (whether it be religious or some other group that offers communal support, help and care) can cut stress, boost immunity, improve your odds of recovering from illness and even reduce chronic pain. Some researchers have even found that regular churchgoers tended to have lower blood pressure and higher 'good' HDL cholesterol than those who don't worship regularly.

Try the following strategies to help tap into your own higher sense of purpose.

Try meditation Meditating regularly can actually lower your blood sugar and increase your body's resistance to stress. Take a class to learn how or simply spend 10 minutes a day breathing slowly and deeply and clearing your mind by letting your thoughts flow by without dwelling on them.

Reconnect with your religion You may already belong to a faith community or hold cherished religious or spiritual beliefs. But if you've let this dimension of life languish, it may be time for a personal revival, whether you choose to attend religious services or pray on your own.

Express yourself through music or art These are great ways to stay focused in the moment.

Lose yourself in nature It's hard not to appreciate the beauty of the natural world when bushwalking, hiking through a lush forest or swimming in the ocean off a pristine beach.

Give back Volunteering is a great way to give back and restore faith in yourself and others. If you don't want to do it formally, look for small ways to help others. Perhaps older neighbours could use a hand with looking after their garden or shopping for food, for example.

Safeguarding your health

Heart disease, cancer, diabetes, osteoporosis—few can stand up to the advice outlined in the previous chapter. Follow even just a few of the steps, and you'll be well on your way to reducing your risk for most major diseases. But while you're at it, think about how to protect yourself against threats lurking outside your body, from germs and toxins to spoiled food, all of which can make you mildly sick, or much worse. Whether you're at home, travelling or in a hospital, this advice can help you stay disease free.

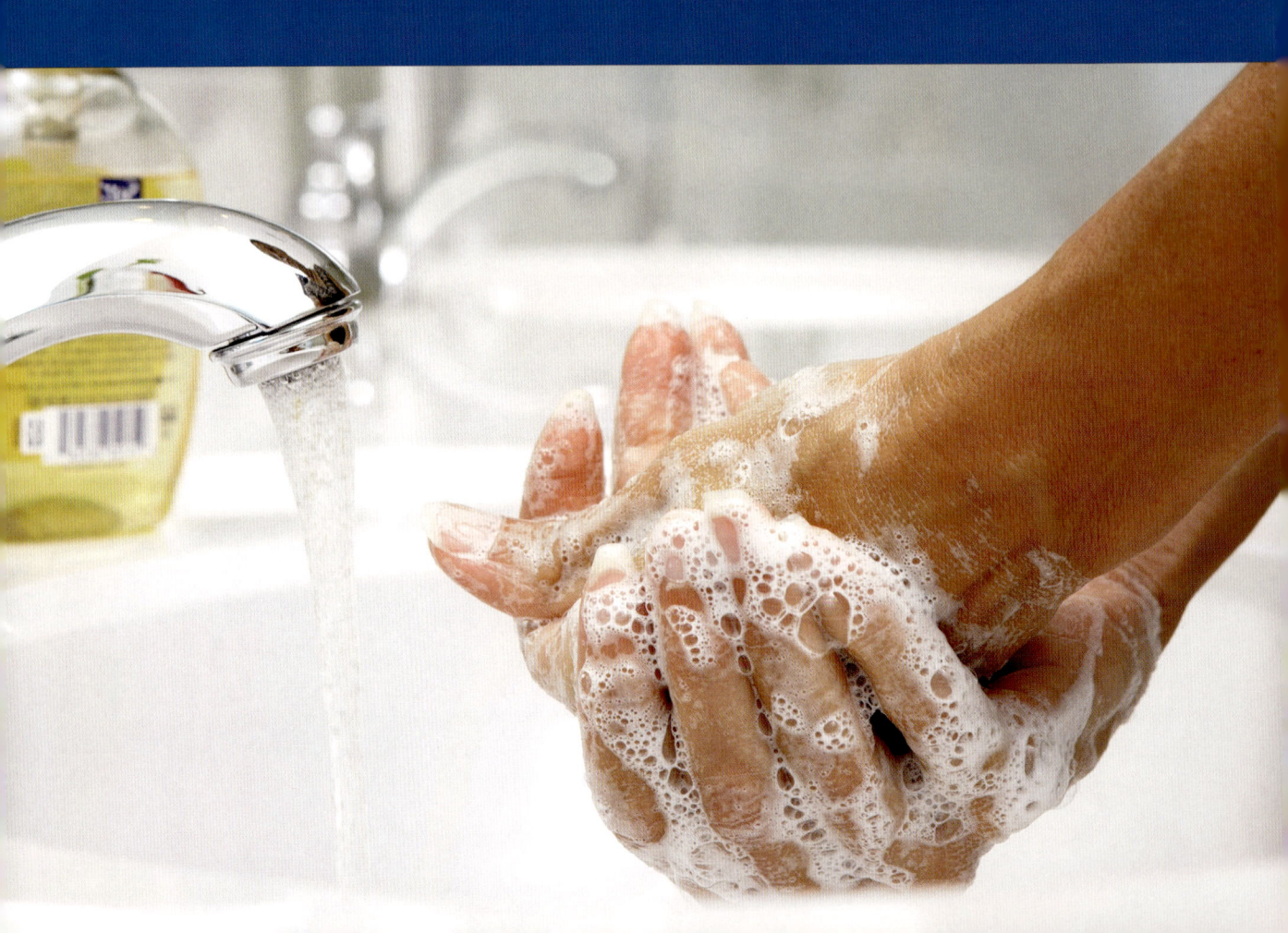

Create a healthy home environment

Your house could well be a haven for more than just yourself and your family. Allergens such as dust and mould, as well as toxic gases, are all found in most homes in varying degrees. Experts estimate that people spend around 80 to 90 per cent of their time indoors, and most of that at home, so why not make your home environment as healthy as possible? No home can ever be truly 'clean', which is not usually a problem, but make sure you address any major issues within the home that may threaten your health, to avoid making you or your family unwell. Here are the three top priorities you need to focus on:

1. Clear the air

HELPS PREVENT: Allergy and asthma attacks; chronic bronchitis; lung cancer and nervous system, developmental and reproductive disorders; and may even prevent death
Modern homes are well sealed, so you'd think they'd be practically pollution-free. In fact, just the opposite is true: indoor air is often more polluted than the air outside. Take these steps to ensure that the air you breathe isn't undermining your efforts to live a healthy, disease-free life.

What to do
Wage war on dust Dust and dust mites trigger allergy and asthma attacks, but dust itself is a 'repository of pollutants', according to experts who have studied it extensively. It's a carrier of countless toxins, including pesticides, flame retardants, volatile organic compounds—VOCs, (emitted as gases by everything from paints and varnishes to cleaning products)—and more. If you live in a dusty house these contaminants enter your body every time you breathe or eat food to which the particles have adhered. You also absorb the dust through your skin.

Battling dust doesn't necessarily mean vacuuming more often—in fact, vacuuming raises clouds of dust and other allergens, even if you use a vacuum cleaner fitted with a HEPA filter. Instead, replace carpets with hard flooring wherever possible and dust with a damp mop. (For more tips on counteracting dust problems see 'Allergies', starting on page 96.)

Minimise mould If you have a stuffy nose, irritated throat, coughing and wheezing, it could be attributable to a mould allergy. You may not even realise that your home has become a mould repository, but old carpets, damp garages and even stacks of old newspapers are very likely to harbour it. Here's how to prevent mould and mould-related health problems:

- Go to a hardware shop and buy a hydrometer to measure the humidity in your home. Aim to keep indoor humidity levels between 40 and 60 per cent. Use a dehumidifier in humid areas such as the kitchen, and run the airconditioner during hot, humid weather.
- Make sure that exhaust fans in your kitchen, bathroom and laundry area are functioning properly and are vented to the outside.

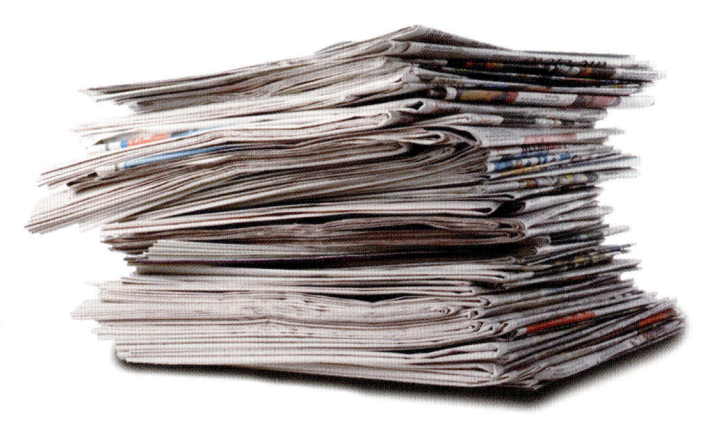

- Fix any leaky roofs, windows or pipes.
- Repair air ducts if you find a buildup of mould, dirt or moisture inside, or if insects or rodents have taken up residence in them. Keeping air filters clean and fixing leaks are the first steps—not duct cleaning, which may not even help.
- Remove mould with a bleach solution made using a cup of bleach added to 4 litres of water.
- Add mould inhibitors to paints before starting a painting project.
- Avoid carpeting your bathrooms or kitchen.

Go green when building or remodelling
Furniture, paints, adhesives, ceiling tiles, drywall and carpeting are major sources of VOCs such as formaldehyde. These compounds have been linked with fatigue, concentration problems, sore throats, runny noses and even cancer. Most of these products are available in VOC-free forms; ask your contractor the next time you're renovating or building a new house.

2. Fight germs in key places

HELPS PREVENT: Viral and bacterial infections
Charles Gerba, a microbiologist and professor at the University of Arizona in the US, notes that 'if you have the right germs in the right place and the right amount, you can get sick from anything you touch'. You'll never get rid of all the germs in your house for the simple fact that bacteria are by far the most numerous organisms on Earth—so it's pointless to think that you can. Instead, choose your battles strategically.

What to do
Microwave your cellulose kitchen sponges
The humble kitchen sponge, or squeegee, may contain more germs than any other object in your house. When US researchers tested common methods of disinfecting sponges—soaking them in bleach or lemon juice, microwaving, or washing them in the dishwasher—they found that microwaving a sponge for a minute destroyed the most germs, followed by using the dishwasher. So don't even bother soaking them.

Scrub the sink After the sponge, the kitchen sink is the second dirtiest place in your house (even worse than the toilet). Keep a spray bottle of cleaner handy and clean the sink after each use, then wipe and rinse clean with hot water.

Beware of mixing chemical 'cocktails' In your enthusiasm for being clean, make sure you never mix bleach with an ammonia-based product, as this creates toxic vapours that can seriously damage your lungs and eyes.

Before ripping up your carpet, read this

Wooden floorboards are popular floor coverings, and are recommend to reduce allergy and asthma symptoms, but many floor finishes used in the 1950s and 60s contain polychlorinated biphenyls (PCBs), which can retard development in foetuses and young children, as well as contribute to your cancer risk. As people rip up carpet in older homes and refinish floorboards, those chemicals are released into the air. In one US study, researchers detected PCBs in the indoor air of a third of homes tested. The highest concentrations in homes and in the blood of their residents were found in places in which the floorboards had just been sanded and refinished. If you're planning to refinish your floorboards, use a process that captures the dust so it doesn't go into the air, and make sure you and your family vacate the house during that time.

Buy a new chopping board Older chopping boards, regardless of whether they are made of wood or plastic, are great hiding places for bacteria, including salmonella, due to deep knife cuts. If yours has seen better days, buy a new one (and choose wood). When researchers smeared bacteria onto plastic and wooden cutting boards, they found that the bacteria grew deep within the pores of the wooden boards. And while that may sound revolting, those bacteria stayed there and didn't reemerge, so they were harmless unless the board was scarred by a knife. The plastic boards, however, retained germs on their surface for hours. Clean wooden chopping boards in a sink of hot soapy water and microwave them for 1 minute (if they fit in) every few days to completely destroy any remaining germs.

Protect your toothbrush Store it at the opposite end of the bathroom from the toilet. When you flush, droplets containing bacteria are propelled through the air, landing on anything nearby. (It's also a good idea to put the toilet lid down before you flush.) Store your toothbrush in an upright position after each use so the water drains away from the bristles; don't store a wet toothbrush in a closed case. And don't let the bristles of family members' brushes touch. If you're still worried about germs, dunk brushes in an antimicrobial mouthwash. Studies show that a 20-minute soak can eliminate germs. Don't re-use the disinfection liquid or soak more than one brush in it at a time. If you've had a cold or flu, replace your toothbrush after you recover to prevent reinfection.

Change nappies on a change table Every time a baby's nappy is changed on the living room couch or floor, bacteria are transmitted to surfaces in the room, no matter how careful you think you're being. Wash your hands thoroughly with soap and water after every nappy change.

Get rid of communal lolly jars or biscuit tins Given that only 67 per cent of people who say they wash their hands actually do, and that only a third of those people use soap, you can imagine the number of germs living in communal vessels.

Wipe down 'sick' surfaces You can't go overboard disinfecting every surface in your house, but even if you did, it wouldn't make much difference. If a family member has been sick, though, it might make sense to wipe down surfaces that everyone touches all the time— doorknobs, light switches, the computer keyboard and mouse, the remote, the telephone— with disinfectant. Disinfectants don't kill all viruses (they mainly work against bacteria), but they may kill some. Experts recommend a solution of 1 part bleach to 10 parts water, which effectively kills bacteria and some viruses. Leave it on the surface for 10 to 20 seconds before wiping dry.

Wash laundry well Even laundered items can be problematic. Sharing towels, for instance, is one way antibiotic-resistant staph infections are spread. Think about it: if you wash undergarments in one load and handkerchiefs in the next, you're blowing your nose in what was in your underwear.

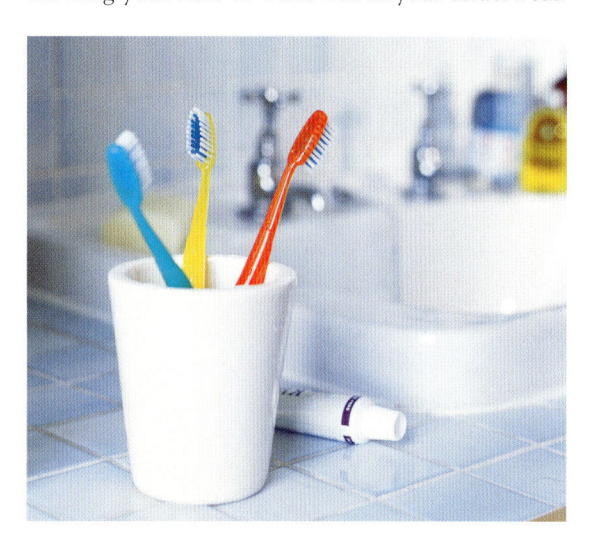

Make your underwear the last load, and at least once a month, run a hot cycle with bleach to clear out germs in the machine. Wash your hands after sorting laundry and before transferring wet items to the dryer. Otherwise you could transfer the bacteria on the laundry to your mouth, nose and eyes, not to mention the clean laundry.

3. Keep your food safe

HELPS PREVENT: Diarrhoea and food poisoning
Food should make you healthy, not sick. If you're careful about how you handle the food you cook, you'll be much less likely to come down with diarrhoea, vomiting or worse. Don't rely on your senses to judge safety—you can't see germs on food, and a food can smell perfectly OK even when it's contaminated.

What to do

Thaw properly The best option is to defrost items in the fridge overnight. But if you're in a hurry, put the frozen item in a plastic bag and immerse it in cold water, changing the water every 30 minutes. Otherwise, use the microwave oven on the defrost setting, but be ready to cook the food as soon as it's thawed.

Use a meat thermometer Poultry should reach 75°C; beef roasts, at least 65°C; pork, minced meats and poultry, 70°C; and casseroles, 75°C.

Shop in the right order Buy nonperishables first, fruit and vegetables next, then meats and poultry and, finally, frozen food.

Take your fridge's temperature Most fridges come with a built-in thermometer, but if yours doesn't, pick up an appliance thermometer from a hardware shop and check that the fridge is at 5°C or below and the freezer at -18°C or below.

Purge your pantry Any highly acidic canned foods such as tomatoes, grapefruit and pineapple should be stored for no longer than 18 months; other canned foods can be kept for two to five years if the can is still in good shape and the label is clearly readable.

Wash, wash, wash *E. coli* from spinach, salmonella from rockmelon ... is nothing safe? Not really. Whether it's a bunch of grapes or an orange you're slicing, always rinse fresh fruit and vegetables first. Remove and toss the outer leaves of lettuce or cabbage, and don't leave cut vegetables or fruit at room temperature for more than an hour.

Travelling disease free

Norovirus has become known as the scourge of cruise-ship holidays, just as viruses caught during plane travel are also known to put a damper on holidays overseas. Don't allow your holiday—or even a business trip—to be ruined by illness or accidents. The goal is to remain disease free whether you're at home or in a four-star hotel in an exotic location. Here are the three key steps to preventing a holiday disaster:

1. Use 'plane' common sense

HELPS PREVENT: Blood clots, respiratory illnesses, stomach complaints, influenza and dehydration
Nothing is more upsetting than catching a virus on a plane en route to your destination—and unfortunately, it's all too common, thanks to packed aeroplanes, germs that settle on every surface you touch and stale recirculated air (the result of airlines trying to save fuel by not

allowing in as much fresh air from outside). Protect yourself with some travel-savvy advice.

What to do
Take the first flight out in the morning Not only is the first flight more likely to be on time (delays haven't started building yet), reducing your stress levels, but the plane will also have been recently cleaned from the previous day.

Take a bottle of water The cabin air in planes is incredibly dry, which puts you at added risk for picking up an infection, since you need moisture in your mucous membranes (nose, throat and eyes) to help repel viruses and bacteria. Avoid salty snacks and alcohol, which are dehydrating, and drink lots of water. Just make sure the water is bottled, whether you take it with you or get it on the plane. The US Environment Protection Agency tested 158 passenger planes and found that the drinking water in nearly 13 per cent was infected with coliform bacteria, the presence of which is often used as a rough indicator of water's general cleanliness.

Stand up and walk every 2 hours Walking around and stimulating your circulation helps to prevent the formation of blood clots in your legs that can occur after sitting for several hours. It's easiest to get up as often as you like if you've booked an aisle seat. If getting out of your seat often is too disruptive, exercise every half an hour by raising your shoulders and shrugging them forward and back, dropping your chin and nodding yes and no, drawing circles with your toes, and pressing up onto the balls of your feet 10 times in a row. And always try to avoid sitting with your legs crossed.

Take your own pillow and blanket Those supplied by airlines are not deep-cleaned often enough. You can buy inflatable pillows and travel blankets from travel shops at most airports.

Buy a pack of antibacterial wipes at the airport Use them to wipe down your seatbelt, tray table and armrests, as well as the button that turns on the light. Take the wipes with you to the bathroom to use when opening the door and flushing the toilet.

2. Pack your suitcase well

HELPS PREVENT: Traveller's diarrhoea, blisters, motion sickness, sunburn and malaria
Sometimes it's the small things like blisters or sunburn that detract from a holiday's enjoyment. Other times it's the not-so-small things, such as a bad case of traveller's diarrhoea that leaves you stuck in a hotel for days. You can prevent a range of health problems by planning in advance.

What to do
See your doctor at least two months beforehand Check with your doctor if you'll need vaccinations for the places you're travelling to and whether malaria tablets are advisable (if they are, start taking them as directed before leaving the country). If you're travelling to areas where the water quality is questionable, putting you at risk for traveller's diarrhoea, it's also a good idea to ask your doctor to write a prescription for an antibiotic, then fill the prescription before you go. For example, a 200-mg dose of rifaximin (Xifaxan)—not available in all countries, so your doctor may prescribe something similar—taken with the first meal you eat upon reaching your destination and followed by 200 mg twice a day with meals, prevents diarrhoea in 72 to 77 per cent of people who take it.

Take insect repellent and insect-blocking clothes Mosquitoes aren't just annoying; the mosquitoes in certain parts of the world can transmit diseases such as malaria and dengue fever. Ticks can cause tick-borne encephalitis. Use an insect repellent on any exposed skin to repel mosquitoes, ticks and fleas. Choose one that contains DEET or a newer pesticide called picaridin. Also take clothes to wear when the mosquitoes are out in force, including long-sleeved shirts, long pants and closed shoes. If you're heading into really heavy mosquito territory, apply insect repellent containing permethrin to clothing, shoes, tents, mosquito nets and other gear (but not your skin). It keeps working even after five washes.

Screen out the sun Whether you're skiing in the Swiss Alps or embarking on a long-awaited cruise of the Pacific, keep in mind that countries near the equator and at higher elevations receive more UV rays than other parts of the globe. Plus, snow and light-coloured sand reflect the sun, increasing your risk of sunburn. Even if you're not heading to the beach, use a high-SPF sun lotion (30 is plenty) that blocks both UVA and UVB rays, and reapply it every couple of hours.

Pack thongs for the shower If you plan to use the hotel pool or public showers, slip some rubber thongs into your suitcase to protect your feet from athlete's foot. If you're planning to visit any rocky beaches, take some aqua shoes along.

Be ready for blisters Blisters seem innocent enough, but if one becomes infected you have a bigger problem, especially if you have diabetes. Take shoes that are already broken in, along with a packet of moleskin (sold in pharmacies) and some travel scissors. As soon as you feel a 'hot spot' developing, cut a piece of moleskin large enough to cover the area and stick it on to prevent a full-blown blister developing.

Prevent Delhi belly You can reduce the risk of traveller's diarrhoea by taking the usual precautions—avoiding tap water or ice, eating unpeeled raw fruit and vegetables, and so on. And you could pack some Pepto-Bismol (available in New Zealand and South Africa; Australians can only buy this preparation while travelling abroad), which can even be used to prevent diarrhoea. Studies show it can cut your risk by 65 per cent. Take two 262-mg tablets at each meal and at bedtime. Do this daily for up to three weeks.

Before you go

In addition to getting flu vaccine and, depending on your age and health status, pneumonia vaccine, make sure your tetanus immunisation is up to date (you need one every 10 years). Also check which vaccinations are recommended for the areas you're travelling to. You can search www.cdc.gov/travel/contentvaccinations.aspx by your destination country (this US website has useful information for all travellers, regardless of where you live). The only ones required are yellow fever vaccine for travel to certain countries in sub-Saharan Africa and tropical South America, and meningococcal vaccine for travel to Saudi Arabia during the religious festival, the Hajj.

Don't forget the Dramamine Dimenhydrinate (Dramamine) and cyclizine work well to reduce nausea and vomiting from motion sickness. The trick is to take either well before you board a ship or begin a winding car ride.

Take steps against altitude sickness This can occur if you move rapidly from sea level to more than 1800 m. To avoid it, move higher gradually (for instance, spend the night at 1200 m before continuing to your destination), slowly integrate physical activity (that 8-km hike should wait a couple of days, until you've had a chance to acclimatise), and avoid alcohol and heavy meals. If you're prone to severe altitude sickness, talk to your doctor; there are medications you can take ahead of time to help prevent this problem.

3. Keep your hands clean

HELPS PREVENT: Diarrhoea, intestinal bugs and colds and other viral illnesses
Next time you embark on a cruise, consider that in 2007 there were 23 outbreaks of noroviruses, which cause 'stomach flu', on 19 cruise ships, affecting about 3000 passengers and crew members. Most involved person-to-person transmission, making hand washing, which studies find removes 99 per cent of the virus particles, crucial. No matter where you go or what you're doing, hand washing should be your number-one strategy for avoiding infections.

What to do
Wash with soap and hot water Wash long and often. Plain soap and hot water are fine; you don't need an antibacterial soap. Just make sure you wash for at least 20 seconds, which is about the time it takes to sing the happy birthday song twice at normal speed. (It's not essential for you to sing out loud, though!)

Use antibacterial hand wipes and gel sanitisers Whenever you have access to soap and water, wash your hands—it's more effective at removing germs than antibacterial products because it physically rinses them away. Hand sanitisers aim to kill germs but don't kill all of them. Still, for times when you can't wash your hands, alcohol-based antibacterial gels and towelettes are a lot better than nothing. Use a sanitiser containing 99.5 per cent ethanol, which studies find is more effective against noroviruses than any other concentration or type of alcohol-based cleaner.

Leave taps and door handles untouched Just think about how many people use public toilets in a day. Then consider how many of them washed their hands before leaving the toilet facility (far fewer than you might think). It's not the toilet seats in these facilities you have to worry about, it's the taps and door handles that are the dirtiest areas, so use a paper towel or hand wipe to turn the water on and off and to open the door when you exit.

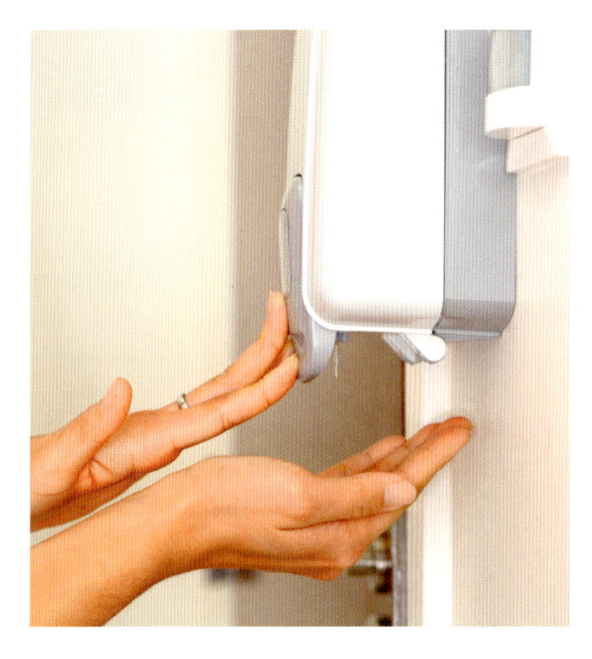

4. Protect your physical safety

HELPS PREVENT: Accidents and injuries
You're more likely to come down with a virus or other infection on the road than to get hurt in an accident, but it can happen. Traffic accidents are a leading non-natural cause of death for tourists. And throwing your back out trying to haul your suitcase through the airport isn't any fun, either.

What to do
Forget about motorcycles and mopeds Just visit a local hospital and witness all the tourists who have sustained moped injuries while on holiday. You'll be much less likely to decide to rent a scooter, no matter how cute and fun they look. Use public transport, rent a car or hire a driver if you're not comfortable driving on strange roads. If you do rent a car, get a large one—it reduces your risk of sustaining injury if an accident does occur.

Wear a seatbelt If the car or taxi doesn't have a working seatbelt, look for another form of transport. It's not worth the risk.

Don't cram too many people into the car Less developed countries are notorious for overfilled buses and cars. If you don't have room to sit comfortably and a seatbelt to click over you, or if the bus or van seems so top-heavy it might tip over, organise another ride, if possible.

Use rolling luggage It saves straining your back. And always lift with your legs, not your back.

Guard against heat exhaustion and heatstroke Whether it's Jamaica in July or Kuala Lumpur in February, the heat indexes of some countries can start your blood boiling. Drink plenty of fluids (not soft drinks as they do not rehydrate), wear light-coloured lightweight clothing and a wide-brimmed hat, retire to your hotel room or anywhere that has airconditioning during the hottest part of the day, slather on plenty of sunscreen, and skip the alcohol at lunchtime.

Avoiding germs where you can

Call it the revenge of the germs. Less than a century after the introduction of antibiotics, the world is facing an onslaught of highly resilient bacteria—some of which are impervious to all but the most powerful of medications—not to mention viruses that have the potential to mutate, leading to another global pandemic. Short of wearing a spacesuit, here are the two key steps you can take to protect yourself:

1. Prevent staph infections

HELPS PREVENT: Potentially deadly infection from MRSA and other staph bacteria
Staph is one of the most common types of bacteria on the planet. The infections aren't always serious; often they cause only minor skin problems. But methicillin-resistant *Staphylococcus aureus* (MRSA), a common strain of staph, can be fatal because it's resistant to even the most powerful antibiotics. Some MRSA infections are relatively harmless, but in the elderly or those with weakened immune systems, they can cause real trouble. People at increased risk include

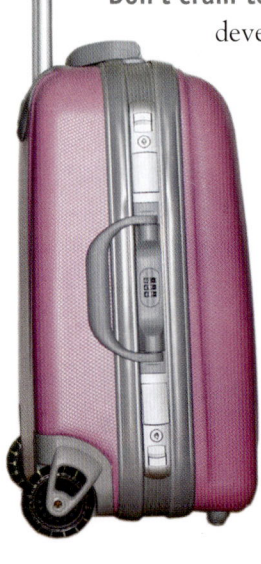

those who have recently had a stay in hospital, people who live in long-term care facilities and anyone who participates in contact sports such as football and wrestling.

What to do
IN EVERYDAY LIFE
Wash your hands It's an often-repeated recommendation, but keeping your hands clean by washing with hot water and soap for at least 20 seconds is the best way to prevent MRSA. If there is a MRSA outbreak in your workplace or school, try using an antiseptic cleanser called Hibiclens (available from most pharmacies). It contains chlorhexidine, which eradicates bacteria that proliferate on the skin.

Shower regularly This is particularly important after working out. Always use soap or another suitable skin cleanser.

Cover scrapes and cuts with a dressing Keep an area of broken skin covered until it's had a chance to heal, to keep out staph bacteria.

Keep your distance Meaning steer clear of other people's wounds or bandages.

Protect yourself from the avian flu

So far, there's no need to worry about contracting avian flu from people. It's spread from animals to people, not from person to person. But if you're travelling to a country that has had outbreaks of the disease, make sure you avoid direct contact with chickens, ducks or geese; poultry farms; live-animal markets; and surfaces that may be contaminated with poultry faeces.

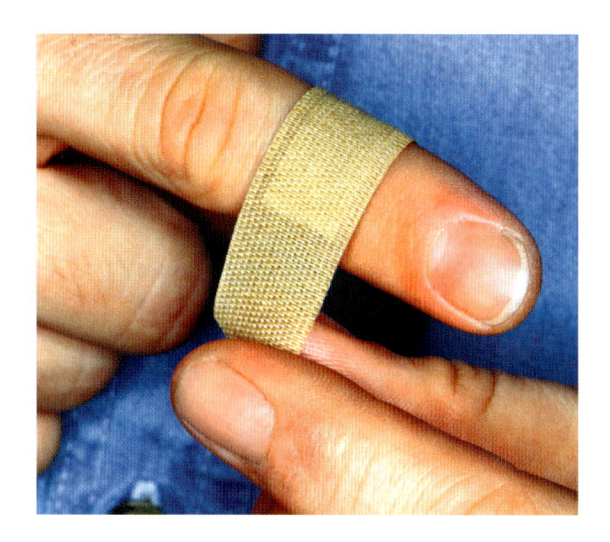

Neither a lender nor a borrower be Don't share towels, razors, makeup, combs or brushes. Even mobile phones and unwashed clothing can harbour staph bacteria.

Create a barrier Use a towel or your clothing as a barrier between your skin and any gym equipment. And wipe all equipment with an antibacterial solution or wipe before and after using it to avoid coming into contact with someone else's body fluids.

Keep a little polite distance between you In team situations it's tempting to hug, slap or engage in other body-to-body contact, which can readily spread bacteria, so try to avoid it wherever possible (without causing offence).

Use the hot setting Washing gym clothes and towels in hot water will help to kill bacteria.

IN A HOSPITAL
Make a few enquiries Before you check in, ask what the hospital does to control hospital-acquired infections, and about its surgical infection rates and infection-control policy. If you're not happy with the responses

—particularly if the person you ask is reluctant to provide full and reliable information—consider finding another hospital, if that's an option.

Pick the right surgeon Ask your surgeon about his or her infection rate—they'll know what it is. Even if you don't fully understand the answer, you should get a good sense of how seriously the surgeon takes infection prevention. And don't be afraid to seek a second opinion if you're not happy with a particular surgeon's infection rate or you'd simply like to make a comparison.

Shower pre-op It's very important to cleanse your skin thoroughly before any operation.

Stop smoking Give up smoking for at least four days before you're admitted to hospital. People who smoke have three times the risk of infection compared to nonsmokers, probably because smoking interferes with the delivery of oxygenated blood throughout the body, affecting the immune response to bacteria.

Check your blood sugar If you have diabetes, your risk of infection is much higher than it is for someone without diabetes. Try to keep your blood sugar levels as stable as possible before being admitted to hospital and make sure they're checked regularly while you're there.

Remain vigilant Request that hospital staff who enter your room—even your doctor—wash their hands or use alcohol-based wipes before touching you. One study found that simply increasing hand washing among intensive care unit (ICU) staff by 25 per cent led to a 25 per cent drop in hospital-acquired infections in the ICU. Also ask your doctor or nurse to wipe off their stethoscope before using it on you. Stethoscopes can also be contaminated with MRSA.

2. Protect yourself from flu

HELPS PREVENT: Complications from flu, hospitalisation and even death from the virus
You may not think of the flu as deadly, but it kills thousands each year (most of them elderly). And

---

Influenza epidemics

During a serious outbreak of influenza it's vital to know when to worry and what to do. Occasionally, a major mutation in the virus that causes flu produces a strain that isn't covered by vaccination. Sometimes this can cause serious illness, as with avian influenza, and sometimes the illness is milder, as with swine flu. To protect yourself during a pandemic, the Australian Government advises you take the following precautions:

- Cover your mouth and nose with a disposable tissue when you sneeze or cough, then dispose of the tissue in a bin and wash your hands (and encourage others to do the same).
- Wash your hands regularly with soap and water or an alcohol-based product.
- Do not share personal items.

If you become sick, take the following precautions:

- Stay at home and avoid contact with others.
- Contact a doctor or hospital by phone rather than in person.
- Rest, drink plenty of fluids, take painkillers such as paracetamol or ibuprofen, gargle with a glass of warm water to ease a sore throat, and use saline nose drops or spray or a decongestant to help clear a stuffed nose. Antibiotics are not effective against flu because it is caused by a virus and antibiotics fight bacteria.

that's just the regular flu. Experts say it's only a matter of time before the big one hits—a flu pandemic reminiscent of the 1918–19 pandemic that killed about 50 million people in nearly every country on Earth, no matter how isolated. The strategies following will help protect you whether there's a flu outbreak close to home or anywhere else in the world.

What to do

Get vaccinated The effectiveness of flu shots varies from year to year, providing anywhere from 40 to 90 per cent protection against the strains of flu that are prevalent that year. But even 40 per cent protection is much better than no protection. If a flu virus suddenly mutates and a pandemic strikes, you'll get at least a little boost from having had a flu shot. If you're 65 or older, also ask your doctor for a pneumococcal vaccine to protect against pneumonia.

Wash and wipe Flu viruses are not like little winged insects; they don't fly from your nose to someone else's. They're usually spread from hand to mouth: someone covers their mouth when they cough, gets the virus on their hands, then uses the phone. An hour later, you pick up the phone, transfer the virus to your hands, rub your eyes and you become infected. Wash your hands as often as possible during flu outbreaks and wipe down surfaces with alcohol-based wipes or solution. This is a good idea outside of cold and flu season, too. You'll find you get sick less often.

Dress like a surgeon You don't need the gown, but the mask could be helpful, especially when you're on a plane full of people coughing and sneezing. Buy an N95 face mask (the standard face mask for flu protection, available from pharmacies), which filters out about 95 per cent of particles the size of the influenza virus.

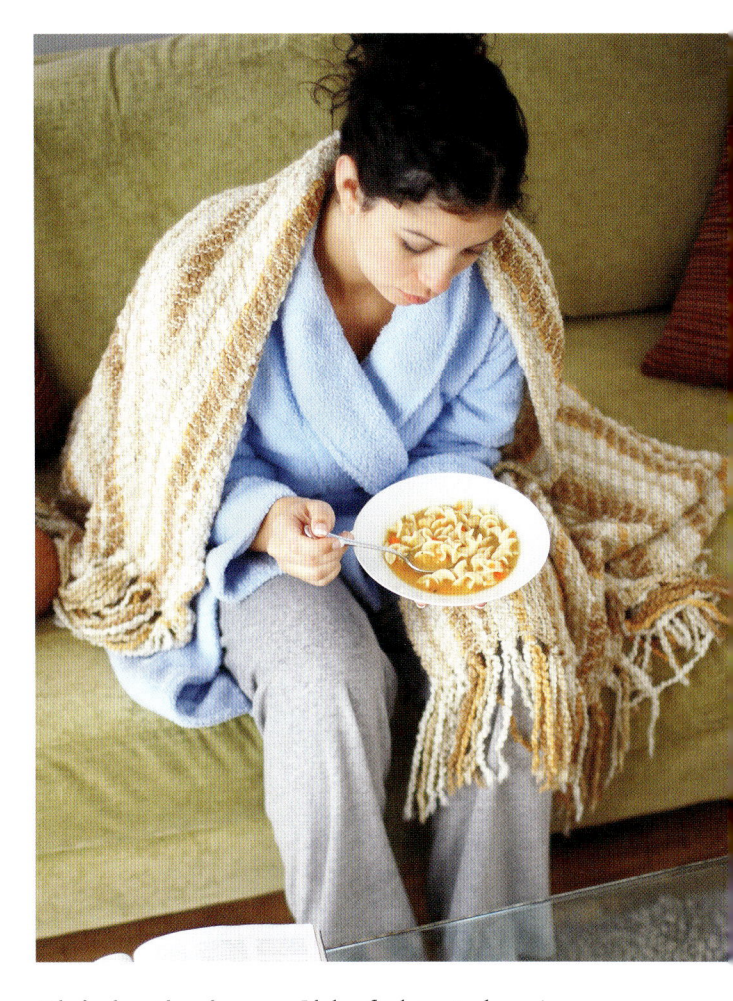

Minimise the damage If the flu hits, it doesn't have to be a death sentence. At the very first sign of the flu, ask your doctor for a prescription for one of the antiviral flu medicines, zanamivir (Relenza) and oseltamivir (Tamiflu). They can cut the flu short by a little over a day. Meanwhile, take paracetamol to bring down fever and stay hydrated with lots of clear liquids and herbal tea.

Keep everything clean If you're taking care of someone who's unwell, wipe down surfaces they've touched with antimicrobial solution; launder all sheets, towels and clothing in hot water with bleach, if possible; and bathe yourself and the patient often.

DISEASE AND MAJOR SYMPTOM PREVENTION

Find out how to protect yourself with prevention plans for more than 75 diseases and major symptoms, and enjoy a long healthy life.

Acne

60% The relative reduction in blemishes when people with acne used benzoyl peroxide from a pharmacy for four months.

Blackheads and bumps, pimples and cysts are a rite of passage for 90 per cent of teenagers. But studies show that up to 54 per cent of adults get acne, too. It's caused by everything from genetics to stress to hormones, and can initiate skin changes that clog pores, cause inflammation and provide acne bacteria with the perfect breeding ground. If you're prone to acne, these strategies can help prevent flare-ups, whether you're 14 or forty-four.

Key prevention strategies

Open your pores with products containing salicylic acid, resorcinol or lactic acid These ingredients are also called alpha-hydroxy acids and beta-hydroxy acids. Available in dozens of pharmacy gels and creams, they work by preventing pores from clogging by breaking down the thick, gunky mix of skin cells and excess oil that starts the whole acne cycle. Some even act as gentle chemical peels to unblock pores that are already clogged. In one very small US study of people with acne, salicylic acid was better than benzoyl peroxide for reducing the volume of pimples.

Stop bacteria with benzoyl peroxide This inexpensive, over-the-counter remedy is a proven bacteria stopper that fights acne's top culprit, the bacteria *Propionibacterium acnes*. Its advantage over oral antibiotics and most antibiotic creams and gels is that it even works on strains of *P. acnes* that are resistant to the most widely used antibiotics for acne, such as tetracycline and erythromycin. Some experts estimate that bacteria are antibiotic resistant in at least half of all cases of acne.

In one UK study of 649 people with acne, 60 per cent of those who used benzoyl peroxide for 18 weeks saw a significant reduction in acne, while only 54 per cent of volunteers who got the oral antibiotics saw an improvement.

Help for sensitive skin

Retinoid creams can be irritating, especially for people with sensitive skin. Here's a gentler alternative: a prescription cream containing azeleic acid (brand names include Azelex and Finacea). In one German study, an alcohol-free azeleic acid gel reduced blemishes by 70 per cent after four months. Researchers also report that the cream can be just as effective as benzoyl peroxide and caused less irritation.

Benzoyl peroxide comes in several strengths; higher strengths are more likely to cause redness, irritation and even peeling. Start with a low dose and move up until you're happy with the results.

Ask about a retinoid cream Prescription-strength creams and washes containing the vitamin A derivatives adapalene (Differin), tazarotene (Tazorac), isotretinoin (Isotrex gel) or tretinoin (Retin-A) speed the shedding of dead skin cells so they can't clog your pores. They may also cool inflammation, easing redness and swelling. When researchers reviewed studies involving 900 people with acne, they found that tretinoin reduced the number of pimples by about 54per cent. In another study, tazarotene produced similar results. Other research suggests that retinoids may clear up 70 per cent of blemishes.

Combine a pore-opening cream with an antibiotic cream It's more effective than using an antibiotic cream alone. Your doctor can prescribe a combination cream that contains both an antibiotic and benzoyl peroxide. Another good duo is benzoyl peroxide plus an alpha- or beta-hydroxy acid or some types of retinoids. In a US study of 517 people with severe acne, 53 per cent of those who used both of these creams saw the number of blemishes cut in half after 12 weeks, compared to 35 per cent of those who used benzoyl peroxide or the retinoid adapalene alone. Benzoyl peroxide can inactivate tretinoin, so use them separately.

Prevention boosters

Light therapy It works by killing bacteria and possibly reducing oil production. There are many types, including combined blue-red light therapy and pulsed-dye lasers. In one study, 85 per cent of people who had four sessions of light therapy over eight weeks saw acne improve by at least 50 per cent, and 20 per cent of study volunteers had a 90 per cent improvement. Results can last up to three months in some people.

Low-dose oral contraceptive pills For women whose acne persists after trying many treatments, oral contraceptives could help. They can clear up skin by changing the hormone balance in a way that reduces the production of oil. It's recommended only for women aged 35 years and younger, who have healthy blood pressure levels, don't smoke and don't get migraines with auras.

▶ WHAT CAUSES IT
Heredity and hormones. The combination causes the production of excess oil by sebaceous glands in your skin, plus a buildup of dead skin cells. Together they clog pores, creating a breeding ground for acne-causing bacteria, which, in turn, trigger an inflammatory response.

▶ SYMPTOMS TO WATCH FOR
Tiny dark spots (blackheads) or small bumps (whiteheads). If clogged pores become infected or inflamed, they turn red; white pus inside may be visible. Larger bumps may signal clogs and a buildup of oil deep within pores. If these become infected, they're called cysts and can leave scars.

▶ LATEST THINKING
Experts have said for years that highly sugary and fatty foods don't cause acne, but research suggests that diets generally high in sugar and refined carbohydrates could play a role. In a study of 43 young men with acne, those who followed a low-glycaemic diet—involving foods that have a gradual impact on blood sugar levels—had 23 per cent fewer blemishes after 12 weeks. Aim to get plenty of fruit and vegetables, and choose wholegrain products when you eat foods such as rice and pasta.

Allergies

58% The percentage of people who rated stinging nettle as effective in relieving their allergy symptoms.

Allergies appear to be seriously on the rise—hay fever, food allergies and allergies to dogs, cats or dust mites—and it's not your imagination. The incidence of allergies—including adult-onset allergies—has risen in developed countries. The reasons for this include too much time spent indoors, higher levels of pollutants and overly clean environments in our childhoods that led to confused immune systems. People with allergies are three times more likely to develop asthma and to have sinusitis. Find out how to avoid an allergy attack.

Key prevention strategies

Wage war on dust and dust mites Think of dust as a repository for almost every allergen you can think of: dust mites, pet dander, cockroach droppings, pesticides and pollution blown in from outside, just for starters. Modern homes are allergen traps. You'll need to make a serious effort to reduce allergens enough to make a noticeable difference, so start with these approaches:

- **Think solid surfaces** Opt for hardwood, laminate, tile and vinyl for your floors, and as much non-upholstered furniture as possible. Carpets and fabrics harbour dust mites and attract pet dander, and grow mould when wet. One study found that the dust on walls, uncarpeted floors and bookshelves had little impact on the overall level of dust mites in the home compared to the dust found on carpets, upholstered furniture, doonas and mattresses and pillows.
- **Dry steam clean your carpets** Vacuuming around the home does little to remove allergens. In fact, on old carpets, it may just bring more pet dander and dust mites to the surface. But dry steam cleaning, also known as vapour steam cleaning—not the same as regular steam cleaning—can reduce the number of dust mites for up to eight weeks. You can have it professionally done or buy a machine and do it yourself. Afterwards, finish up by using a vacuum cleaner equipped with a HEPA filter.

A shot at permanent relief

The way to permanently prevent allergy attacks is to 'reboot' your immune system with immunotherapy—yes, allergy shots. The shots, which you receive over a period of several months or years, contain increasingly larger doses of the substance to which you're allergic. Over time, your immune system learns to tolerate the allergen.

- **Encase your bedding** Always use hypoallergenic covers on your pillows, mattress and bed base. They prevent dust mites from accumulating in your bed. Wash all covers in hot water (60°C) once a week and dry them in a tumble-dryer on the highest heat setting to kill dust mites. If you don't use pillow covers, choose feather pillows, which studies find harbour far fewer dust mites than synthetic pillows do, probably because of the tighter weave on the covering, to stop feathers from escaping.
- **Vacuum your mattress—top and bottom** A Brazilian study compared dust mite bodies on the lower mattress surface (including the bed frame) and upper mattress surface and found more than three times as many dust mites on the lower surface. So flip the mattress monthly, vacuum each side and wipe down the bed frame with hot soapy water. If you're interested in more hard-core cleaning, find out where your mattresses can be sent for sterilising. Once a mattress has been sterilised, make sure you keep it wrapped in hypoallergenic coverings.
- **Clear out clutter** All those knick-knacks and piles of magazines lying around are magnets for dust and mould.

If you can't part with your pet, use an air purifier The truth is, there's scant proof that air purifiers can lessen allergy symptoms very much for most people. Buy if you buy one with a HEPA filter, use it in the bedroom and keep your pet out of the room, you will create a friendlier environment for your respiratory system. These filters remove airborne particles, including those coated with pet dander. One study on using air filters in the bedroom found that they significantly reduced cat allergens. Another study evaluating the benefits of whole-house air cleaners fitted with HEPA filters found that they reduced levels of dog allergens by 75 per cent when the dog was allowed in the room and 90 per cent if the dog was kept out of the room.

Rinse your nasal passages daily Just as a rain shower rinses pollen from the air, a saline rinse washes allergens from your nasal passages. One study found that rinsing three times a day during allergy season eased congestion, sneezing and itching and reduced the amount of antihistamines participants needed.

To make your own saline rinse, mix ½ teaspoon salt, ½ teaspoon bicarbonate of soda and 500 ml warm tap water. To get it into your nose, use an infant ear bulb-syringe or a neti pot,

> 'Carpets and fabrics harbour dust mites and attract pet dander.'

Prevent allergies in children

Whether you're just thinking about having children, are pregnant or already have children in the house, these measures may help to reduce their risk of contracting allergies in the first place.

During pregnancy

1. **Follow a Mediterranean diet** That means one rich in whole grains, fruit and vegetables, and fish, with olive oil used as the primary fat. In one study, children whose mothers followed such a diet were 82 per cent less likely to have wheezing and 45 per cent less likely to have the skin rashes that predict childhood allergies.

2. **Take 1000 mg of fish oil a day** There is some evidence that supplementing with this anti-inflammatory fat can reduce the risk of allergies in young children. Check with your doctor first.

3. **Take a probiotic supplement** Children whose mothers take supplements of these beneficial bacteria during pregnancy—and those who received probiotics as infants—appear to be less likely to develop eczema, an itchy skin condition that is a common precursor of allergies in children.

During childhood

1. **Feed children plenty of fruit, vegetables and fish** Researchers who followed nearly 500 Greek children from the time their mothers were pregnant until the children turned six found that diets high in these foods significantly reduced the risk of allergies and asthma. The children who ate fruit and vegetables at least twice a day were 74 per cent less likely to develop allergic rhinitis than those who ate them less often.

Fruit and vegetables popular in Crete include grapes, oranges, apples, tomatoes, eggplants, cucumbers, green beans and zucchini. Eating an average of 60 g of oily fish daily also helped. Margarine, on the other hand, made allergies more likely, probably because hydrogenated oils trigger inflammation.

2. **Get a pet** Some studies suggest that exposing your infant to a cat or dog during the first year can help prevent allergies to common airborne allergens such as dust mites and pollen.

3. **Breastfeed for four to six months** This is the amount of time required to reduce the risk of all allergies in your child, probably by providing important immune system support.

4. **Hold off on cereal** Studies find that children who don't eat solid foods until they're six months or older may be less likely to develop food allergies. Discuss this with your doctor or an early childhood nurse.

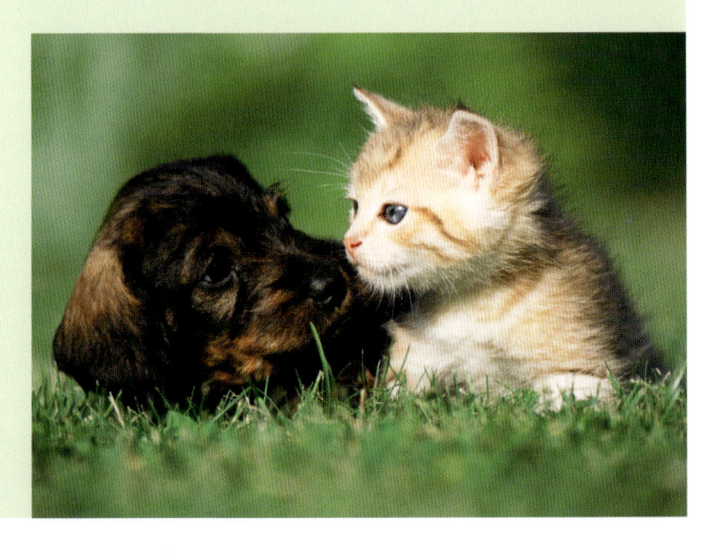

available from most health food shops and pharmacies. Lean over a sink and turn your head so that your left nostril points downwards. Gently flush your right nostril with 250 ml of saline, which will drain out through your left nostril. When you're finished, gently blow your nose. Repeat with the other nostril.

Prevent attacks with stinging nettle You may experience fewer allergy symptoms when you take this herb daily. In one study of volunteers who took 300 mg a day of freeze-dried nettle leaf capsules, more than half of the 69 participants said it relieved their allergy symptoms, and nearly half said it worked better than an allergy medication. Another potentially helpful natural remedy to try is quercetin. Follow the directions on the product packaging.

Prevention boosters

Eat yogurt every day US researchers at the University of California found that people who ate about 250 g of yogurt containing live, active cultures every day had half as many days with allergy symptoms during hay fever season as people who didn't eat yogurt. The researchers aren't sure why yogurt helps, but it probably affects the immune system's response to allergens.

Eat more apples and drink more tea Apples with the skin on and green or black tea are excellent sources of quercetin. This powerful anti-oxidant checks the release of inflammatory chemicals from mast cells, the immune cells responsible for your run-of-the-mill allergic reaction. Other good sources of quercetin include raw onions and red grapes.

Up your vitamin E intake You'll find this vitamin in spinach, wheatgerm, almonds, sunflower seeds and kumara (orange sweet potatoes). A German study on the dietary habits of 1700 adults with and without hay fever found that those who ate foods rich in vitamin E had a 30 per cent lower incidence of hay fever than those whose diets were low in vitamin E.

Shut the windows A warm spring breeze seems just the thing to freshen up your house, but the problem is that it's filled with pollen. Keep the windows closed and turn on the airconditioner if the inside air temperature gets too warm.

▶ WHAT CAUSES IT
Your immune system overreacts to irritants such as dust, pollen, dander, mould, food proteins or insect venom, releasing inflammatory chemicals that trigger allergy symptoms.

▶ SYMPTOMS TO WATCH FOR
A runny nose and itchy eyes, particularly during high-pollen seasons; sneezing; hives (an itchy, red rash) and/or trouble breathing after eating certain foods, such as peanuts or shellfish; and red, dry itchy skin.

▶ LATEST THINKING
UK researchers have discovered a protein called p110delta that plays a key role in triggering allergy attacks. Medications targeting it could prevent allergies, leaving existing allergy medications—which mostly reduce symptoms once the allergic reaction has occurred—way behind.

Alzheimer's disease

60% The difference in Alzheimer's risk between those who eat oily fish at least once a week and those who don't.

Alzheimer's disease was barely a dot on the horizon 50 years ago, because few of us lived long enough to develop it. But with life expectancies creeping into the mid-seventies or older, we're facing a potential epidemic of dementia. The good news is that scientists are learning more about it all the time. In the past decade, they've identified numerous biological and lifestyle risk factors for Alzheimer's, opening the door to potential preventive strategies.

Key prevention strategies

Eat at least one meal of oily fish per week You may know that salmon is heart healthy, but it could be just as good—or even better—for your brain. This added benefit is probably due to the omega-3 fatty acids, especially a type called DHA, which your brain is largely made up of. Low levels of omega-3s are linked to memory and learning problems, and even Alzheimer's disease.

DHA is thought to guard against the accumulation of beta amyloid proteins, which are the substances responsible for the sticky brain lesions, known as plaques, that are the hallmarks of Alzheimer's disease. Fish fats also counter inflammation, which may contribute to protein buildup in the brain. When scientists added DHA to the diets of mice bred to develop Alzheimer's disease, the mice had lower levels of brain plaques than those mice who didn't get the DHA.

One population study suggests that eating fish once a week or more even after the age of 65 can reduce your risk of developing Alzheimer's by 60 per cent compared to someone who eats less fish. If you don't like fish, talk to your doctor about taking 1000 to 2000 mg of fish oil daily.

Exercise your brain Every time you challenge your brain to learn new information or attempt a new task

> **DRUGS THAT PREVENT DISEASE**
>
> That same daily aspirin that some people take to protect themselves from heart attack may protect them from Alzheimer's disease, too. In one study, people who took a nonsteroidal anti-inflammatory drug (NSAID), such as aspirin or ibuprofen, every day for two years or more were 80 per cent less likely to develop Alzheimer's than those who took an NSAID less often. Even people who took an NSAID for a month to two years reduced their risk by 17 per cent. Talk to your doctor about whether or not you should take a daily aspirin as there are potential side effects to consider.

(whether it's playing chess or just brushing your teeth with your non-dominant hand), you create new connections between brain cells, in effect strengthening your brain. Research suggests that daily mental stimulation could reduce Alzheimer's risk by as much as 47 or 75 per cent, depending on which study you look at. So get out those crossword puzzles and sudokus, and think about learning a new language or a musical instrument, too.

Walk 3 km a day At a brisk pace, this should take you no more than 30 minutes, the amount of time required to cut your risk of Alzheimer's by 50 per cent, according to a Canadian study of about 10,000 people. Exercise probably has numerous benefits, including increased blood flow to the brain and increased production of a chemical called brain-derived neurotrophic factor (BDNF)—a sort of fertiliser that encourages nerve cells in the brain to multiply and create more connections with each other.

Check the scale If you're obese, your risk of Alzheimer's is nearly twice that of someone whose weight is normal. For example, an analysis of several studies concluded that one in five cases of Alzheimer's disease in the US was related to obesity. The link? For starters, carrying extra body fat—particularly around your waist—bumps up your risk of heart disease and diabetes, both of which make people more vulnerable to Alzheimer's. What's more, the fat itself releases inflammatory chemicals that may contribute to brain inflammation—and Alzheimer's.

Prevention boosters

Eat your spinach Despite what Popeye believed, it won't make your muscles strong, but what it could do is help you maintain healthy brain function. Spinach is an excellent source of folate, a B vitamin that helps keep levels of homocysteine—an amino acid—in check. This amino acid damages blood vessels and doubles the risk of Alzheimer's disease. Another B vitamin to look for is niacin. Studies find that a diet containing at least 17 mg of niacin (vitamin B_6) a day reduces the risk of Alzheimer's disease by 70 per cent compared to a diet low in niacin. You can get 14 mg from a 100-g serve of cooked liver, 10 mg from 1/2 cup of peanuts and 13 mg from 85 g of chicken breast. Other great sources of B vitamins are legumes (beans, peas and lentils), fortified grains, wholemeal breads and nuts.

Got the gene?

Researchers have identified at least 20 genes and genetic abnormalities linked to Alzheimer's disease. The best known is the ApoE gene, which affects the concentration of apolipoprotein Apo(E) in the blood. Apo(E)'s job is to help remove excess cholesterol from the blood and carry it to the liver for processing. While you can be tested for the gene, there's nothing you can do if you have it. Instead, live your life as if you do have it by following our tips here for reducing your overall risk.

Have a glass of wine, with food, on most days One of the best studies of dementia in the world, the Canadian Study of Health and Aging, found that drinking a glass of wine a day reduced the risk of Alzheimer's disease by 62 per cent in women and 51 per cent in all participants when men were included with the women. The benefit is probably due to something in the wine itself, since the protection afforded by wine was far greater than that from spirits or beer. However, it's important to remember that drinking more than this amount can be detrimental to your health.

Start drinking pomegranate juice The risk of developing Alzheimer's is 76 per cent lower in people who drink this juice at least three times a week compared to those who drink it less than once a week, probably because of the high levels of anti-oxidants, called flavonoids, in pomegranates. These anti-oxidants neutralise free radicals—damaging molecules that attack cells and contribute to the formation of brain plaques. Pomegranate juice has already been shown to help prevent an Alzheimer's-like disease in mice.

Wear a helmet Protect your head while cycling, rollerskating or motorcycling, and avoid heading the ball during soccer matches or colliding with the head of another player during football games. There's fairly good evidence that sustaining a moderate or severe head injury increases your risk of Alzheimer's disease (up to 3.5 times as much if the injury is severe).

Prevent high cholesterol Although the theory is still controversial, population, animal and laboratory studies suggest a link between high cholesterol levels in midlife and Alzheimer's disease. High cholesterol levels interfere with the breakdown of the amyloid precursor protein (APP), which plays a major role in the development of Alzheimer's disease. (Follow the tips starting on page 214 for ways to keep your cholesterol under control.) There is also

Check your pressure

The link between Alzheimer's disease and heart disease grows clearer every year. New evidence suggests that high blood pressure may hasten the development of Alzheimer's in people with early memory loss. US researchers following 5092 Utah women with mild dementia for three years found that those with systolic blood pressure readings (the top number) higher than 160 mmHg declined 100 per cent faster than those with normal blood pressure. Those who also had angina, and/or had had a heart attack before their diagnosis, declined even faster. The good news is that a study in the same group of women found that taking medication to reduce high blood pressure reduced the risk of Alzheimer's. Check your blood pressure once a week; if it's higher than 120/80 mmHg, see your doctor. You may need to exercise more, change your diet or take medication to bring it down to the normal range.

some evidence that using cholesterol-lowering statin medication may help prevent Alzheimer's, though it's too soon for doctors to start prescribing these medications just for that reason. The link between statins and Alzheimer's prevention may actually be unrelated to their ability to lower cholesterol and may instead result from their ability to reduce inflammation.

Drink some coffee If you enjoy a cup of coffee in the morning, don't give it up—it may be protecting your brain. According to recent research, caffeine appears to help protect the so-called blood–brain barrier from the harmful effects of high cholesterol, possibly reducing the risk of dementia. Other studies suggest that caffeine can help shore up memory in older people.

Take steps to prevent diabetes Men who develop diabetes in midlife increase their risk of Alzheimer's disease by 150 per cent, according to one study. The risk remained no matter what their blood pressure, cholesterol levels or weight and is probably linked to low levels of insulin. Interestingly, the risk was highest in people who did not have the so-called Alzheimer's gene. (See also 'Diabetes', starting on page 164, to find out how to prevent diabetes.)

Watch out for depression A study of 486 people found that those who had experienced depression severe enough to seek medical help were two and a half times more likely to develop Alzheimer's than those who had never suffered from the condition. Those whose depression occurred before the age of 60 had a risk four times higher. One theory is that depression results in the loss of cells in two areas of the brain that also are linked to Alzheimer's disease. (See also 'Depression', starting on page 160, to find out more.)

▶ WHAT CAUSES IT

Advancing age is the greatest risk factor, although an early form of the disease is linked to a genetic mutation. It's not clear what causes Alzheimer's, but it is associated with protein clumps, called amyloid plaques, in the brain, along with 'tangles' of brain cells. It's likely that these interfere with processing in the brain.

▶ SYMPTOMS TO WATCH FOR

Memory loss, difficulty planning or completing everyday tasks, forgetting simple words, or substituting unusual words in writing or speech; getting lost in familiar places; showing poor judgement, such as wearing shorts outdoors when it's freezing; having difficulty with abstract tasks such as adding up a column of numbers; putting things in unusual places; mood changes; and loss of initiative.

▶ LATEST THINKING

People with Down syndrome usually develop Alzheimer's disease by the age of forty. Now researchers suspect that people without the syndrome who get Alzheimer's may develop a small number of the same chromosomal abnormalities throughout their lifetimes. If true, it could one day mean new options for prevention, diagnosis and treatment.

Anxiety

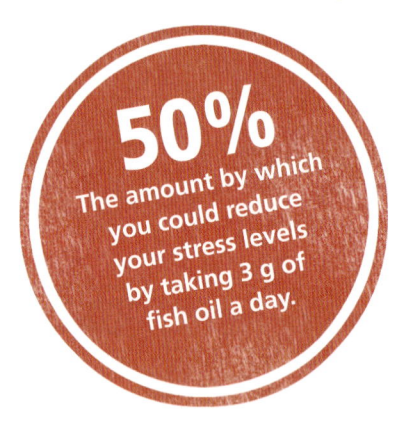

50% The amount by which you could reduce your stress levels by taking 3 g of fish oil a day.

No matter what the cause, chronic anxiety is bad for your health. It makes your heart beat faster than it should and even makes your blood stickier, increasing your risk of a heart attack or stroke. If you're predisposed to anxiety, try these strategies to help you stay calm and quieten your mind.

Key prevention strategies

Talk to someone Preferably a therapist trained in cognitive behavioural therapy. In this form of therapy, you learn to separate worry from reality and put your fears into better perspective. Studies find that, as a treatment for anxiety disorders, it works better than medication; other research finds that it can help prevent a full-blown anxiety disorder if it's employed early on.

Take a walk 'Feelgood' hormones are released during exercise, and one is the neurotransmitter known as gamma aminobutyric acid, or GABA. Studies find low levels of GABA in people with some anxiety disorders, particularly panic disorder. They also find that exercise, even yoga, can increase GABA levels. One study had 15 people walk for 30 minutes, then gave them a medication simulating a panic attack. Six had panic attacks after exercising, compared to 12 who had them when given the medication after resting.

Breathe calmly Many of the symptoms of an anxiety attack are caused by hyperventilation—when you take such short breaths that you never fully release the carbon dioxide in your lungs. As the carbon dioxide builds, you don't have enough room in your lungs to bring in fresh oxygen, making you dizzy and light-headed. Learning to breathe properly when you feel anxiety building can help stem the release of stress hormones that underlie hyperventilation.

Your best bet is to take a class in relaxation: contact your local community centre, or talk to your doctor. Until then,

> **DRUGS THAT PREVENT DISEASE**
>
> If your heart races, your hands sweat and your mouth turns dry when you have to speak in front of people, talk to your doctor about taking a low dose of a beta-blocker. These medications, which include metoprolol (Lopressor or Toprol-XL) and propranolol (Inderal), block the effects of the stress hormone adrenaline, soothing the jitters of performance anxiety with few negative side effects.

try to focus deliberately on your breathing when you feel anxious. Take one deep breath as slowly as possible (count to five as you breathe in), watching your stomach (not your chest) inflate. Hold your breath for a few counts, then let it out, again counting to five. Repeat this five times.

Prevention boosters

Rediscover religion A study of 718 adults found that women who had stopped attending religious services were three times more likely to have an anxiety disorder than those who still attended. The link may be related to the social interactions women get from being part of a church, synagogue or mosque.

Supplement with kava This herb is a member of the black pepper family. Numerous studies attest to its ability to calm anxiety, but check with your doctor before taking it. Kava can interfere with how your body metabolises certain medications and, in large amounts, could cause liver damage.

Sip tea As if sipping tea weren't calming enough, UK researchers recently discovered that people who drink tea several times a day recovered faster from stressful situations designed to increase heart rate and blood pressure. The tea drinkers' blood also showed lower levels of stress hormones. Anti-oxidants in tea may attach to the same receptors in the brain that anti-anxiety medications target.

Take brewer's yeast Brewer's yeast is an excellent source of biotin, also called inositol or vitamin B_7. In one study, supplementing with 12–18 g of inositol worked just as well as the antidepressant fluvoxamine (Luvox) for reducing the intensity and frequency of panic attacks. To prevent the attacks altogether, start taking a B-vitamin supplement that contains 12–18 g of biotin. Besides brewer's yeast (try sprinkling a tablespoon over cereal or yogurt), peanut butter is also a good food source.

Take 3 g fish oil daily There's intriguing evidence that fish oil can help relieve depression, and now it seems it may reduce stress as well. After three months, study participants who took 3 g of fish oil a day reported feeling half as stressed as those who took a placebo, but check with your doctor before taking any supplement.

▶ WHAT CAUSES IT
Just about anything in life can cause anxiety. But if your anxiety is excessive or irrational and it disrupts your life, you may have a condition known as generalised anxiety disorder.

▶ SYMPTOMS TO WATCH FOR
Restlessness, difficulty concentrating, irritability, trouble falling asleep, obsessive thoughts about something specific, racing heartbeat, shortness of breath and unusual sweating.

▶ LATEST THINKING
In people who have experienced a traumatic situation, such as child abuse, war or rape, intervention through counselling and other approaches can prevent an anxiety disorder developing.

Arthritis

30% The reduction in arthritis risk in women who exercise for an hour a week.

If you've ever seen people hobbling on arthritic hips or knees, or struggling to simply hold a butter knife with stiff, aching fingers, you know how this disease can interfere with life. But osteoarthritis—in which the shock-absorbing cartilage between joint bones wears away—isn't inevitable. Everything from genetics to joint injuries to age-related changes in cartilage-protecting enzymes plays a role. But there's also plenty of evidence that you can cut your risk significantly.

Key prevention strategies

Lose weight If you're carrying excess weight around your middle, hips or buttocks and thighs, here's yet one more reason to shed a few kilos: you'll put less pressure on your joints and thereby lower your risk of arthritis. Australian researchers maintain that osteo-arthritis risk goes up 36 per cent for every 5 kg over your healthy weight range. Lose just 500 g, on the other hand, and you'll put nearly 2 kg less stress on your knees. Losing 5 kg if you're obese can cut your odds of developing arthritis over the next 10 years by 50 per cent.

Losing weight benefits not only your knees but your hips, too. When US researchers at the Harvard Medical School checked the weight and health histories of 568 women with osteoarthritis, they found that women with a higher body weight were twice as likely to need hip replacement surgery.

Exercise for at least an hour a week Until recently, doctors and scientists thought that a lifetime of exercising made people more vulnerable to arthritis, since studies showed a higher risk of joint problems among ageing athletes. But now researchers say that joint injuries, not exercise itself, account for the difference. In fact, there's growing evidence that exercise can prevent problems by building up muscles that protect joints.

In one Australian study of middle-aged and older women, those who got at least 2.5 hours of exercise per week cut their odds of developing arthritic joints by about 40 per cent. Exercising for just an hour a week lowered risk by about 30 per cent. And stretching exercises help, too.

Add strength training Strengthening your muscles by using any form of so-called resistance training (using light hand weights, elastic bands, or machines at the gym or doing home exercises that use your own body weight as resistance—think knee bends) may shield joints from damage. In one study, women with stronger thigh muscles had a 55 per cent lower risk of developing knee arthritis and an amazing 64 per cent lower risk for arthritis of the hips than women with weaker thigh muscles.

Getting stronger helps if you already have arthritis, too. When Tufts University researchers tested a gentle, at-home strength-training program for older men and women with moderate to severe knee osteoarthritis, the results surprised and pleased study volunteers. After 16 weeks, exercisers had 36 per cent less pain and 38 per cent less disability. (See the at-home exercise routine you can try on your own, starting on page 110.)

Experts say gentle strength training can also dampen the pain and disability of rheumatoid arthritis (RA), which occurs when the immune system attacks the tissues that protect bones. In a study from Finland, people with mild RA who followed a home strength-training program for two years saw pain decline by 67 per cent and disability drop by 50 per cent.

Prevention boosters

Don't smoke Women who smoked cigarettes raised their risk of developing RA by 30 per cent in one US study of 121,700 nurses. Smoking doubled the risk of the disease in another study of 30,000 women. According to Swedish researchers, tobacco smoke may provoke immune-system changes that lead to an attack on joints. The good news is that women who had quit smoking had no extra risk after about 10 years.

Get more vitamin D If you're running low on the 'sunshine vitamin', your joints may be at risk. Vitamin D, produced by your skin upon exposure to the sun, may help keep the immune system healthy and protect joints from wear-and-tear damage by strengthening nearby bone, too. When researchers studied men and women whose knees showed signs of osteoarthritis, those who took in above-average amounts of vitamin D from food and supplements were in better shape eight years later than those who didn't.

'Tobacco smoke may provoke immune-system changes that lead to an attack on joints.'

Are glucosamine and chondroitin worth it?

This dynamic duo is taken by more people with osteoarthritis than any other 'joint' supplement. But a collection of recent research casts doubt on how well they work. Here's what you need to know to help make a choice:

What are they? Both are components of human cartilage, the smooth covering on knee bones and other joints that acts as a shock absorber. In osteoarthritis, cartilage softens, cracks and wears out, allowing knee joints to rub together.

Glucosamine is thought to be involved in cartilage growth; supplements are derived from the shells of crabs and lobsters. Chondroitin gives cartilage its elasticity; supplements are usually derived from animal cartilage.

The claim Proponents say that glucosamine and chondroitin relieve pain by maintaining cartilage so that joint bones don't grind against each other.

The research There's a lot of conflicting data out there. Belgian researchers recently found that glucosamine had no effect on pain or joint deterioration in people with osteoarthritis in their hips. And a large US study of 1583 people with osteoarthritis found that this combination didn't ease joint pain any better than placebos did. But when researchers looked at the 20 per cent of study participants with moderate to severe arthritis pain, they found a benefit: 79 per cent of those taking the supplements (they took 500 mg of glucosamine plus 400 mg of chondroitin three times a day) had at least a 20 per cent reduction in pain, compared to 54 per cent taking placebos.

What about joint protection? Other studies suggest that these supplements may help maintain 'joint space'—the distance between bones. (More joint space means less grinding, less damage and less pain.) In a Belgian study of over 300 women with osteoarthritis, those who took glucosamine for three years showed no narrowing of the space between knee bones, while those taking a placebo saw the gap grow smaller. The glucosamine group also reported a 14 per cent improvement in pain and stiffness from the beginning to the end of the study, while the placebo group was a little worse by the end of it.

Are these supplements safe? Yes. Long-term studies have found only mild side effects such as intestinal gas and softer bowel movements.

What should I take? The US Arthritis Foundation suggests this pair may be worth a try. Take a supplement containing 500 mg of glucosamine and 400 mg of chondroitin sulfate three times a day. Try it for at least six weeks (some experts recommend three months) to see if you're getting any noticeable benefit. If not, stop taking them.

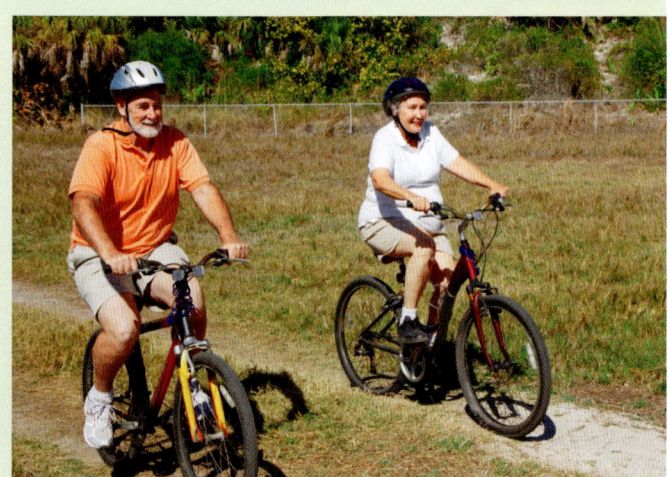

Vitamin D may protect against RA as well. When US researchers at the University of Iowa followed 29,368 women aged 55 to 69 for 11 years, they found that women who got less than 5 mcg, or 200 IU, of vitamin D from food or supplements were 33 per cent more likely to develop the disease.

The Australian National Health and Medical Research Council (NHMRC) recommends that younger adults (19 to 50 years) get 5 mcg, or 200 IU, a day of vitamin D. This rises to 10 mcg, or 400 IU, a day for adults aged 51 to 70 years, as older adults are less able to make their own vitamin D after skin exposure to sunlight, and 15 mcg, or 600 IU, a day for people over seventy. However, some experts believe that higher doses than this would bring more benefit. The safe upper limit is thought to be 80 mcg, or 3200 IU, a day.

You'll probably need to take a supplement to get therapeutic benefits. Unless you're eating oily fish such as salmon or sardines every day (100 g of either contains about 9 mcg, or 350 IU, of vitamin D), it's very hard to get enough from food. (A glass of skim milk, another good source, has just 2.5 mcg, or 98 IU.) And while your body makes vitamin D from skin exposure to sunlight, if you can't see your shadow, the amount of sunlight exposure probably isn't enough. To check your vitamin D status, ask your doctor for a blood test at the end of winter, when most people's levels are at their lowest.

Eat colourful foods If it's red, orange, blue or green, chances are it's packed with anti-oxidants—compounds that neutralise rogue molecules called free radicals, which are thought to interfere with cartilage repair and rebuilding. Mangos, peaches, oranges and watermelon are all rich in beta-cryptoxanthin, an anti-oxidant and one of a pair of compounds that lowered the risk of arthritis by an impressive 20 to 40 per cent in a UK study of 25,000 people. The other anti-oxidant, zeaxanthin, is found in spinach, sweet corn, peas and orange capsicums. People with the highest blood levels of both of these anti-oxidants cut their arthritis risk by 50 per cent.

Vitamin C is joint friendly too. Eating plenty of strawberries, oranges, red capsicums and broccoli—all good sources—could help slow the development of knee pain if you already have osteoarthritis, according to Boston University researchers in the US. In one study, people who got the most vitamin C were three times less likely to have arthritic knee pain than people who got the least.

▶ WHAT CAUSES IT

For osteoarthritis, cartilage breakdown is the cause. Injuries, extra weight, genetics and muscle weakness can all contribute. Over time, cartilage may wear through in spots so that bones rub against each other, creating intense pain. Rheumatoid arthritis happens when your immune system attacks the lining of your joints (the synovium), leading to intense pain, swelling and joint deformities.

▶ SYMPTOMS TO WATCH FOR

Pain, stiffness, tenderness and swelling in joints. Osteoarthritis most often affects the knees, hips, hands and spine. Rheumatoid arthritis usually begins in small joints in the hands and feet, then spreads to larger joints. In addition to pain and swelling, rheumatoid arthritis can cause fever, tiredness and weight loss.

▶ LATEST THINKING

If you have a type of knee arthritis in which the wear and tear is harming the middle of your joint—called medial-knee arthritis—special innersoles in your shoes could help. Lateral-wedge innersoles are thinnest at your instep and widest at the outer edge of your foot, realigning your feet and lower legs in a way that can reduce some of the twisting that wears down knee joints. Your doctor can tell you which type of knee arthritis you have.

Exercises for arthritis prevention

These moves strengthen key muscles that act as shock absorbers for your joints in your legs and arms, helping to protect you against arthritis. Start with 500-g weights and an exercise band. Ask your doctor if this program is right for you, and then exercise for 10 minutes three times a week. As you become stronger, do more repetitions, increase the weight and switch to an exercise band with greater resistance.

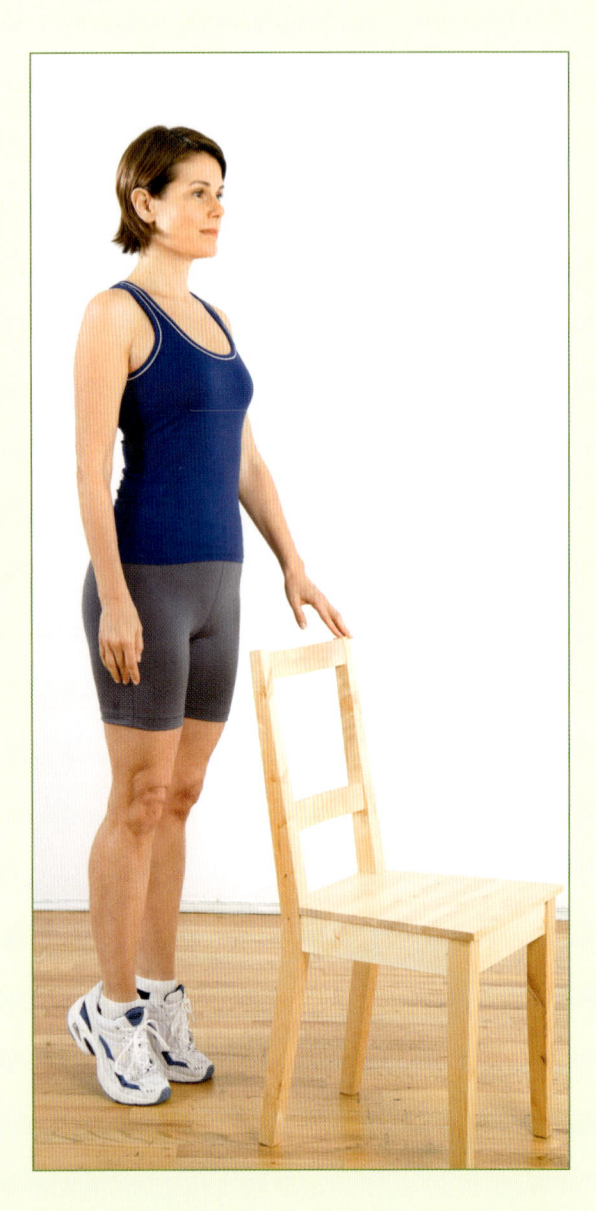

Calf strengthener

Stand facing a chair back or table with your feet a few centimetres apart and hold on to the chair or table for balance. Rise onto the balls of your feet, then lower. Repeat until your calves feel tired. If this becomes easy after a few weeks, add weight: use a small backpack with a 2-kg weight in it (such as a dumbbell). To make it even harder, do the exercise (without the backpack or weight) with one foot on the floor and your other knee bent so that the foot is raised.

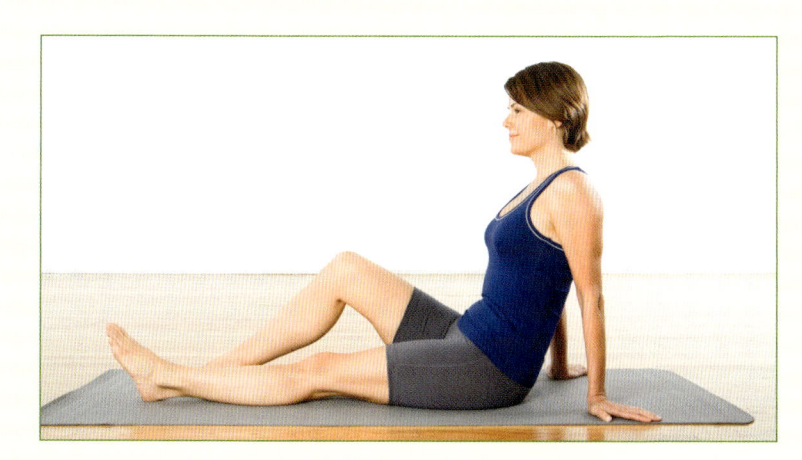

Quadriceps toner

1 Sit on the floor with your left leg straight in front of you and your right leg bent. You can support your back by sitting against a wall or by putting your hands slightly behind you.

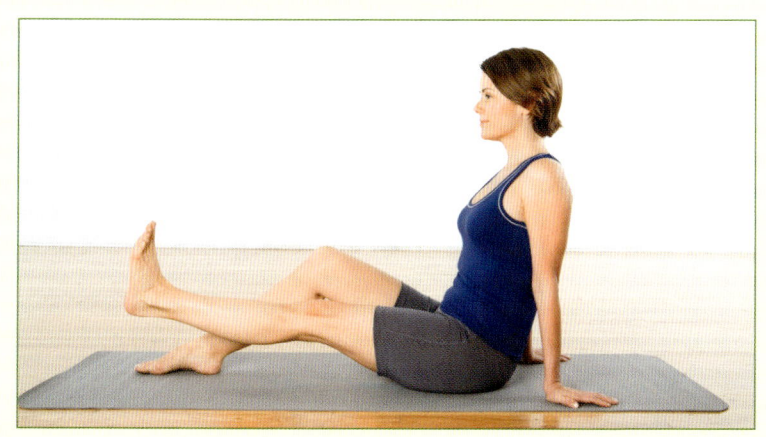

2 Keeping your abdominal muscles tight, lift your left leg off the floor. Lower and repeat until your leg feels tired. Switch legs and repeat.

Hip flexor builder

1 Lie on your back on the floor, bend your right knee, keeping your right foot on the floor.

2 Tighten the quadriceps muscle in your left thigh, turn your leg outward slightly, and raise it as far as you can (but not above your right knee). Lower and repeat until the muscle feels tired. Switch legs and repeat.

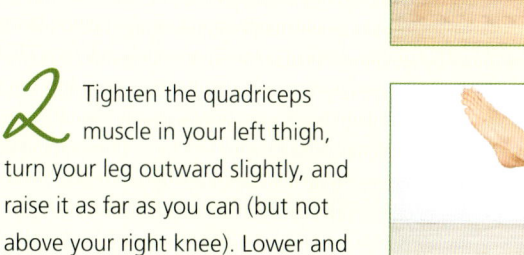

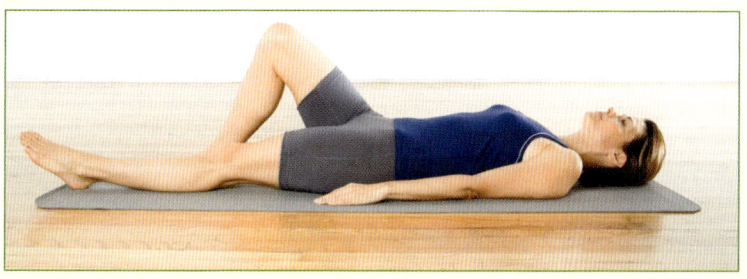

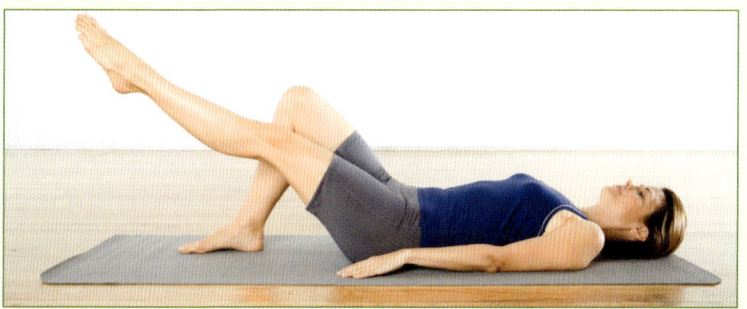

Hamstring builder

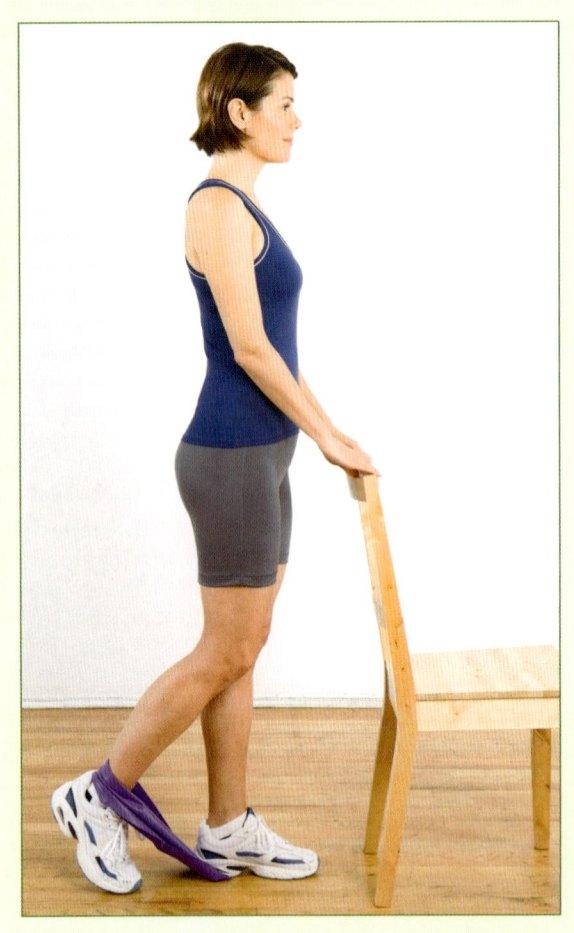

1 Knot an exercise band to make a medium-sized loop. Stand facing a table or sturdy chair that you can use for support. Put one end of the loop under your left foot and the other around your right ankle.

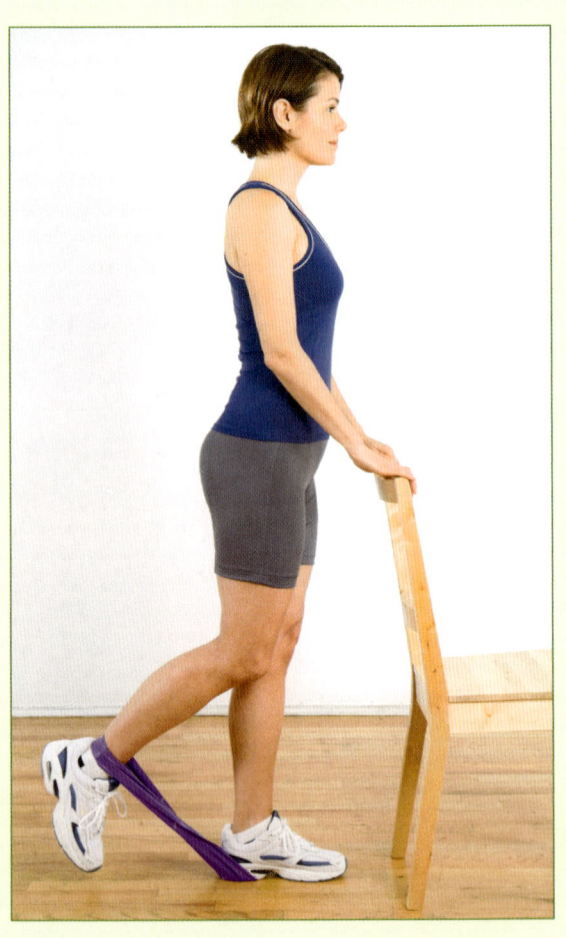

2 Bend your right knee and raise your foot behind you, pulling against the resistance of the band. Don't let your back arch. Repeat until the back of your thigh feels tired, then switch sides.

Foot builder

Spread a hand towel in front of a chair. Sit down and put one bare foot near the back edge of the towel. Keeping your heel on the towel, use your toes to gather the fabric and pull it under your foot. Keep going until you've gathered all you can. Repeat with your other foot.

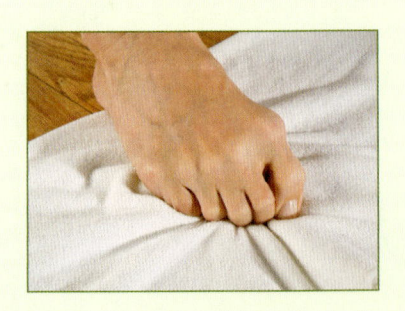

Arthritis | 113

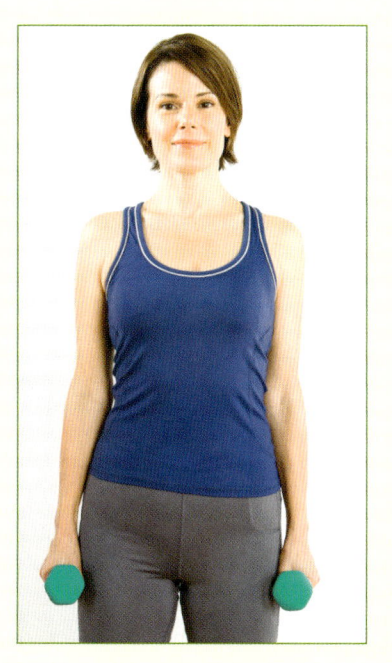

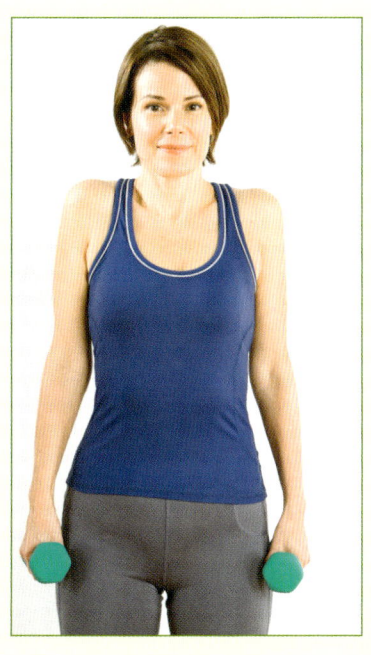

Shoulder shrug

Stand and hold a pair of light-weight dumbbells (start with 500-g weights) at your sides. Keeping your arms straight, shrug your shoulders upward, then relax. Repeat 20 times.

Shoulder strengthener

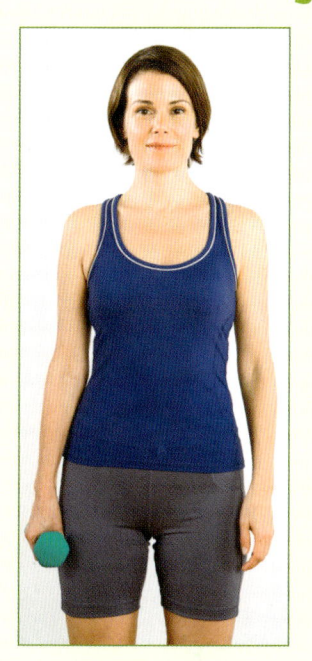

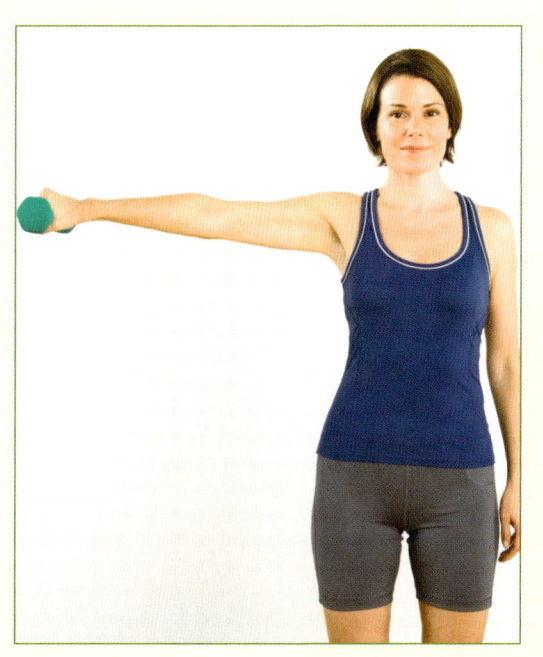

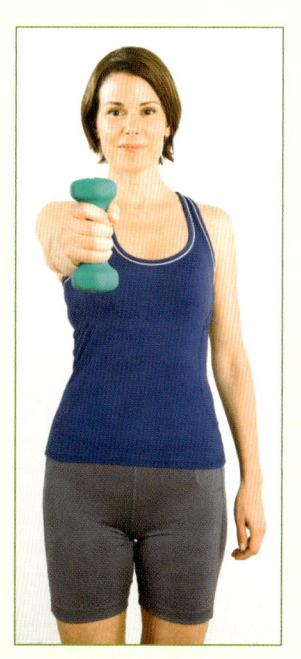

Hold a dumbbell in your right hand, with your arm down at your side. Lift the weight straight out to the side, then rotate your elbow joint and swing it slowly out in front of you as far as you comfortably can. Slowly swing your arm back to the side. Repeat 5 to 10 times, then switch hands.

Asthma

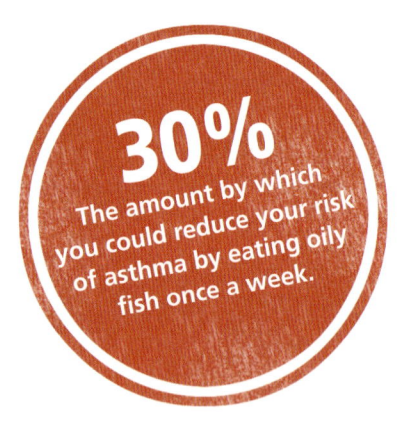

30%
The amount by which you could reduce your risk of asthma by eating oily fish once a week.

Asthma is on the rise in most developed countries, and one widely believed reason for this is that children today are not exposed to germs and dirt the way earlier generations were, so their immune systems haven't learned to react appropriately. Studies also find that adults raised on farms are much less likely to have asthma. Still, there's plenty you can do to prevent attacks if you already have asthma.

Key prevention strategies

Allergy-proof your house More than half of all homes have at least six detectable allergens, and the remainder have at least three. And here's a really sobering statistic: more than a third of homes in the US were found to have levels of mouse allergens high enough to contribute to asthma. And it's probably safe to assume that the situation isn't so different in Australia, New Zealand or South Africa. The bottom line here is that the higher the allergen levels are in your house, the more likely you or your children are to have asthma. Following are some suggestions for targeting the most common asthma-causing allergens. (Find more tips on allergy-proofing your house, see 'Allergies', starting on page 96.)

MOUSE ALLERGENS

- Damp-mop your floor daily. It's not enough to simply sweep the floor, as the highest levels of mouse 'urinary proteins' are found on kitchen floors and can only be removed with washing.
- Seal all cracks and holes in walls and doors, around window frames, and in the attic if you have one or the roof space if it's easily accessible, as well as around wiring entrances to all electrical outlets and light switches and fixtures—they're perfect entry points for mice. If the cavities are too large to fill with caulk, stuff them with steel wool, which repels pests.
- Keep all food in sealed containers. Cardboard boxes aren't good enough; mice can easily gnaw through them.
- Use mousetraps. There's a wide variety, including humane traps that keep the mouse contained until you find it, before setting it free away from your home.

Got the gene?

Because asthma and allergies, such as hay fever and eczema, tend to run in families, it's been long suspected that certain genes make some people more susceptible. Now we're finding potential culprits for this: a variant in the gene ORMDL3 seems to increase the risk of asthma in children by 60 to 70 per cent.

COCKROACH ALLERGENS
- Store open boxes of food in the refrigerator, not a pantry.
- Make a natural spray with 60 ml eucalyptus or peppermint oil for every 400 ml water. Then spray it around your kitchen, outside, around water pipes—anywhere you've seen cockroaches or suspect they may be gaining entry.
- Sprinkle a thin layer of boric acid where you've seen the insects.
- Kill them with poisoned bait (a concoction of flour, cocoa, ground oats, boric acid and plaster of Paris should do it). For every cockroach the concoction kills directly, 20 or 30 more will die from eating poisoned faeces.

Check the scale Gained a few kilos lately? Noticed your asthma is getting harder to control? It's not a coincidence. You're 66 per cent more likely to have persistent asthma symptoms if you're obese than if your weight is in the normal range. This may have to do with inflammatory chemicals released from fat cells.

Researchers are beginning to study the effects of weight loss on asthma symptoms. In one small Italian study, 12 obese women with asthma who had stomach-reduction surgery, and who lost a significant amount of weight as a result, saw a 31 per cent improvement in scores that measure shortness of breath and an 18 per cent improvement in scores that measure the use of rescue medication compared to women who didn't have the surgery or lose weight.

Draft your own asthma plan with your doctor A major reason for uncontrolled asthma is the lack of a personalised asthma plan. These plans provide information about how and when to use daily and emergency medications and a peak flow meter to monitor lung function. They also tell you when it's time to seek emergency medical care or call your healthcare provider. Studies find that using these plans significantly reduces asthma attacks and deaths from asthma. It's a good idea to make a list of questions to ask your doctor before you start out, and the following questions are a good place to start when you're developing your plan:
- When should I call you?
- When should I seek emergency care?
- When is quick-relief medication not enough?
- When, if ever, should I increase my use of inhaled steroids?
- When, if ever, should I start taking oral steroids?

'You're 66% more likely to have persistent asthma symptoms if you're obese.'

Once developed, the plan should be reviewed and updated annually, and given to family members and others who might need to know what to do in the event of an emergency.

Prevention boosters

Learn to use your inhaler properly About one-third of people with asthma don't know how to use their inhaler properly. This lack of understanding can increase the risk of asthma attacks, hospitalisation and even death. Ask your pharmacist to show you.

Prevent asthma in children

Believe it or not, asthma prevention actually begins in the womb. Here's what you can do to reduce the risk of your child developing asthma:

1. **Quit smoking** The link between exposure to secondhand smoke in childhood and asthma is strong and undeniable.

2. **Follow the right diet while pregnant** That means one high in foods rich in vitamin E (wheatgerm, sardines, egg yolks and nuts) and zinc (red meat and shellfish). These nutrients influence lung and immune system development. At least two studies find that low levels during pregnancy can increase the risk of allergies and asthma in children. Also include fatty fish such as salmon, trout or sardines twice a week, or take a daily fish-oil supplement after checking with your doctor, especially if you are taking blood thinning medication. Studies find that getting the healthy fats in fish and fish oil during pregnancy reduces the baby's risk of asthma, possibly by leading to healthier immune system development. Skip fish sticks, however, which can actually increase the risk of asthma in your child, perhaps because of the high levels of inflammatory trans fats some brands contain.

3. **Give children allergy shots** If your child has allergies, treatment with immunotherapy—either injections or under-the-tongue drops—may help protect him or her from developing asthma.

4. **Breastfeed for four to six months**

5. **Hold off on solids** Current advice advocates that babies should be at least six months old before eating cereal or other solid foods.

6. **Skip acid-blocking medication while you're pregnant** Researchers find that taking medications such as H2 blockers like cimetidine (Tagamet), famotidine (Pepcid) and ranitidine (Zantac) or proton-pump inhibitors like omeprazole (Prilosec or Probitor) and esomeprazole (Nexium) during pregnancy increased the risk of asthma in infants by more than 50 per cent.

7. **Limit exposure to dust mites** UK researchers who followed 120 children from birth to eight years found that those who were breastfed and had limited exposure to dust mites due to the use of mattress protectors and pesticides were 76 per cent less likely to have asthma and 87 per cent less likely to have allergies by the age of eight. (See pages 81 and 96 for more on dust mites.)

Use a peak flow meter If you have trouble recognising the early signs of worsening asthma, this small, inexpensive device may help (available from pharmacies or online). Peak flow meters measure your lung function, providing an early warning of an impending asthma attack. Using it daily, and adjusting your medication based on the results, can help keep you attack-free.

Use hypoallergenic mattress and pillow covers One study found that these covers not only reduced the number of dust mites in beds but also enabled children with asthma to cut their dose of inhaled steroids by at least 50 per cent.

See an allergy specialist You may be likely to have fewer problems controlling your asthma and less severe symptoms if your care is provided by an allergy specialist instead of a GP. As you'd expect, a specialist is going to have more in-depth knowledge and will be on top of cutting-edge treatments.

Serve salmon twice a week A study of the dietary habits of 13,000 adults found that those who ate oily fish once a week were 30 per cent less likely to have asthma than those who ate it once a month or less often, and about 36 per cent less likely to have asthma symptoms such as wheezing. One explanation may be the anti-inflammatory benefits of oily fish such as salmon and sardines. Asthma is first and foremost an immune system disease, in which immune cells overreact to triggers by pumping out inflammatory chemicals that narrow airways.

Stay away from traffic Diesel exhaust (think trucks and buses) can cause serious problems for people with asthma. Just walking along busy streets can significantly reduce lung capacity and increase inflammation in people with asthma, probably because of tiny particles of dust and soot in the exhaust that are inhaled deep into the lungs and absorbed into the blood.

Take an aspirin every other day Check with your doctor first, but if it's fine to do so, taking a small dose (75 mg) of aspirin every other day could cut your risk of developing asthma by 10 per cent if you're a woman and you're not obese. Men generally require a higher dose (300 mg), but the resultant benefits are also higher— a risk reduction of 22 per cent.

▶ WHAT CAUSES IT

A combination of genes and environment leads to an overly sensitive airway that reacts to triggers such as airborne pollutants, allergens or cold air by releasing inflammatory chemicals. These lead to constriction of the muscles surrounding, and swelling in the lining of, the bronchial tubes in the lungs, often accompanied by extra mucus production.

▶ SYMPTOMS TO WATCH FOR

Shortness of breath, coughing, chest tightness and wheezing.

▶ LATEST THINKING

According to Australian researchers, brief, regular exposure to ultraviolet (UV) light, found in sunlight, can suppress certain immune reactions, including those that trigger asthma symptoms—at least in mice. But wait for a UV light therapy to be developed, since too much sun exposure can lead to skin cancer.

Back pain

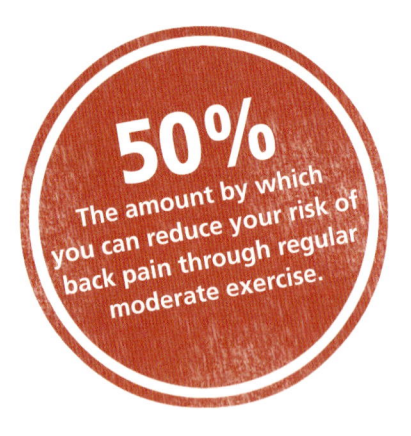

50% The amount by which you can reduce your risk of back pain through regular moderate exercise.

The reason that back pain is such a common complaint could be because humans were not designed to walk upright. It turns out that the same evolutionary change in our spines that allowed us to walk on two limbs also made it easier for vertebrae (the bones encasing the spinal cord) to crush and strain the soft discs between them. Unfortunately, we can't change our evolutionary heritage, but what we can do is guard ourselves from the effects of this design weakness.

Key prevention strategies

Get yourself off the couch or out of the chair If you're sitting around all day (which in itself is bad for the back), you're not getting exercise, the one strategy known to prevent back pain. Exercise helps keep extra weight off, strengthens abdominal and back muscles that support the spine, and increases the flow of oxygenated blood to the muscles and the vertebrae and other bones that keep your back properly aligned.

Don't worry about what kind of exercise you do; a major review of studies found that no single activity is best, nor is there any clear evidence as to how often and for how long you should work out—it may in fact vary from person to person. We always recommend that you get at least 30 minutes of moderate exercise (walking fast enough so you're slightly out of breath) at least four or five days a week.

Perfect your posture Surprisingly, that doesn't mean sitting up straight. Scottish researchers used specialised scanning (MRI) to evaluate three sitting postures in 22 volunteers. The participants either hunched forward, sat ramrod straight or leaned back slightly. The researchers found the greatest risk of vertebral movement, which can lead to misaligned spinal discs, in people who sat up straight and the least in people who leaned back slightly. So find a chair that provides good back support but also allows you to lean back just a bit.

Mind your mattress

Tempted by a fluffy, pillow-top mattress? Resist. Studies find that firm mattresses provide more support for your back, resulting in less back pain. Your mattress shouldn't be as hard as a granite slab, though; choose one that's medium-firm for the best back-health outcome.

Here are some other posture pointers:
- **Sleep on your side or back, not your stomach** Sleeping on your stomach increases the curve of your lower back, pulling it out of normal alignment.
- **Stand in front of the mirror and straighten up** Memorise how it feels when your entire body—from your ears to your ankles—forms a straight line.
- **Check your workstation** Even when leaning back slightly in your chair, put both feet flat on the floor and keep your eyes level with your computer monitor without bending your neck.
- **Walk with your stomach pulled in** Don't allow your lower back to arch. Hold your head high.
- **Walk lightly** If you literally pound the pavement, you're sending shock waves throughout your body, creating extra stress on your joints, including your pelvic and spinal joints. Have someone watch (and listen) to how you walk. If they observe that you're walking 'too hard', practise walking heel-toe, heel-toe instead of landing on your whole foot. This will cushion each step and distribute your weight more evenly.

Lift like a pro Most physiotherapists and orthopaedic surgeons recommend that you bend and lift in the following ways:
- **Light objects such as a piece of paper** Hold on to a nearby chair or table for support. Then lean over the object, slightly bend one knee and extend the other leg behind you. Push up with your bent leg after you've picked up the object.
- **Heavy objects such as a grocery bag or laundry basket** Stand in front of the object, bend at the knees and lift with your leg muscles. Don't bend at your waist, and don't rely on your arm strength alone for lifting heavy weights.
- **Luggage** Stand right next to the suitcase, bend your knees, grasp the handle and then straighten up.

Treat stress and depression You may think that depression is all in the mind, but in reality it's often all in the back. Chronic pain such as back pain can lead to depression, but it can also work the other way around, according to studies. If you've lost interest in your normal activities, find yourself sleeping significantly more or less than usual, have considered hurting yourself, or have other symptoms of depression, see your doctor immediately. (See also 'Depression', starting on page 160, for more advice.)

'The better your spinal stability, the less likely you are to develop back pain.'

If you've ever suddenly found yourself flat on your back and unable to move without excruciating pain after a stressful event, you're not alone. At least 11 studies find a significant relationship between stress, anxiety and back pain. We can't recommend avoiding all stressful situations in life, but we can recommend learning better ways to manage your stress. Here are some of our favourites:

- **Take up a repetitive hobby** such as knitting, crocheting, sewing or woodcarving.
- **Learn to meditate** Classes are available in most communities.
- **Volunteer** Helping others in need quite often puts your own issues and problems into better perspective.

Prevention boosters

Try Pilates or see an exercise physiologist There's no evidence that one is better than the other for preventing future episodes of back pain. They can develop a program of exercises for you that addresses impairments in flexibility and strength, and may help you enjoy a more active lifestyle. Pilates focuses on strengthening your core muscles—all the muscles that surround your spine and abdomen—that play a role in stabilising your back. But if you already have back problems, make sure you let your Pilates instructor know this before you begin classes.

Work out with an exercise ball Researchers in California tried an experiment on 20 sedentary office workers. Half of them exercised twice a week for 10 weeks with inflatable, oversized balls, also known as stability balls (available online and in specialty sports shops), which are designed to strengthen the core muscles. The other half did nothing. The people who used the ball showed major improvements in spinal stability; the muscles they developed in their abdomen and back acted like a thick belt around the waist to support the spine. The better your spinal stability, the less likely you are to develop back pain. The sizes of stability balls can vary considerably; so make sure to try a few, and choose the right size for your height.

Bike basics

Cycling is great exercise, but hunching over the handlebars can wreak havoc on your back. Try tilting the front of the bike seat down 10 to 15 degrees. It relieves pressure on your spine, in turn reducing back pain, according to a UK study of 40 recreational cyclists. Also take your bike into a bike shop and ask the technician to make sure the seat is at the right height and that the frame itself is the right size. And don't let your shoulders ride up around your neck when leaning on the handlebars; try to draw your shoulders down and back.

Wear flatties When you wear high heels, you throw your body weight forward, which exaggerates the curve of the lower back, making your back muscles work harder.

Set your alarm to get up and move When you're sitting for a long time at the computer, in the car or on a train, set an alarm on your watch or mobile phone to remind you to move every 20 minutes. If you can, get up and walk. If you're stuck in the car, shift your weight from one buttock to the other in a rocking movement and flex your legs to the extent you can. On long car trips, try to stop and walk around at least every hour.

Clean out your 'carryall' Large bags may be great for carrying around a lot of stuff, but they can cause untold problems for your back, especially if you sling a bag over one shoulder. They make your gait lopsided and pull your neck and shoulder—and hence your back—out of alignment. The best option is a 'bumbag', which puts the weight evenly on your hips. If that's not an option for you, try a daypack or a bag slung across your body, each of which tends to distribute the weight more evenly across your shoulders or chest. And also regularly empty out unnecessary clutter in handbags and daypacks. Regardless of what you're carrying, a bag shouldn't weigh more than 10 per cent of your body weight.

Use a step stool It will keep you from reaching too high, which could pull or strain a back muscle. If the stool has a low step, you can also place one foot on it (occasionally switching feet) to relieve your back a bit while you're washing dishes.

Counteract low kitchen benches Benchtops should be designed at the right height for the people using them, but tall people often end up leaning over to wash dishes or prepare meals. Put a stool or small stepladder in front of your legs and lean the front of your legs against it. A study by Japanese researchers found that this simple change significantly reduced lower-back strain.

Quit smoking Smoking narrows arteries, thereby impeding blood circulation and reducing the amount of oxygen-rich blood that gets to the spine and back muscles, among other areas. A lower blood supply interferes with the ability of bone and muscle to repair itself, which spells disaster if you've got back troubles.

▶ WHAT CAUSES IT
Strained muscles or ligaments or the breakdown of the discs between the vertebrae.

▶ SYMPTOMS TO WATCH FOR
Spasms, pain that may or may not radiate down the leg; numbness in your legs and restricted function; pain worsening at night; and bladder or bowel problems.

▶ LATEST THINKING
You may one day be able to blame chronic back pain, in part, on genes. Norwegian researchers believe that there is at least one genetic variant that increases susceptibility to back pain.

No-back-pain daily routine

A strong, supple back is one that's less likely to be injured. Simply doing this series of easy exercises every day can help to protect against back pain. They strengthen and/or lengthen the back muscles, abdominal muscles (which provide support for your back), and even the hamstrings at the back of your legs, which help minimise stress on the lower back. Start slowly then build up to the number of repetitions suggested.

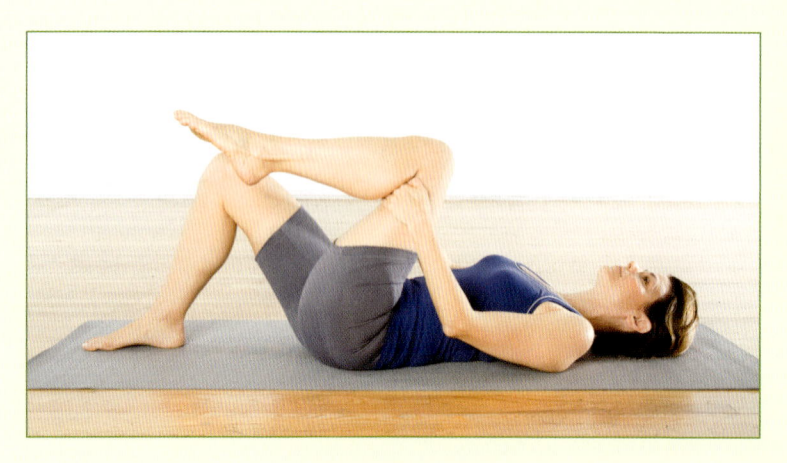

Hamstring stretch

1 Lie on your back, with your knees bent and right foot flat on the floor. Draw up your left leg, keeping your hands under your left thigh.

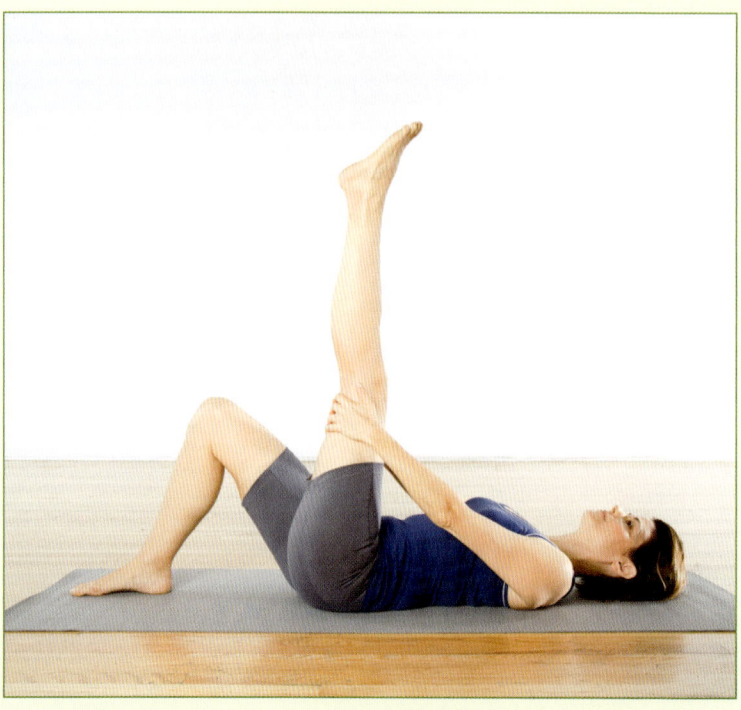

2 Straighten your left leg until you feel a comfortable stretch. Keep your entire back on the floor. Hold for 15 seconds, then return to the starting position. Repeat four times on each side.

Back pain | 123

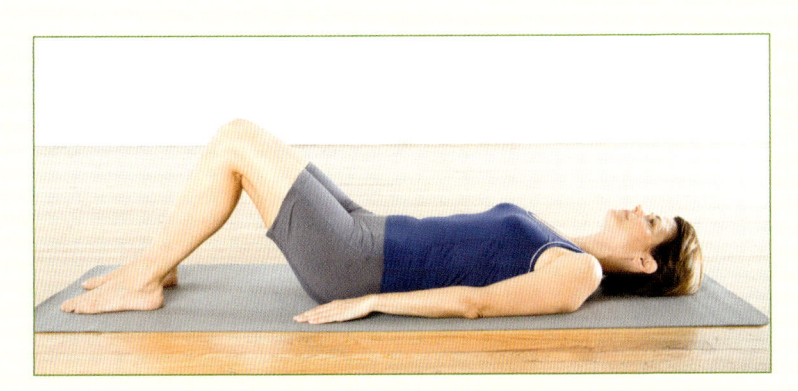

Knee-to-chest stretch

1 Lie on your back, with your knees bent and feet flat on the floor, arms by your sides.

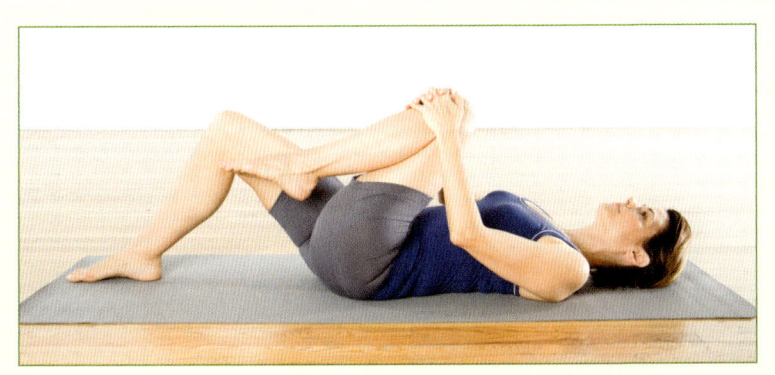

2 Using both hands, pull one knee towards your chest until you feel a comfortable stretch in your lower back. Hold for about 15 seconds. Return to the starting position and repeat with other leg. Repeat four times on each side.

Pelvic tilt

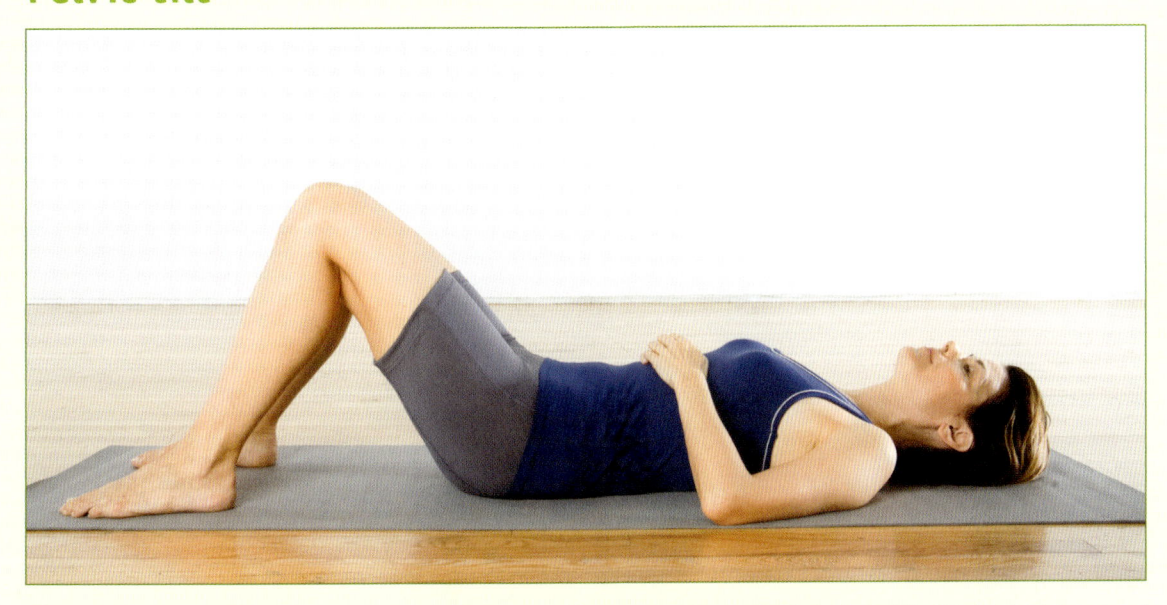

Lie on your back, knees bent and feet flat on the floor. Tighten your abdominal muscles and gently press your lower back into the floor. This is a small motion, mostly felt and not seen. Hold for 5 seconds. Repeat 10 times.

Back rotation

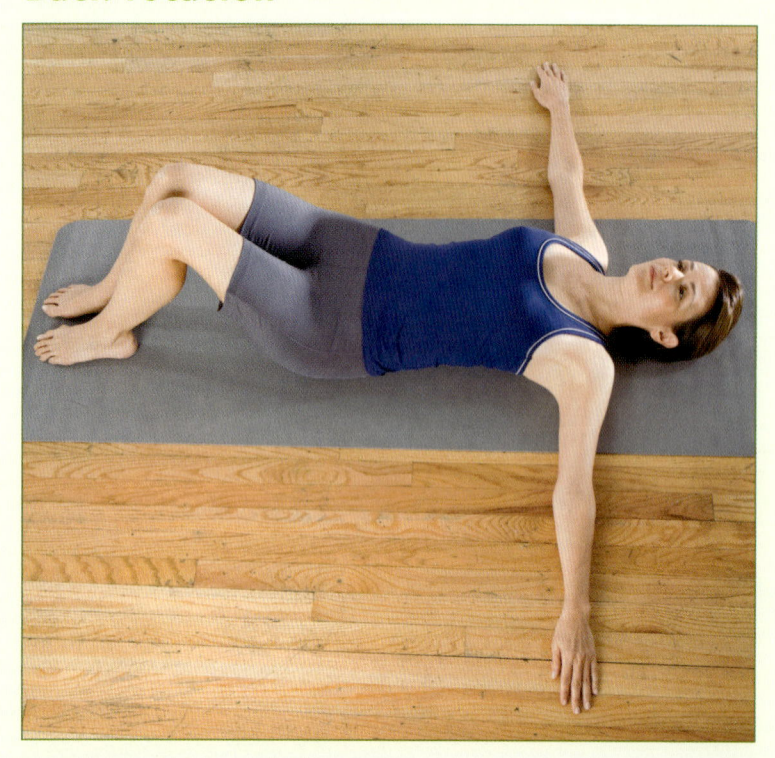

1 Lie on your back, with your knees bent, feet flat on the floor and arms out to the sides.

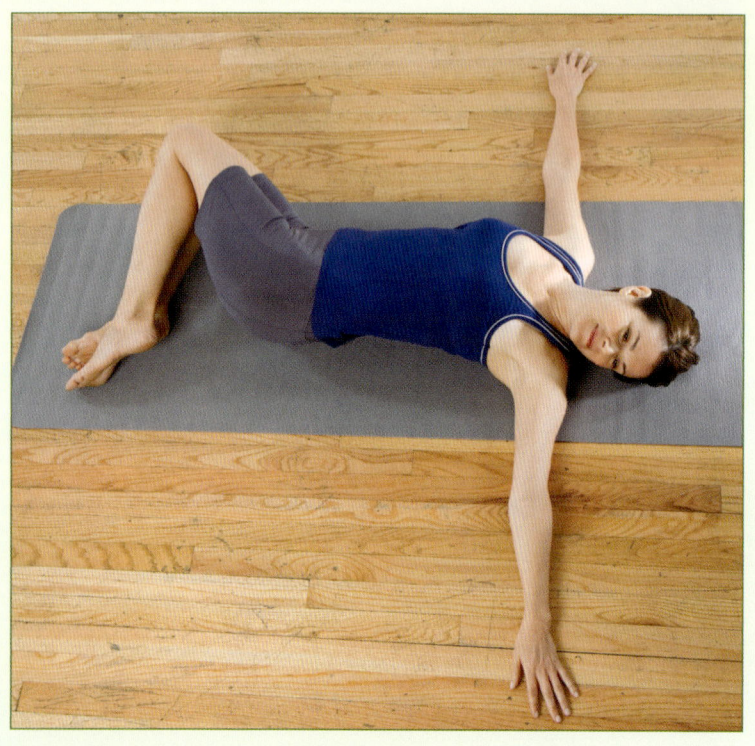

2 Keeping your shoulders on the floor, turn your head to the left and let your knees drop to the right until you feel a comfortable stretch. Hold for 15 seconds. Repeat four times on each side.

Back extension

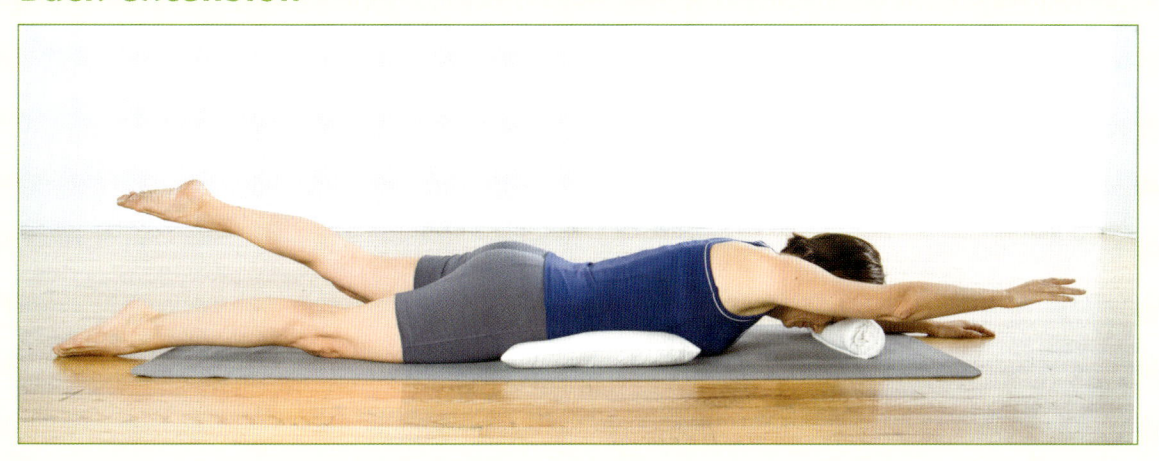

Lie face down with a thin pillow under your stomach and a small rolled towel under your forehead. Tighten your buttocks, then lift your right hand and left leg about 10–20 cm off the floor. Hold for 2 seconds, then lower and repeat on the other side. Continue for 2 minutes.

Halfway sit-up

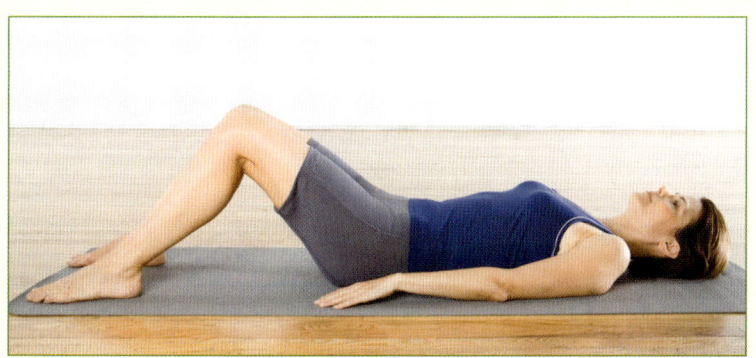

1 Lie on your back with your knees bent and feet flat on the floor. Tuck your chin to your chest and stretch your arms out in front of you.

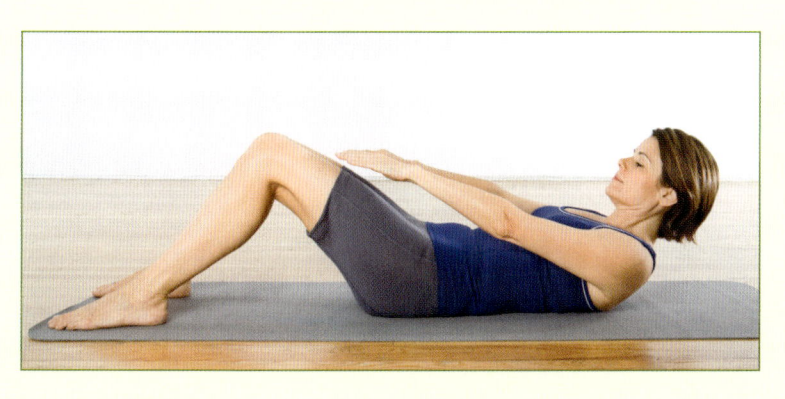

2 Using your abdominal muscles, slowly curl your upper body forward, lifting one vertebra off the floor at a time, until your shoulders clear the floor. Hold for 3 seconds. Slowly lower yourself to the floor one vertebra at a time. Repeat 10 times.

Hip bridge and roll down

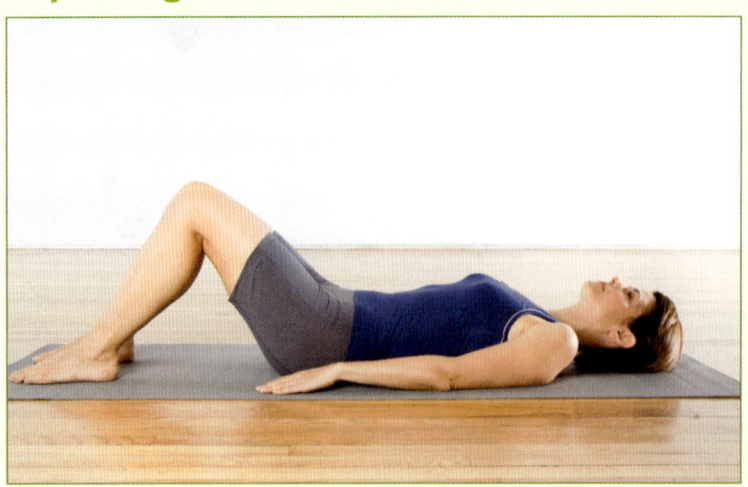

1 Lie on your back with your knees bent and your legs about hip-width apart.

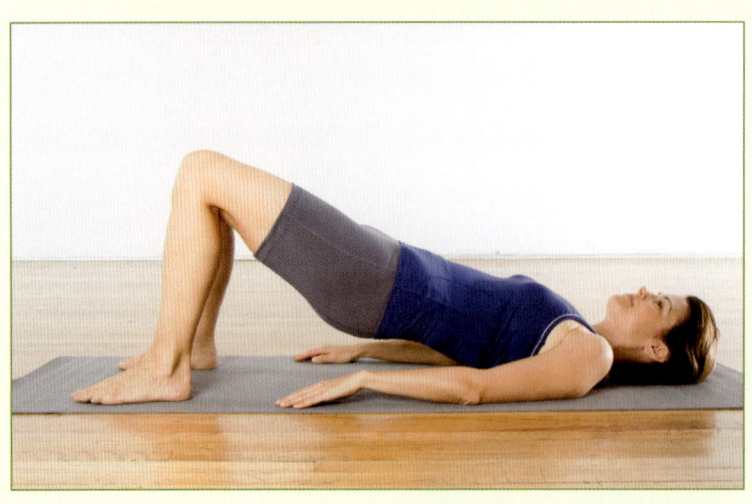

2 Tighten your abdominal muscles and lift your hips until your body forms a straight line from knees to shoulders. Hold for 5 seconds.

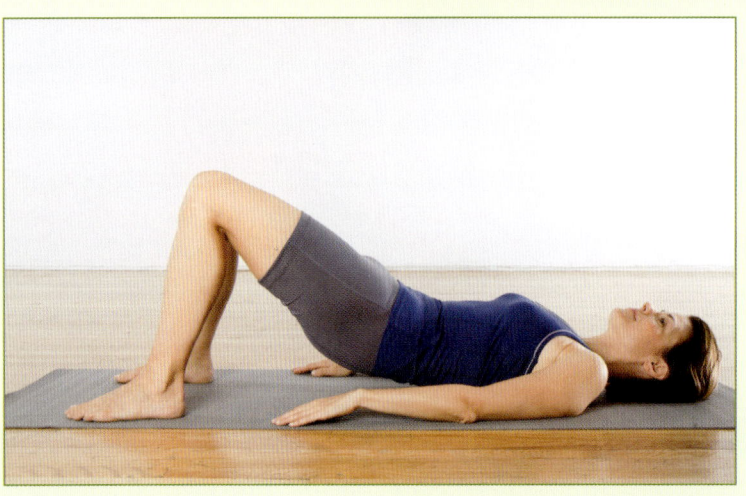

3 Slowly roll your spine back down to the starting position, touching one vertebra at a time to the floor, starting near your shoulder blades and ending with your tailbone. Repeat 10 times.

Cat stretch

1 Get on your hands and knees on the floor.

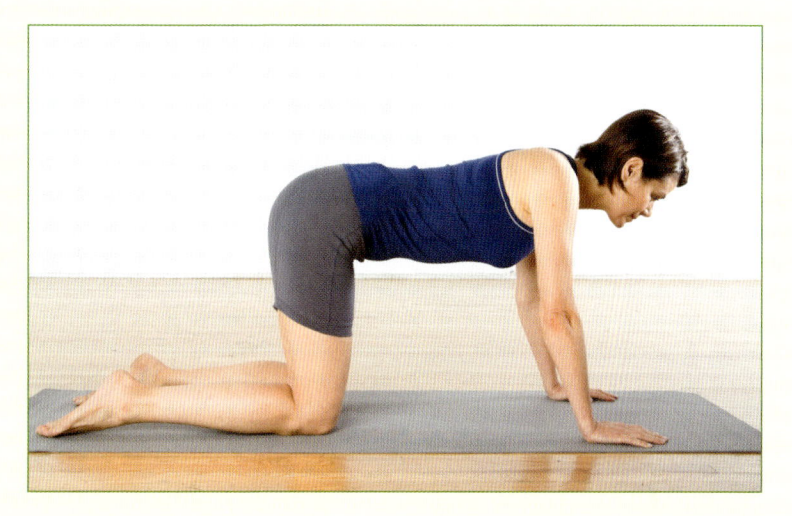

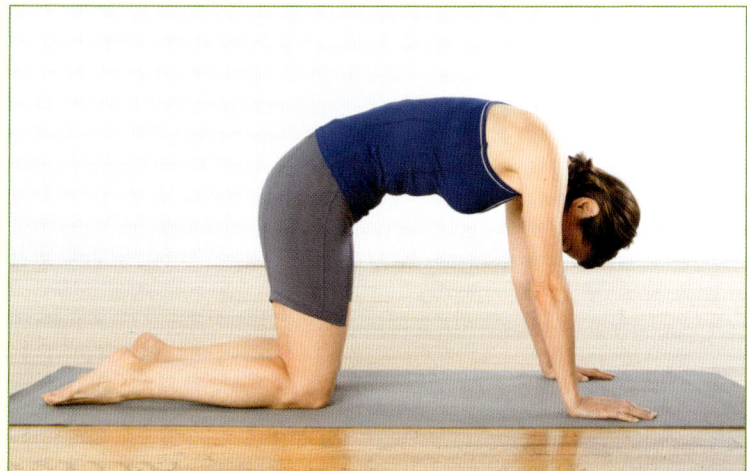

2 Drop your head, tuck your tailbone under and raise the middle of your back. Hold for 5 seconds, then return to the starting position.

3 Raise your head and hips and allow your back to sag towards the floor. Hold for 5 seconds. Return to the starting position. Repeat 10 times.

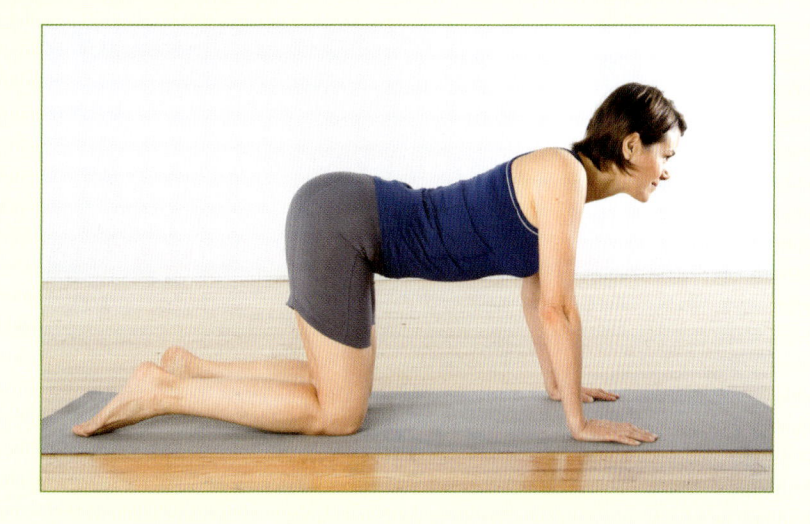

Benign prostatic hyperplasia

50% The amount by which you could reduce your risk by exercising vigorously 2 hours a week.

As men age, their prostate gland is likely to enlarge, which could lead to symptoms such as difficulty urinating or urinating too often. However, while nearly 80 per cent of men have benign prostatic hyperplasia (BPH) by the time they turn 80, only about a third develop symptoms.

Key prevention strategies

Eat more vegetables When researchers compared the diets of 6000 men with BPH to 18,000 men without it, they found those who got about 10 serves of vegetable a day were 21 per cent less likely to have BPH. Ten serves may sound like a lot, but if you start with a vegetarian omelette for breakfast, snack on a dozen baby carrots with low-fat dip and have a large spinach salad for lunch, you're halfway there. Your best bet, the study found, is vegetables high in vitamin C and the anti-oxidant lutein, such as capsicums and spinach. Also pay special attention to onions. Men who eat several portions of onions a week are far less likely to develop BPH than those who don't.

Discover linseed (flaxseed) and soy Both are sources of hormone-like plant compounds called phyto-oestrogens. These help guard against BPH by blocking an enzyme that converts testosterone into a different form—one that triggers prostate growth. Phyto-oestrogens also counteract the effects of oestrogen (yes, men have oestrogen, too), which also fuels prostate cell growth. Researchers think one reason why men living in Western countries have higher rates of BPH than those living in Asian countries is that they eat lower amounts of phyto-oestrogen-rich foods.

DRUGS THAT PREVENT DISEASE

Finasteride (Proscar), prazosin (Minipress), tamsulosin (Flomaxtra) and terazosin (Hytrin) are medications used to treat BPH. Finasteride blocks the enzyme that converts testosterone to dihydrotestosterone (DHT); DHT—three times more potent than testosterone—causes cells in the prostate to grow. Low doses can reduce the risk of BPH worsening over time and also reduce the rate of prostate cancer by 30 per cent. Prazosin, tamsulosin and terazosin belong to a family of alpha-blockers that relax the muscles in the prostate gland, bladder neck and urethra, reducing or even reversing some of the symptoms of BPH. Using finasteride with an alpha-blocker provides more benefit than using a single agent, but they all have side effects.

Linseeds are easy to add to your diet: buy them ground (store ground linseeds in the fridge) and sprinkle them on practically anything, from cereal to yogurt to salad. You can also add ground linseeds to meatballs and baked goods.

For soy, you don't have to rely on tofu. Try snacking on soy nuts or soybeans in the pods, known as edamame (available frozen), and using soy milk in your cereal or in smoothies.

Burn off some kilojoules every week A study involving 1000 men who were followed for nine years found that those who burned the most kilojoules each week through physical activity were half as likely to develop BPH as those who barely moved off the couch. Two hours a week of swimming laps burns about 5275 kilojoules—putting you in the 50 per cent risk-reduction zone based on this study. Other good options include running for 2 hours or walking for a minimum of 4 hours each week.

Check your cholesterol levels Here's something you probably didn't know: reproductive hormones such as testosterone are largely made of cholesterol. There is some evidence that men with high levels of LDL ('bad') cholesterol are more likely to have BPH.

Prevention boosters

Forgo unhealthy snacks Cutting out sugary snacks and simple carbohydrates such as doughnuts, white bread and potato chips is a good way to lose weight and also guard against high blood sugar levels. Men who are very obese (defined as a body mass index of 35 or higher) are three and a half times more likely to develop BPH than men of normal weight. Men with high blood sugar levels are three times more likely to develop BPH than men with normal levels.

Stop at one beer Cutting back on alcohol intake is a good idea. Men who have two or more drinks a day are 30 per cent more likely to develop BPH than those who have less than one a month.

Reach for low-fat or fat-free options If you're getting more than 38 per cent of your energy from fat, you're not only eating a very high-fat diet, you're also about 30 per cent more likely to develop BPH than someone who consumes fewer than 26 per cent of his energy from fat.

▶ WHAT CAUSES IT
Overgrowth of prostate tissue spurred by hormones such as oestrogen and testosterone. Age is the most common risk factor; 40 per cent of men aged 60 and older have it, and 90 per cent of men aged 80 and older.

▶ SYMPTOMS TO WATCH FOR
Increased need to urinate, particularly at night; weaker urine stream; burning sensation during urination; problems starting to urinate and dribbling.

▶ LATEST THINKING
Men with fast-growing BPH may be more likely to develop prostate cancer, particularly if they have metabolic syndrome.

Bladder cancer

30% The amount your bladder cancer risk drops within four years of quitting smoking.

Most men worry about prostate cancer, but few think about bladder cancer—the second most common cancer in middle-aged and elderly men. Women can be affected, too, although less commonly. About one in five cases of bladder cancer occur after exposure to certain chemicals used to make dyes, paints, textiles and other products, most of which you would have been exposed to 30 to 50 years before the cancer developed. There's not a lot you can do about that if you fall into that category, but there's a surprising amount you *can* do to prevent bladder cancer from other causes.

Key prevention strategies

Quit smoking If you smoke, your risk of developing bladder cancer is two to four times higher than someone who has never smoked. In fact, researchers estimate that two-thirds of all cases of bladder cancer are related to smoking. The longer you smoke and the more cigarettes you smoke, the greater your risk.

Don't try to quit on your own. Studies prove that you're more than twice as likely to be successful if you combine nicotine replacement products such as gum or nasal spray with some form of organised support, such as a counselling program or a telephone quit line. (See page 62 for more advice on how to quit.)

Get your water tested If you're drinking well water with high levels of arsenic, your risk of bladder cancer just went up. Arsenic levels should be less than 10 mcg per litre. If you drink from a well, you can have the water tested by a private company.

Munch on raw broccoli and cauliflower Cruciferous vegetables such as broccoli, cauliflower, cabbage, buk choy and brussels sprouts are filled with isothiocyanates. These anti-oxidants inhibit enzymes that make certain chemicals in the body more likely to cause cancer. One study found that eating three or more serves a month cut bladder cancer risk by about 40 per cent. Cooking destroys the enzyme needed to produce isothiocyanates, reducing available amounts by 60 to 90 per cent, so eat these vegetables raw as often as possible.

Prevention boosters

Eat foods rich in selenium This trace mineral is a powerful anti-oxidant linked with lower rates of several cancers, including bladder cancer. In your body, selenium comes into direct contact with bladder cells, where it is thought to prevent damage from free radicals (the unstable molecules that wreak havoc on DNA) and reduce levels of cancer-causing toxins. In one 12-year study of nearly 26,000 people, those with the lowest blood levels of selenium were more than twice as likely to develop bladder cancer compared to those with the highest levels.

Selenium is found in numerous foods, including brazil nuts (the best source by far), wholemeal flour, barley and fish, including tuna. Most people don't need selenium supplements; check with your doctor if for some reason you'd like to supplement.

Switch to skim milk and low-fat yogurt High levels of saturated fat (found in full-fat dairy products, not to mention fatty meats and cheese) more than doubled the rate of bladder cancer in a large Spanish study. Other studies find the overall amount of saturated fat in your diet increases your risk, so opt for low-fat dairy foods and trim cuts of red meat, and your risk will drop.

Brazil nuts are rich in selenium, which is linked to lower rates of bladder cancer.

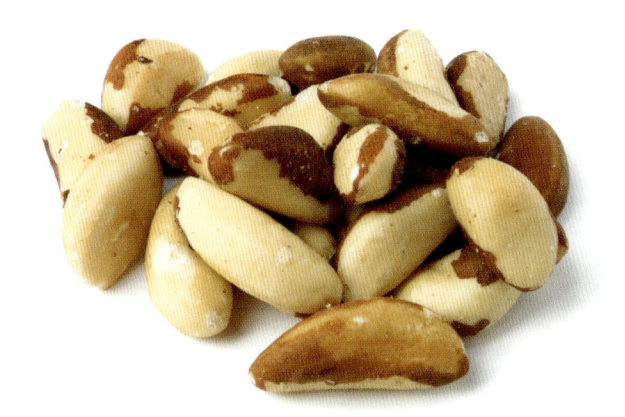

▶ WHAT CAUSES IT

Most often, toxins coming into contact with bladder cells. Over time, they can affect the DNA in these cells, leading to cancer. These toxins can come from the food you eat and the water you drink, tobacco by-products, and environmental and occupational chemicals. Other causes include infection with certain parasites (schistosomiasis).

▶ SYMPTOMS TO WATCH FOR

Blood in the urine, pain during urination, frequent urination or feeling that you need to urinate but can't, and abdominal pain.

▶ LATEST THINKING

Surgery to remove just the tumour, followed by chemo-therapy and radiation therapy, may be just as effective as removing the entire bladder for most stages of bladder cancer.

Breast cancer

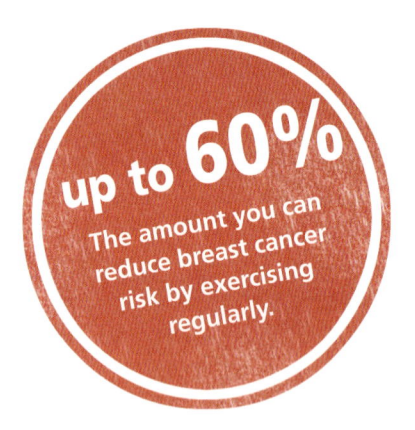

up to 60%
The amount you can reduce breast cancer risk by exercising regularly.

Breast cancer is the most common cancer in women and the most common cause of cancer deaths in women, but it has a reasonable cure rate, especially when caught early. It's also the only cancer with two medications approved to prevent it (for women at high risk). However, most women don't need to take medication to prevent breast cancer.

Key prevention strategies

Limit hormone replacement therapy (HRT) after menopause

Giving breast cells extra oestrogen is like pouring petrol on a fire. It makes the cells divide faster, raising the risk that some will mutate during division, producing a cancerous cell. Your immune system can typically destroy a few cancerous cells, but if you're taking oestrogen, those mutated cells could quickly overwhelm your natural defences. One study found that undergoing HRT for just three years resulted in a fourfold increase in risk of one of the most dangerous types of breast cancer.

Researchers suspect that the nearly 7 per cent drop in breast cancer diagnoses in the US between mid-2002 and mid-2003—after 20 years of increasing rates—was due to the fact that millions of women stopped taking HRT in 2002, the year a major report showed that the most commonly prescribed hormone medication increased the risk of breast cancer, heart disease and stroke, especially if taken in the long term.

Researchers don't think HRT causes the cancer; instead, it enables microscopic cancers that might have faded away or remained tiny for decades to roar to life.

Skip the chocolate mud cake
Here's another good reason to say no to decadent desserts and over-sized portions: every 5 kg you gain after menopause bumps up your breast cancer risk by 1 per cent. The major

---

DRUGS THAT PREVENT DISEASE

If the threat of breast cancer is a real worry for you, talk to your GP. A simple quiz can determine your five-year and lifetime risk of breast cancer. If it's at least 60 per cent higher than that of other women your age, you may be a candidate for chemoprevention (taking one of two medications—tamoxifen or raloxifene—for five years). The Australian Government doesn't pay for this expensive treatment. These medications mimic oestrogen in the body, preventing the real thing from affecting breast cells. Studies find that either medication reduces breast cancer risk by a staggering 49 per cent in high-risk women. If you're 35 years or older, you can calculate your own risk of developing breast cancer at www.cancer.gov/bcrisktool.

reason appears to be that fat cells release chemicals that can convert other hormones such as testosterone, which both men and women have, into oestrogen. On the other hand, if you're postmenopausal and you lose 5 kg or more and keep the weight off—and you don't take HRT—your risk is 57 per cent lower than that of women whose weight stays the same (and is presumably a bit higher than it should be).

Schedule that mammogram Breast cancer screening using mammography is the best way to reduce deaths from breast cancer, especially in women aged 50 to 69 years, but also in women aged 40 to 49, and those 70 and older. In the 50 to 69 group, for every 10,000 women who are screened, up to 20 deaths from breast cancer will be prevented over a 10-year period. But mammography isn't foolproof. There is a chance that the test will either miss a cancer (false negative) or suggest a cancer where there is none (false positive), leading to extra tests and anxiety. The chance of a misreading is higher in younger women because their breast tissue is denser, making it more difficult to interpret X-ray changes. Your GP can help you weigh up the pros and cons of having a mammogram every two years after the age of forty.

Prevention boosters

Limit alcohol intake A glass of wine with a meal is good for your heart, but it can very slightly increase your risk of breast cancer—probably not enough to really worry about. If you have more than one drink a day, however, you should worry. About 4 per cent of breast cancers are thought to be linked to this level of alcohol intake, and the more you drink, the higher the risk. Researchers think it's because alcohol increases oestrogen production.

If you decide to have more than one standard drink of alcohol a day (which is not recommended), you can hedge your bets by taking a daily supplement containing at least 400 mcg of folic acid. This B vitamin helps repair mistakes that cells make when they divide and might erase the increase in risk caused by the alcohol.

Keep moving Regular physical activity for at least 30 minutes a day, five days a week, can reduce your risk of breast cancer. The reason is that the more physically active you are, the lower your body fat, which in turn lowers breast cancer risk.

WHAT CAUSES IT

High circulating levels of hormones such as oestrogen are the main disease drivers. After menopause, obesity and weight gain drive up hormone levels and thereby increase risk. The longer you live, the more oestrogen and environmental toxins you've been exposed to and the greater your likelihood of developing the disease. The one-in-eight statistic you may have heard only applies if you live to be 90 or older. Inherited genetic mutations account for only about 5 to 10 per cent of breast cancer cases.

SYMPTOMS TO WATCH FOR

A lump or thickening in or near the breast or in the underarm area; tender nipples; changes in how the breast or nipple looks, including the size or shape; scaly, red or swollen skin on the breast, nipple or areola (the dark area surrounding the nipple); a nipple that turns inward; or nipple discharge.

LATEST THINKING

Even if you carry mutations in the genes BRCA1 and BRCA2, the 'breast cancer genes', your risk of developing breast cancer by the age of 70 is far less than once thought. Instead of the 80 per cent risk often cited, new research from the US finds a risk of between 36 and 52 per cent.

Bursitis and tendonitis

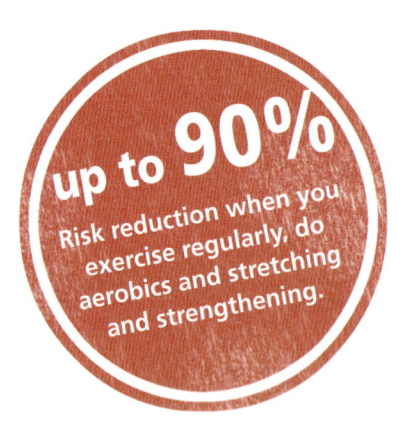

up to 90% Risk reduction when you exercise regularly, do aerobics and stretching and strengthening.

Doing the same movements over and over again can end in tendonitis, which is caused by inflammation of a tendon, a tough band of tissue that connects bones to muscles. Unfortunately, tendons lose some of their elasticity with age, making the condition more likely. Overuse of a joint can also cause bursitis, or inflammation of the fluid-filled sacs that cushion pressure points where muscles and tendons move across the bone. You can even get a form of tendonitis by leaning on your elbows too much.

Key prevention strategies

Get moving Exercise is an important part of a healthy, balanced life, but for some conditions, such as bursitis and tendonitis, it's an essential element requiring the right approach.

- **Revamp your exercise routine** Overuse or misuse of joints and muscles causes the majority of tendonitis and bursitis cases. But that doesn't mean you should stop exercising; instead, follow our tips for injury-free movement.
- **Book a session or two with a personal trainer** This way you can evaluate your regular work-out and identify movements that may be putting unnecessary strain on your joints and tendons.
- **Start slowly** Just as it takes a few minutes for the water in your shower to warm up, it takes a few minutes for your muscles and joints to warm up when you start working out.
- **Be consistent** That means exercising several times a week, not just once or twice a month. It also means you shouldn't throw yourself into a competitive basketball game if you haven't played or exercised for a while. Increase exercise by no more than 5 to 10 per cent each week, in terms of either time spent or weight lifted.
- **Switch activities throughout the week** For instance, if you work out with weights twice a week, spend one day on leg exercises and one day on upper-body exercises. If you run three times a week,

Help for 'housemaid's knee'

If you kneel a lot on the job, while cleaning, or when gardening, you're at risk of developing this condition, officially known as prepatellar bursitis. Investing in a thick pair of knee pads, available from home improvement and garden centres, can save you from the pain.

cycle on the other days. If you garden intensively one day, just water the garden or take a walk the next day.

- **Rest** Give yourself at least one day off each week. And if you feel any joint soreness after a work-out, put an icepack on the joint to ward off inflammation.

Stretch and strengthen Range-of-motion exercises and weight-bearing exercises designed to strengthen muscles can reduce strain on joints, helping to prevent overuse injuries. For best results, book a few sessions with a personal trainer or exercise physiologist to identify the best exercises for you based on the activities you do most.

Cut your kilojoule intake As with many conditions related to joints, being overweight increases the pressure on joints, bones and tendons, increasing your risk of injury.

Prevention boosters

Use innersoles or orthotics if you need them A major cause of Achilles tendonitis, an injury to the tendon that attaches the calf muscle to the heel bone, is hyperpronation of the foot—a medical term that simply means your ankles roll in. When you shop for joggers or walking shoes, do it at a sports shop, not a department store, and ask the salesperson to help you find a shoe with the level of support you need.

If your pronation is bad, you may want to see a podiatrist to be fitted for custom orthotics, or start with a basic pair of shoe inserts from a pharmacy to see if they help. In addition, wear the right shoes for the sport you're playing. For instance, if you play basketball, wear high-top sneakers.

Pay attention to pain If your joint feels sore, take some ibuprofen or put an icepack on it. Both can relieve inflammation, possibly preventing long-term damage.

Use a band or brace where you need it Supports for elbows and knees help reinforce and protect tendons during activities. There are many different types available, so check with your doctor or exercise physiologist about which one to choose.

▶ WHAT CAUSES IT
Ageing, repetitive movements and biomechanical problems with joints.

▶ SYMPTOMS TO WATCH FOR
Pain and tenderness near a joint that gets worse with movement. The skin over the area may become red or warm to the touch. Your doctor can tell whether it's bursitis or tendonitis based on where the problem occurs.

▶ LATEST THINKING
The antibiotic ciprofloxacin and others in its family (moxifloxacin and norfloxacin) can cause an inflamed Achilles tendon and even cause tendon rupture. Ask your doctor how you can protect your Achilles tendon if you need one of these antibiotics.

Carpal tunnel syndrome

49% The percentage of people whose carpal tunnel symptoms improved after wearing a wrist splint at night.

It's not always true that hard work never hurt anyone. If your job (or your life) involves typing on a computer for long periods, cutting meat, using sign language or any other repetitive task involving your wrists and hands, you could be in danger of developing carpal tunnel syndrome. Hobbies such as knitting, sewing and guitar playing also put you at risk. The condition is caused by inflamed tendons or ligaments in the wrist that put pressure on a nerve running through the base of your palm. It's marked by numbness, tingling and pain in the hand and fingers. If it gets bad enough, you may even have trouble picking up your coffee cup. Prevent the pain with the following suggestions.

Key prevention strategies

Embrace proper ergonomics Good posture can help you avoid carpal tunnel syndrome. That means sitting up straight and not letting your shoulders roll forward, which puts pressure on nerves in the back and arms, and not rounding your lower back or thrusting your chin forward—all common postural mistakes we make at the computer that squeeze the muscles in the neck. That in turn can affect muscles and nerves in your hands, wrists and fingers. It's also important to keep your wrists relatively straight—not bent up or down. If you're sitting at a keyboard, follow the advice in 'Type smart', on page 138.

Warm up and take breaks Flex your fingers up and down 10 times whenever you've been away from your computer or haven't been using your hands for more than 5 minutes. It's also important to give your wrists a rest. Take a 30-second break every 20 minutes, and schedule a 5-minute

Carpal tunnel as a symptom

Studies find much higher rates of carpal tunnel syndrome in people with rheumatoid arthritis, hypothyroidism, Type 1 diabetes, fibromyalgia and certain other conditions. In fact, some experts think that carpal tunnel syndrome may actually be the first symptom of these diseases. Other conditions that can cause it include multiple myeloma, non-Hodgkin's lymphoma and acromegaly—a disease in which the bones grow very long. If you have any of these diseases or conditions, managing them with lifestyle changes and medical treatments may reduce your risk of carpal tunnel syndrome, or improve symptoms if you already have it. Pregnancy and menopause also increase the risk, suggesting that hormones may also play a role.

stretching break every hour (keep a full water jug at your desk; drinking throughout the day will force you to take breaks to go to the toilet).

Vary your tasks If you just spent 2 hours typing, switch to drafting an outline using a pen and paper (the fatter the pen, the better), meet with colleagues or read a hard-copy report.

Use a wrist splint Wearing a splint that keeps your wrist in a neutral position can help prevent the kind of damage that turns into carpal tunnel syndrome. In one study, 63 people with early signs of carpal tunnel wore custom-fitted wrist–hand splints nightly for six weeks. After six weeks, about half reported that their symptoms improved, with scores on a test measuring pain severity dropping from an average of 7.24 to 4.43. Even if you don't wear the splint every night, slip it on when you feel the first painful twinges.

Perform gentle stretching Try the exercises starting on page 139, as they tone and stretch muscles and ligaments in your hands and wrists to help guard against injury.

Prevention boosters

Use the right tools Product designers have caught on to our need for more ergonomically correct tools, such as hammers, screwdrivers or can-openers. Toss your old tools and kitchen implements and restock with tools that distribute the force of your grip across the muscle between the base of your thumb and your little finger, not the centre of your hand. If you use tools that vibrate (such as a motorised saw or knife), add shock absorbers to reduce vibration or wrap the vibrating part in a towel.

Check your risk of metabolic syndrome This condition is marked by three of the following factors: low HDL ('good') cholesterol, a waist measurement greater than 88 cm (for women) or 102 cm (for men), high blood pressure, high triglycerides, and insulin resistance. When researchers studied 107 people, they found that 75 per cent of those with metabolic syndrome also had carpal tunnel. The more severe the metabolic syndrome symptoms, the more severe the carpal tunnel. Metabolic syndrome also increases your risk of diabetes, and studies find that people who

▶ WHAT CAUSES IT

Repetitive hand movements, particularly if you have to pinch or grip something while your wrist is bent. This inflames the nine tendons in the carpal tunnel, a narrow passageway that runs from the forearm through the wrist. These tendons enable you to flex your fingers. When they become inflamed, they put pressure on the median nerve, which also runs through the tunnel and supplies feeling to several fingers.

▶ SYMPTOMS TO WATCH FOR

Pain, numbness and tingling in the affected hand and/or fingers, especially the thumb and index and middle fingers. The pain and numbness may be worse at night; sometimes it's bad enough to wake you up. You may find you have trouble holding objects tightly and have weakness in your thumb.

▶ LATEST THINKING

Perhaps we need to stop pinning the blame for carpal tunnel syndrome on work. One study found that people who used a keyboard for 4 hours or more a day were significantly *less* likely to have carpal tunnel than those who used it for an hour a day or less. Other risk factors include rheumatoid arthritis, hypothyroidism, Type 1 diabetes and non-Hodgkin's lymphoma. Pregnancy and menopause also increase risk.

have diabetes are much more likely to have carpal tunnel than those who don't have diabetes. (See also 'Diabetes', starting on page 164, for prevention tips, and page 210 for preventing high blood pressure and avoiding metabolic syndrome.)

Type smart

Practise smart ergonomics at work, and you'll be less likely to end up with carpal tunnel syndrome.

- **Adjust your chair** The idea is that you sit with your spine against the chair back, your shoulders relaxed, your elbows along the sides of your body, your wrists straight and both feet flat on the floor or propped on a footrest.
- **Keep materials used for typing at eye level** so you don't have to drop or twist your neck.
- **Change the setting on your keyboard** (usually found in the software that comes with the keyboard, if that's applicable) so you can gently tap the keys instead of having to pound them.
- **Keep your wrists flat while typing** A wrist rest under the keyboard can help, but don't rest your wrists on it while typing.
- **Make sure the surface supporting the keyboard is at least 75 cm wide** This is necessary to accommodate both the keyboard and mouse. Don't put the mouse on a higher or lower level than the keyboard.
- **The keyboard should be between 70–75 cm off the floor** If you can type with your elbows bent at a 90-degree angle, it's at the right height. Pull it close to your body to maintain that 90-degree angle.
- **Use a computer table** This piece of custom-built furniture is thinner than a regular desk, which allows plenty of thigh clearance.
- **Place the monitor directly in front of you** Position the top of the screen at eye level or below. You should be looking down slightly as you type.

Get treated for depression A UK study found that 14 per cent of adults with carpal tunnel syndrome had symptoms of major depression, while 22 per cent had depression or some other psychological condition, such as an anxiety disorder. (See also 'Depression', starting on page 160; for treatment, talk to your doctor.)

Drop a few kilos If you're overweight, your risk of carpal tunnel syndrome is twice that of someone of normal weight.

Do the downward dog Oddly enough, yoga may help protect your wrists. Firstly, it can help you manage stress, which may contribute to carpal tunnel syndrome. It can also strengthen your wrist grip. In one study, people who participated in twice-weekly yoga sessions for eight weeks saw their grip strength increase by 25 mmHg, and pain in the carpal tunnel region of the wrist dropped by nearly half on a scale that measures pain.

Bump up your Bs Vitamin B_6 is essential to healthy nerves. While this vitamin has primarily been studied for relieving the pain of carpal tunnel, it's worth increasing your intake from food sources—brown rice, salmon, chicken thighs, some breakfast cereals and macadamia nuts are among the best sources—or you may want to take a supplement to help prevent pain.

Exercises for hands and wrists

Repetitive wrist and hand motions can lead to painful carpal tunnel syndrome. Take regular breaks to do preventive exercises. Perform each one before you begin work, once an hour while you're doing a repetitive task such as typing and at the end of the day before you go home. Hold each move for 5 seconds. When you're done, repeat the routine 10 times, then stand with your arms relaxed by your sides for 10 seconds.

Fist flex

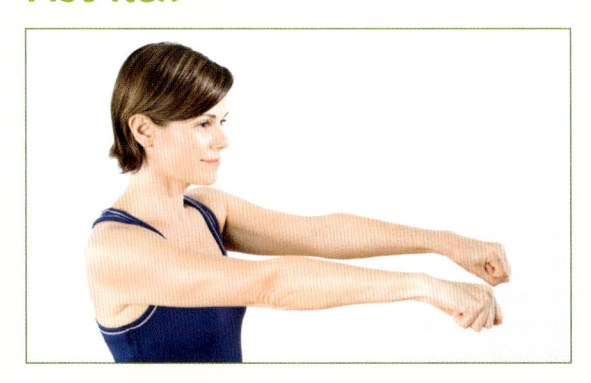

1 Hold your arms straight out in front of you, then make fists with your hands and squeeze as tightly as you can.

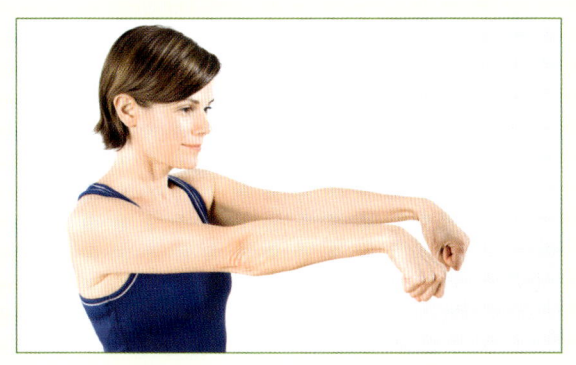

2 Keeping your hands in fists, bend your wrists down at a 90-degree angle.

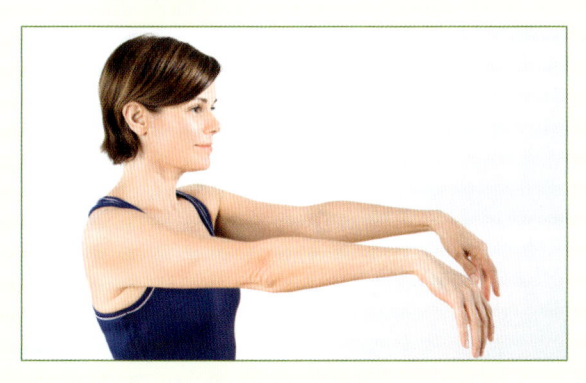

3 Straighten your wrists out and then let your relaxed fingers hang down.

Wrist extender

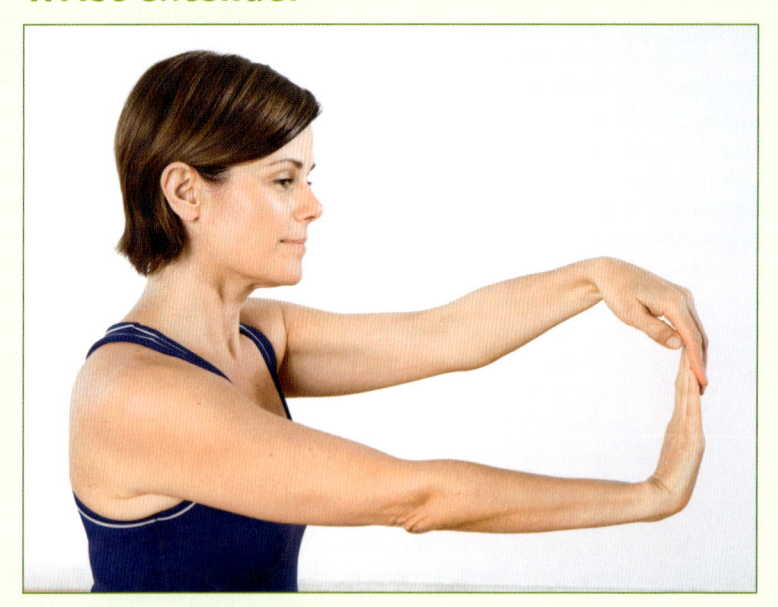

Hold your right arm out in front of you. With your left hand, gently pull back your fingers until you feel a stretch in the bottom of your forearm. Ultimately your wrist should be bent at a 90-degree angle so your fingers point straight up. Repeat with the left arm.

Muscle strengthener

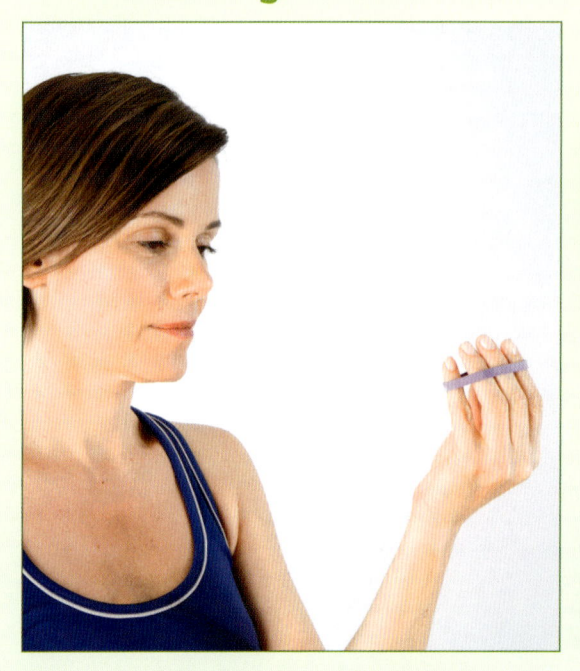

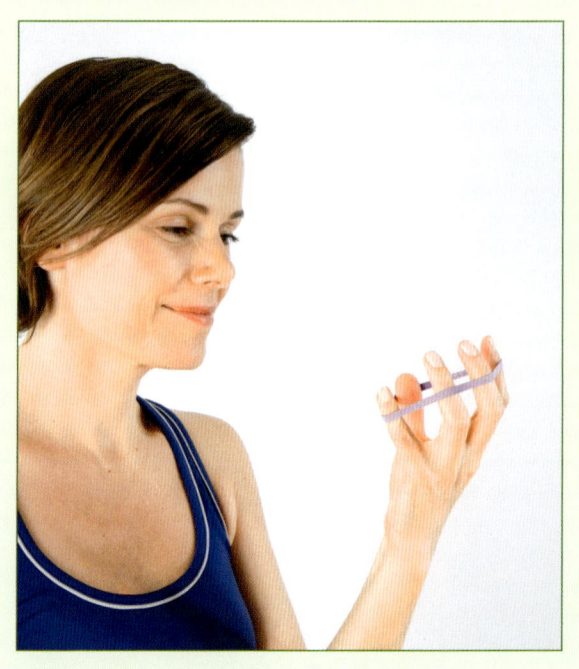

1 Place a thick rubber band around your slightly separated fingertips, near the top.

2 Slowly spread your fingers, then close them, keeping a steady resistance against the rubber band. Repeat this exercise 10 times.

Carpal tunnel syndrome

Forearm stretch

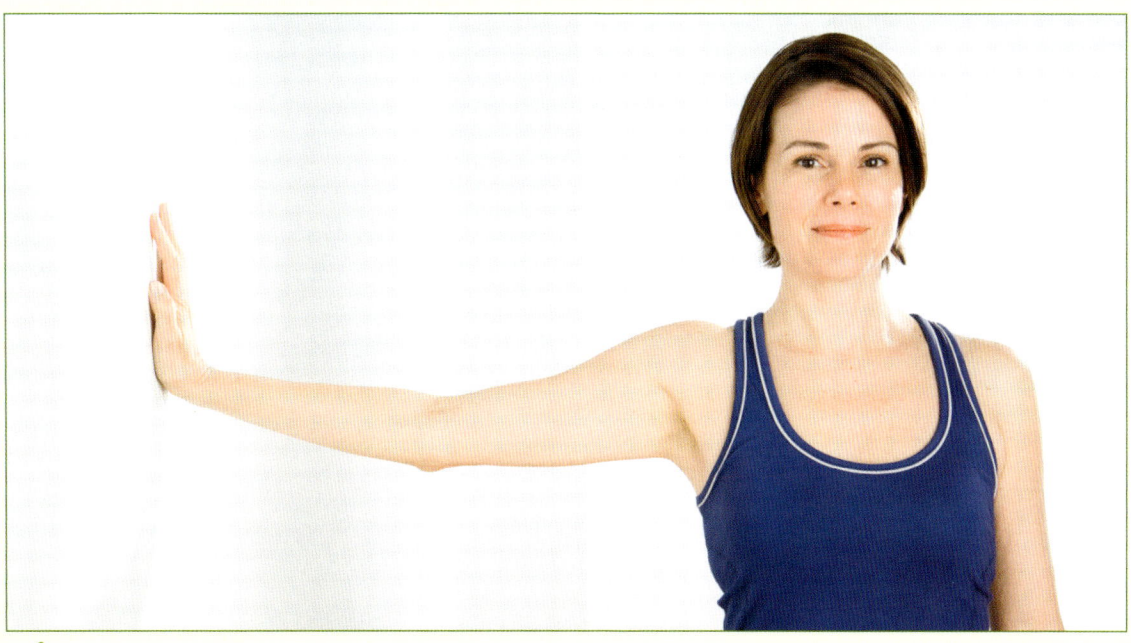

1 Press your right hand against a wall, with your fingers open. Firmly press the palm of your hand into the wall.

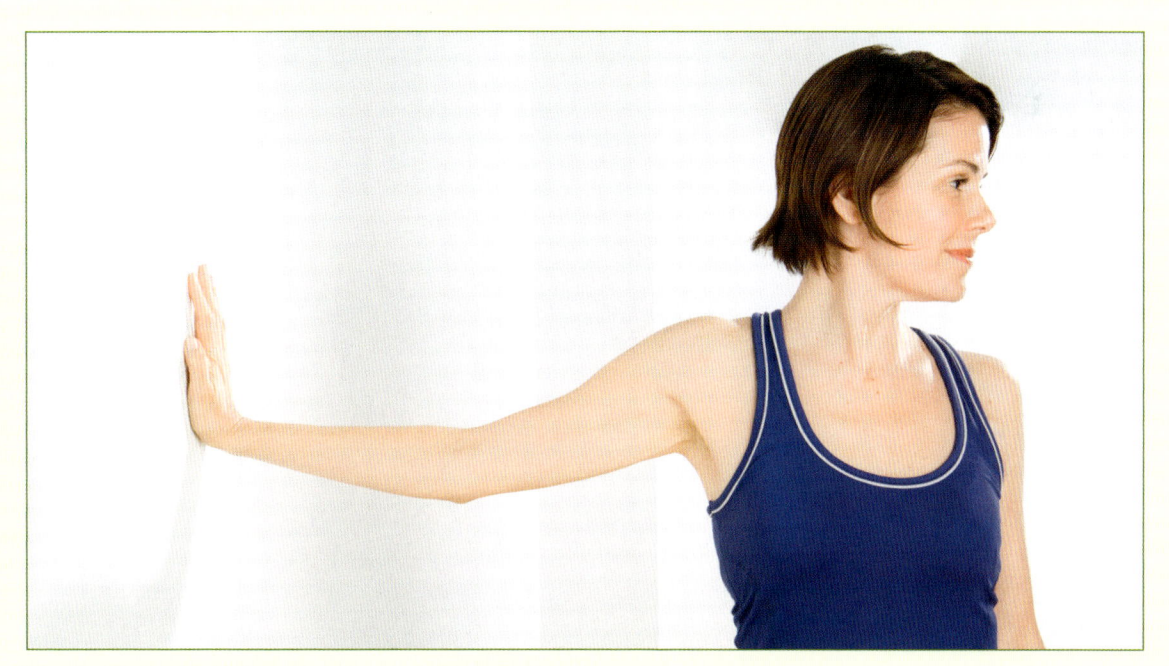

2 Slowly bring the tip of your right shoulder blade forward, turning your head to the left, until you feel a stretch in your arm.

Cataracts

66% The potential drop in your risk of cataracts if you shield your eyes by wearing a broad-brimmed hat and sunglasses.

When the lenses in your eyes grow cloudy, you know you've got cataracts. Your vision becomes blurred, driving at night can become difficult due to headlight glare, and colours become muted. The painter Claude Monet had cataracts and was forced to choose colours by reading the labels on tubes of paint. Cataract surgery can replace clouded lenses with artificial ones, but taking steps to prevent getting cataracts in the first place is a much better option.

Key prevention strategies

Enjoy a spinach salad with hard-boiled eggs, red capsicum and sunflower seeds Getting plenty of the anti-oxidants lutein and zeaxanthin, as well as vitamin E, cuts cataract risk by 16 per cent according to a Harvard School of Public Health study of over 23,000 women. Other studies show that getting plenty of vitamin C also provides protective benefits.

Your body stores lutein and zeaxanthin in high concentrations in the lenses of your eyes, where they seem to work like sunglasses to filter out harmful ultraviolet rays. Anti-oxidants, including vitamins C and E, also seem to protect proteins in the lens from damage by destructive oxygen molecules known as free radicals.

Eating just seven serves of fruit and vegetables a day plus two serves of nuts is enough to provide your body with plenty of these important nutrients. Top sources of lutein and zeaxanthin include dark green vegetables such as spinach, broccoli and zucchini, as well as eggs and corn. For vitamin E, try tahini, sunflower seeds, hazelnuts, almonds and whole grains. Good sources of vitamin C include red and green capsicums, brussels sprouts, orange juice and strawberries.

Keep your blood sugar low and steady Diabetes raised cataract risk 80 per cent in one study of 6000 people. Experts suspect that high blood sugar damages proteins in the lens of your eye. Even high to normal blood sugar and prediabetes increase your odds. In a UK study, people with a prediabetic condition called impaired fasting glucose had double the normal risk. If you have diabetes, work with your doctor to keep your blood sugar under control. If you're at risk, follow all the steps in the entry on 'Diabetes', starting on page 164, to keep your blood sugar levels healthy.

Wear sunglasses and a broad-brimmed hat When scientists checked the eyes of nearly 900 US fishermen, they found that those who spent the most time in the sun were three times more likely to have cataracts than those who spent the least. But wearing sunglasses and a broad-brimmed hat reduced the risk by two-thirds. Experts suspect that solar radiation alters proteins in the eye's lens, causing it to cloud.

Inexpensive sunglasses can be just as good as expensive ones; just look for a label that says the lenses protect against 99 per cent of UVB and 95 per cent of UVA rays—or 'UV absorption up to 400 nm'—and you're covered.

Quit smoking Smoking cigarettes doubles your risk for cloudy lenses. Quit and your risk begins to drop, say Swedish researchers who tracked the health of 34,595 women. Light smokers (who smoked 6 to 10 cigarettes a day) completely erased their added risk 10 years after quitting; heavier smokers (over 10 cigarettes daily) who quit needed 20 years to reduce their risk to that of nonsmokers.

Prevention boosters

Lose weight Carrying extra weight can raise your risk for cataracts by as much as 36 per cent, according to a US study of 133,000 people. If you're overweight you're more likely to have blood sugar problems (even if you're not diabetic). You may also have high blood pressure or high triglycerides. Other research suggests that these factors can raise risk by about 80 per cent.

If you use steroid medications, get your eyes tested soon
Oral steroids increase cataract risk; in one study of 2446 people taking steroid medication to treat conditions such as rheumatoid arthritis, asthma, emphysema or chronic bronchitis, lupus and inflammatory bowel disease, those who took 10 mg of steroids per day for a year raised their cataract risk 68 per cent. By 18 months, the risk increase rose to 82 per cent. At higher doses, inhaled steroids may also raise risk. Steroid creams and steroid eye-drops may also push your odds higher. If you're taking steroids long term, have an eye examination and ask how often you need repeat checks.

▶ WHAT CAUSES IT
Sunlight, smoking, a low-antioxidant diet, high blood sugar and other factors seem to deactivate compounds, called alpha-crystallins, that normally prevent proteins in the eye's lens from clumping. Clumped proteins make the lens cloudy, distorting or even blocking the passage of light.

▶ SYMPTOMS TO WATCH FOR
Cloudy or blurry vision, glare or a halo around lights, poor night vision, double vision, colours that look faded and frequent prescription changes in your glasses or contact lenses.

▶ LATEST THINKING
Cholesterol-lowering statin medications have a surprising vision bonus. In a study of 6000 people, published in the *Journal of the American Medical Association*, those who took statins cut their risk for cataracts by 60 per cent. Researchers suspect that statins act as antioxidants, protecting proteins in the lens from damage.

Cervical cancer

70% The percentage of cervical cancers that could be prevented with the Gardasil vaccine.

If you think that medical research moves at a glacial pace, you haven't been paying attention to advances in cervical cancer. As recently as 20 years ago, we didn't even know what caused cancer of the cervix. Now we know it's caused by the human papillomavirus (HPV)—and we also have a newly developed vaccine to prevent infection with that virus. Someday, possibly in the not-too-distant future, cervical cancer will have gone the way of polio, diphtheria and other viral illnesses prevented by vaccination. Until then, here are some key tips for doing all you can to protect yourself.

Key prevention strategies

Get vaccinated We prevent tetanus, whooping cough, meningitis and numerous other illnesses with vaccines; now, for the first time, we can prevent cancer with a series of three shots. The Gardasil vaccine was developed by a team of medical scientists, and prevents infection with four HPV viruses that cause about 70 per cent of all cervical cancers. Ideally, young women should be vaccinated before they become sexually active, which is why Gardasil is recommended for girls as young as 11 (it is licensed for girls as young as 9 years). In reality, any woman can get the vaccine as long as she is not pregnant, but there is no evidence of a benefit in women who have already been infected with HPV.

Have regular Pap smears Cervical cancer is one of the few cancers that can be prevented with regular screening. Pap smears, in which a doctor or nurse scrapes a few cells from your cervix for examination under a microscope, can pick up very early cellular changes that may eventually turn into cancer. Burning, cutting or freezing off those cells can prevent the cancer. In fact, Pap smears are the primary reason cervical cancer rates have plummeted 70 per cent since the 1950s.

You should have your first Pap smear two years after you first become sexually active, then every two years until you turn seventy. Once you turn 70, and have had two consecutive normal Pap smear results, you can stop being screened altogether.

Prevention boosters

Choose a nonhormonal contraceptive If you're worried about cervical cancer, avoid taking oral contraceptives that combine oestrogen with progestin. They're actually classified by the International Agency for Research on Cancer as a cause of cervical cancer. A review of 24 international studies found that the longer you use this form of contraception, the greater your risk. And using birth control pills for 10 years beginning around the age of 20 to 30 nearly doubles your risk of cervical cancer. As soon as you stop using them, your risk drops; after 10 years, it's the same as that of a woman who never used contraceptives. The risk seems to be linked to the fact that women who use birth control pills are more likely to be infected with HPV, possibly because they have more sexual partners than women who use other forms of birth control or because they are not using condoms, which help prevent sexually transmissible infections (STIs). You also need to consider that the Pill reduces your risk of ovarian and endometrial cancer.

Settle on one partner The more sexual partners you have, the more likely you are to become infected with HPV.

Watch your stress levels Being infected with HPV doesn't automatically mean you'll develop cervical cancer; many women, especially those under the age of 30, can shake off the virus as easily as they shake off dozens of other viruses they encounter on a daily basis. But daily stress—from having a difficult boss, problems with your children or spouse, or money worries—can impair your ability to fight off all viruses, including HPV, increasing your risk of long-term infection that could lead to cervical cancer.

Increase your intake of folate Low levels of the B vitamin folate increase the risk that precancerous cervical cells will turn into actual cancer. Folate is found in green leafy vegetables such as spinach and salad greens. Don't take a folate supplement before discussing this with your doctor, as it can mask symptoms of vitamin B_{12} deficiency, which is a serious condition.

▶ WHAT CAUSES IT
The primary cause is the human papillomavirus (HPV), which is spread via sexual contact.

▶ SYMPTOMS TO WATCH FOR
There are no symptoms with early cervical cancer. In later stages, the most common symptoms are abnormal vaginal bleeding (not during your period), such as bleeding after intercourse, or discharge. In the very late stages it may cause pelvic pain.

▶ LATEST THINKING
An interaction between cigarette smoking and HPV may increase the risk of cervical cancer. Carcinogens in cigarette smoke are thought to enable the virus to stick around longer and replicate, making the cervix more vulnerable to cellular changes that can lead to cancer.

Colds

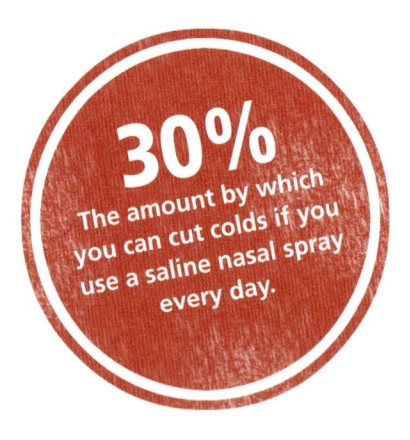

30% The amount by which you can cut colds if you use a saline nasal spray every day.

All you need to avoid sniffling, sneezing and sick days by 45 per cent is hand cleanser and water. Along with sound sleep and good nutrition, hand washing is the best defence against cold viruses, which can survive for up to seven days on light switches, ATMs, doorknobs and other surfaces— and for at least 3 hours on unwashed hands. A strong immune system is your best bet in the fight against viral infection.

Key prevention strategies

Wash your hands frequently Do this even if your hands don't look or feel dirty. Scrubbing five times a day with soap and water reduced the number of upper respiratory infections among Navy recruits by 45 per cent in one two-year US study. A brisk, 10-second scrub rinses away 99 per cent of viruses. This cuts your odds of infection substantially, but not completely; a single viral particle can start a cold. For the best results, wet your hands, lather vigorously for a full 20 seconds, rinse, then dry with a clean paper towel. Use the towel to turn off the tap, too. Any hand cleanser will do— washing works by scrubbing viruses off your skin, not by killing them (and antibacterial handwash doesn't kill viruses).

Walk five days a week Regular exercise invigorates your immune system's natural killer cells and virus-killing antibodies. US researchers from the University of South Carolina found that adults who exercised moderately to vigorously at least four times a week had 25 per cent fewer colds over one year than those who moved less. A brisk 40-minute walk five days a week should do it; in another study, this much

The new cold fighters

Echinacea may be one of the top-selling herbal supplements, but its cold-battling prowess remains controversial. One authoritative German review of 16 clinical trials concluded that echinacea doesn't prevent colds (though other research says it does). And it seems that vitamin C is even less likely to prevent colds. A definitive analysis of 29 well-designed studies involving over 11,700 people concluded that vitamin C has no power to prevent a cold. Instead, you may want to try one of these alternatives:

Andrographis In one well-designed study, volunteers who took two 100-mg tablets a day for three months had half as many colds as volunteers who got placebos.

Probiotics These beneficial bacteria seem to increase production of immune cells where you need them most to fight colds: in the tissues lining your respiratory system. Capsules containing the bacteria *Lactobacillus gasseri*, *Bifidobacterium longum* and *B. bifidum* MF shortened colds by an average of two days in volunteers who took them daily for three months.

exercise halved the number of days volunteers had cold symptoms. But don't overdo it: working out for an hour and a half or more could reduce immunity.

Use a saline nasal spray Moist nasal passages are less receptive to cold viruses than dry ones. In one 20-week US study of military recruits, those who used a saline nasal spray every day had 30 per cent fewer colds and 42 per cent fewer days with runny noses or congestion. Use the spray during winter, when heated indoor air is dry, and also during plane flights.

Prevention boosters

Tame the stress monster In a year-long Spanish study of 1149 university staff, sniffles were twice as likely among people who felt stressed compared to those with the least stress in their lives. And once you catch a cold, stress can make symptoms worse.

Season or supplement with garlic This ancient remedy may help by boosting the activity of your immune system's virus-killing T cells. When 146 women and men took either a garlic capsule or a placebo daily during the cold season, the garlic group caught 24 colds, while the placebo group got sixty-five. Researchers at the UK's Garlic Centre say that garlic takers who did get sick recovered in just a day and a half, while the placebo group had the sniffles for an average of five days. (Other research is less positive about garlic.) If you love garlic, use it liberally. Always let chopped, crushed or bruised garlic sit for 10 minutes before using to maximise levels of its active healing component.

Use alcohol-based hand sanitisers when you can't wash These gels and sprays kill bacteria and some viruses, but don't use them instead of hand washing. Studies show that brands containing 60 per cent ethyl alcohol are powerless against rhinoviruses (which cause colds). Some researchers report that a 70 per cent ethanol sanitiser can be effective.

Hop into a sauna twice a week In an Austrian study, people who did this twice a week for six months had half as many colds as those who didn't use a sauna. The link may be air temperature—at over 27°C, sauna air is too hot for cold viruses to survive.

▶ WHAT CAUSES IT
At least 250 viruses—and possibly hundreds more. The sheer number has made it impossible so far for scientists to develop an effective vaccine. But time's on your side: the human body develops some resistance to each cold virus it encounters, which is one reason we get fewer sniffles as we age.

▶ SYMPTOMS TO WATCH FOR
Sore throat, stuffy and/or runny nose, sneezing, coughing and even a mild fever. It may be the flu if you have chills, body aches, significant fatigue and/or a very high fever.

▶ LATEST THINKING
Perhaps your mum was right: being cold *can* increase your risk of catching a cold, at least according to one study. People exposed to a chill were three times more likely to develop cold symptoms than those who stayed warm, according to a study of 180 people from the Common Cold Centre in Wales. The cold–cold connection is that being chilly constricts blood vessels in the nose, reducing the supply of nutrients to infection-fighting white blood cells. This may allow dormant infections to roar to life.

Colorectal cancer

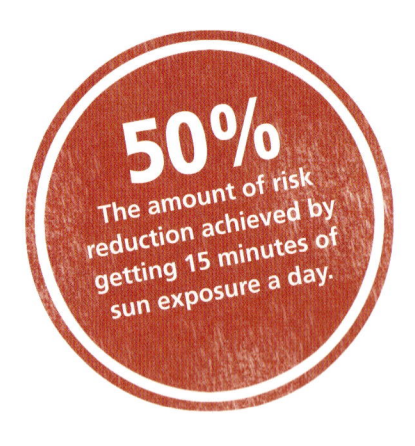

50% The amount of risk reduction achieved by getting 15 minutes of sun exposure a day.

Surprisingly, clinical study reviews have found that high-fibre diets don't protect against colon cancer the way that was once thought. However, although colorectal cancer is the most common cancer in Australia and the second leading cause of cancer deaths, it's also the most preventable cancer in the world after lung cancer. There are many steps you can take to protect yourself against this cancer, many of which, as you might imagine, still involve what you eat.

Key prevention strategies

Get screened Australian recommendations are for all men and women aged 50 and over to be tested for bowel cancer at least every two years (every year if possible), using a bowel cancer testing kit. Often, but not always, bowel cancer leads to microscopic amounts of blood in the stool, which can be detected with special kits. The cure rate for patients who have surgery before bowel cancer has spread is about 90 per cent. As with all tests, there is a risk of missing a cancer or getting a positive result from the kit when no cancer is actually present. To get accurate results from some kits, you mustn't eat red meat, specific fruit and vegetables (for example raw broccoli), vitamin C supplements, and aspirin or anti-inflammatory medications for three days before taking each test sample, so follow the instructions carefully. If your father, mother or a sibling has had bowel cancer, you have a higher risk and should see your doctor to discuss your individual risk; genetic testing and five-yearly colonoscopies may be recommended.

Get out there and exercise An analysis of 19 studies found that men who are physically active reduce their risk of colon cancer about 21 per cent; for women, the

Should you go 'virtual'?

Many doctors agree that virtual colonoscopy, which involves lying on a table and passing painlessly through a CT or MRI scanner to have detailed 3-D images of your colon taken and examined, isn't ready yet as a tool to replace traditional colonoscopy. So it doesn't excuse you from the pre-test bowel-cleansing ritual that no one enjoys. And if the test finds a polyp, you'll need to follow up with a traditional colonoscopy—and repeat the bowel cleansing—to have the polyp removed. If you decide to get virtual colonoscopy, go to a doctor who's very experienced with the procedure; otherwise, the results may not be as reliable as they should be.

benefit of brisk walking, heavy gardening, cycling or swimming, etc., is greater, yielding a 30 per cent risk reduction.

Cut back on red meat Here's a simple equation: the less red meat you eat, the lower your risk of colorectal cancer. Eating 500 g a week (the amount in two large hamburgers) increases your risk by about 30 per cent; every 45 g after that increases your risk by another 15 per cent, according to the American Institute for Cancer Research. (Just for comparison's sake, most people in Western countries eat an average of 1 kg of red meat a week.) There are several possible reasons for the link. Firstly, people who eat a lot of meat tend to eat fewer health-protective fruit and vegetables. But a diet high in fatty red meat also contributes to 'oxidative stress'; in other words, it creates harmful free radicals in the body that can damage cells, DNA and other microscopic components of your digestive tract. Some of those interactions are as dangerous as those caused by radiation, which is why eating plenty of fruit and vegetables is so important, because they contain valuable anti-oxidants that help ward off that oxidative damage. So aim to eat a piece of meat that is no larger than your hand and grill capsicums, onions and pineapple to go with it.

Skip the cold cuts Eating about 60 g of processed meat (about two slices of salami) a day could increase your risk of colorectal cancer by 50 per cent compared to people who eat no processed meat. The culprit may be N-nitroso compounds (NOCs), the result of nitrates used to preserve meat.

Go heavy on fish When you put colon cancer cells in a dish with fish oil or feed fish oil to animals, the number of colorectal tumours drops, along with the overall risk of colorectal cancer. We're not quite sure what goes on in humans, but it appears that people who eat fish once or twice a week reduce their risk by about 12 per cent compared to those who eat it less; each additional serve reduces the risk by another 4 per cent. The link between fish and colorectal cancer prevention may be due to the high levels of selenium and vitamin D in fish, both of which are also prized as colorectal cancer preventives.

Limit yourself to one standard alcoholic drink a day A standard drink contains 10 g of alcohol. The volume of liquid making up a

'Colorectal cancer is one of only two cancers that can be completely prevented through screening.'

standard drink depends on the concentration of alcohol, so look at the label (Australian laws require the label on a product containing alcohol to give the approximate number of standard drinks in the package). Not sure what a standard drink is? It's 100 ml of wine, 300 ml of beer (about a middy) or 30 ml of spirits.

As your body breaks down alcohol, cancer-causing acetaldehyde forms. Alcohol also appears to make cells more permeable to other cancer-causing compounds. An analysis of more than 4600 cases of colorectal cancer among 475,000 participants found that those who drank more than 45 g of alcohol a day increased their risk of colorectal cancer by 41 per cent. The risk increased 16 per cent in those who consumed 30–44 g a day.

Prevention boosters

Eat more legumes Beans, lentils and peas are excellent sources of folate, a B vitamin also known as folic acid. According to a Harvard study of nearly 89,000 women, those with a family history of colon cancer who consumed more than 400 mcg of folate each day lowered their risk by more than 52 per cent compared to women who got 200 mcg a day. You can get almost 300 mcg by eating a cup of chickpeas or cooked spinach, another great source. If you take a multivitamin, you may already be getting enough folate.

Season with garlic About six cloves of garlic a week, whether raw or cooked, can help reduce your risk of colorectal cancer by as much as 31 per cent, according to one University of North Carolina analysis of many studies from the US. The benefit probably comes from allicin compounds in garlic—its active ingredient—that prevent colorectal tumours from forming, possibly by forcing aberrant cells to commit the equivalent of cellular suicide.

DRUGS THAT PREVENT DISEASE

If you're already taking aspirin or another nonsteroidal anti-inflammatory drug (NSAID) such as celecoxib (Celebrex), you may enjoy a happy side benefit: a lower risk of colon cancer. When women take at least 325 mg of regular aspirin twice a week for at least 10 years, their risk of colon cancer plummets by a third compared to women who take aspirin less often. And in a study of people who had already had precancerous polyps removed, those who were taking 400 mg of celecoxib a day were one-third less likely to have the growths return within three years. Unfortunately, it's too soon to recommend taking medications such as these solely to prevent colon cancer, as they can have unwanted side effects.

Statins, the medications prescribed to lower cholesterol, may also lower the risk of colon cancer. A study involving 4000 people found that taking a statin for at least five years cut the risk of colon cancer nearly in half. But as with aspirin and NSAIDs, statins have side effects, and doctors aren't ready to prescribe them unless they're specifically needed to regulate blood cholesterol.

All these medications have one thing in common: they reduce inflammation, which can contribute to cancer development. But they probably work in other ways, too. Researchers around the world are now studying their mechanisms to try to figure out a way to create a medication with all the cancer-preventing benefits but with none of the negatives.

Drink a glass of skim milk every day Just 250 ml a day reduces women's risk of colorectal cancer by 16 per cent and men's risk by 10 per cent, according to an analysis of studies by US researchers at Brigham and Women's Hospital, and Harvard Medical School. Every two additional glasses drops the risk by another 12 per cent. Why? It may be the vitamin D that's added to milk in the US, or its calcium (high calcium consumption is also linked to lower rates of colon cancer). Milk also contains the fatty acid conjugated linoleic acid and the protein lactoferrin, both of which help prevent colon cancer in animals.

Use olive oil, not butter, as your fat of choice Animal fats such as butter are associated with an increased risk of colorectal cancer, probably because diets high in fat lead to increased levels of bile acids in the colon to break down that fat. These bile acids can be converted to cancer-causing compounds. This is another reason to get your protein from sources such as fish, soy or legumes rather than fatty red meat.

Drop a few kilos Being overweight considerably increases your risk of cancer, including colorectal cancer. An analysis of numerous studies found that men's risk jumped 37 per cent if they were overweight or obese; women's risk inched up 7 per cent. Researchers think the higher levels of hormones such as insulin, leptin and insulin-like growth factor in overweight people are to blame. All provide fuel for cancer cells.

Get 15 minutes of sunscreen-free sunshine a day It's your best source of vitamin D, one of the most important vitamins when it comes to preventing colorectal cancer. An analysis of five studies found that getting at least 2000 IU a day from diet, sunlight or supplementation could cut the risk of colorectal cancer in half. How? By detoxifying a dangerous form of bile.

Most people in Australia, New Zealand and South Africa have a low risk of developing vitamin D deficiency, as sunlight triggers vitamin D production in the skin. However, it may still be found in elderly people who are confined indoors; in people who, for religious or modesty reasons, keep most of their skin covered; or those who spend less than 10 or 15 minutes a day in the sun without sunscreen. About 100 g of sardines or salmon has 400 IU and 100 g of chicken livers has 10 IU. If you supplement, aim for 400 IU daily.

WHAT CAUSES IT
Ageing, genetic abnormalities and diseases such as inflammatory bowel disease.

SYMPTOMS TO WATCH FOR
Blood in your stools; narrowing of stools; a change in bowel habits, including diarrhoea or constipation for more than a couple of weeks; cramping, wind or pain; abdominal pain with a bowel movement; feeling that your bowel doesn't empty completely; weakness or fatigue; and unexplained weight loss.

LATEST THINKING
A simple blood test could provide a warning about precancerous colorectal growths. The test, currently under investigation, detects chemical markers of colon cancer that make their way into the bloodstream.

Congestive heart failure

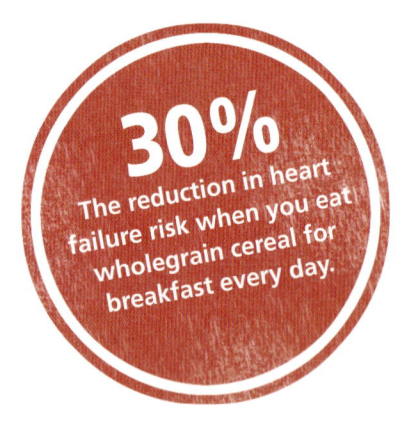

30% The reduction in heart failure risk when you eat wholegrain cereal for breakfast every day.

Heart failure is one of the fastest-growing heart conditions in the world, thanks to everything from the obesity epidemic and rising rates of high blood pressure to the fact that more people are surviving heart attacks and facing life with damaged hearts. When your heart is too weak or too stiff to pump enough blood to the organs and tissues in your body, your lungs can fill with fluid, your kidneys may fail and you become very, very tired. This condition kills 80 per cent of men and 65 per cent of women within six years of diagnosis. Here's how you can take steps to try to avoid it.

Key prevention strategies

Exercise and follow a heart-healthy diet If you think heart failure happens only to other people, consider this statistic: your odds of developing it after the age of 45 are one in five. The biggest contributors are high blood pressure and heart attack, so the best defence is to stay active, and at your next meal, load your plate with fruit and vegetables, and whole grains. Small changes can make a big difference. Simply eating a wholegrain breakfast cereal every morning can lower your risk by as much as 30 per cent.

If you already have heart disease or high blood pressure, talk to your doctor or experts at a cardiac rehabilitation program about what kind and amount of exercise is right for you.

Maintain a healthy weight Every 2 to 4 kg you gain—whatever it takes to raise your body mass index (BMI) one point—increases a woman's risk for heart failure by 7 per cent and a man's by 5 per cent, according to the landmark Framingham Heart Study from the US. Being obese, with a BMI of 30 or higher, doubles your odds. Extra kilos hurt your heart by raising your risk of high blood pressure and diabetes. Excess weight also puts a strain on your heart that can damage muscle.

Check your weight

If you have any health conditions that put you at increased risk of heart failure, stay alert for early signs. Watch unusual weight changes: an increase of 1.5 kg in a day or 2.5 kg in a week could mean you're retaining fluid because your heart is losing its ability to effectively pump blood. Another sign is swollen ankles or calves that make your socks feel tight.

Tame high blood pressure Ninety per cent of people who have heart failure had pre-existing high blood pressure. This results in your heart having to pump harder to force blood through blood vessels in your body. Over time, this can make the chambers of your heart become 'muscle-bound', a condition called left ventricular hypertrophy that interferes with the heart's pumping ability. A 10-point drop in systolic blood pressure (the top number) can cut your risk of heart failure by 50 per cent, according to research.

If you need medication, ask about a diuretic. Studies show they cut heart failure risk more than other, more expensive drugs such as ACE inhibitors and calcium channel blockers.

Ask about ACE inhibitors after a heart attack About one in four men and half of all women who survive a heart attack will be disabled by heart failure within six years. Medications called ACE inhibitors reduce that likelihood. In one study, an ACE inhibitor called ramipril (Tritace) cut heart failure risk by 23 per cent in 9000 high-risk women and men, many of whom had had heart attacks. These medications ease the strain on the heart by relaxing blood vessel walls and lowering blood pressure.

Prevention boosters

Maintain good blood sugar control if you have diabetes If you have Type 2 diabetes, your risk of heart failure is five times higher than normal if you're a woman and nearly four times higher than normal if you're a man. Since people with diabetes often have coronary artery disease or high blood pressure, or may have had silent heart attacks, your doctor may prescribe medications to help guard your heart. But don't overlook the power of blood sugar control. In one study, people with diabetes who kept their blood sugar within a healthy range were half as likely to develop heart failure as those whose blood sugar remained high.

Have grilled or baked fish US researchers at Harvard Medical School tracked the health of 4738 adults and found that those who ate grilled or baked tuna, or other fish, once or twice a week cut their risk of congestive heart failure by 20 per cent. And more is better: those who had fish five times a week cut their risk by 32 per cent. However, you do need to choose a fish rich in omega-3 fatty acids, such as salmon, sardines, trout or mackerel.

▶ WHAT CAUSES IT

Damage or death of heart muscle due to narrowed arteries or a heart attack; high blood pressure, which makes heart muscle grow large and stiff; malfunctioning heart valves (due to a birth defect, infection or heart disease); and heart-rhythm problems.

▶ SYMPTOMS TO WATCH FOR

Breathlessness, especially when lying down; coughing and wheezing; swollen feet, ankles, legs or abdomen; fatigue; lack of appetite; nausea; confusion and memory loss; and rapid heartbeat.

▶ LATEST THINKING

Depression can make heart muscle stiffer, raising the risk of heart failure. US scientists at the University of Maryland School of Medicine found that depression raised levels of chronic inflammation in the body, which stimulated the production of collagen, a protein that can stiffen heart muscle.

Constipation

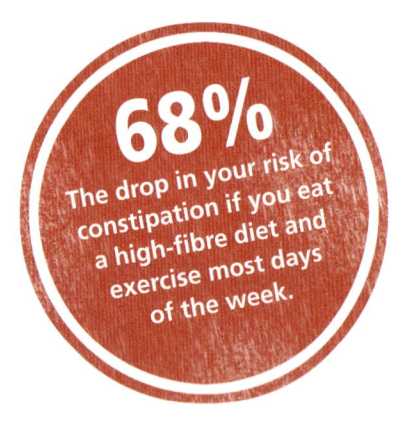

68% The drop in your risk of constipation if you eat a high-fibre diet and exercise most days of the week.

Normal bowel movements range from three a day to three per week, so don't automatically assume you're constipated. If you can't seem to open your bowels when you need to, chances are that you're not eating enough fibre or drinking enough fluids. Anxiety, medications and conditions such as pregnancy and diabetes can also contribute to the problem.

Key prevention strategies

Increase the fibre in your diet Getting at least 20 g of fibre a day could cut your risk of constipation by 46 per cent, according to Harvard School of Public Health researchers who tracked more than 60,000 women. Those who ate less than 7 g a day had the highest constipation rates. Fibre helps by making your stools bulkier and heavier, which allows the muscles in the inner walls of the intestines to move stools towards the rectum with greater ease. Fibre may even make your bowels move faster.

You can get to 20 g by starting the day with porridge or a high-fibre cereal such as Weet-Bix (top with berries and a sprinkling of wheatgerm or ground linseeds for even more fibre), having your sandwich on wholegrain bread, eating a serving of barley or brown rice at dinner, and consuming a wide variety of fresh fruit and vegetables (including legumes) throughout the day. Remember to keep at it, as it can take a few weeks to see an improvement.

Drink plenty of water If you've just started a higher-fibre diet or have been following one and feel constipated, drink plenty of water. If you're taking a fibre supplement, water is even more important. When researchers gave 117 people with chronic constipation a fibre supplement, the group that was also told to drink 2 litres of water a day saw more improvement than those who drank half that amount.

Trying biofeedback

One in three people with chronic constipation gets little relief from standard approaches, say US researchers from the University of Iowa. In a little-recognised, lifelong constipation problem called dyssynergic defaecation, the muscle contractions that should move stools along are weak and uncoordinated, and it's hard to sense when there's stool ready to exit the bowels. The solution? In one study, a biofeedback technique that involves using a pencil-thin rectal probe and artificial 'practice stools' helped 80 per cent of people with this problem learn to push at the right time and overcome constipation.

Take a walk When middle-aged Dutch men and women with chronic constipation took a brisk 30-minute walk every day, researchers found that they didn't have to strain as much during bowel movements and had fewer hard stools. Food also passed more quickly through their intestinal tracts. As a result, the number with constipation dropped by a third. And in a study of 62,036 women, those who exercised every day were 44 per cent less likely to be constipated than women who were active less than once a week.

While you're at it, eat more fibre. These two strategies seem to do more together to prevent constipation than either one can alone: in the study mentioned above, active women who also ate a high-fibre diet were 68 per cent less likely to be constipated than inactive women who ate a low-fibre diet.

Prevention boosters

Eat prunes or sip prune juice Research has confirmed something many of us have experienced first-hand: prunes really get your bowels moving. Studies show that they stimulate contractions of the intestinal wall and seem to make bowel movements wetter, which can make elimination easier. In one US study from Boston University, prunes stimulated the bowels more than any other food tested.

Change your prescription Experts estimate that prescription and over-the-counter medications and remedies are responsible for up to 40 per cent of constipation problems. If you take any of the medications in the list following, and are having trouble with regularity, ask your doctor if you can switch to another medication that doesn't result in the same problem: antacids containing aluminium or calcium, antidepressants, antihistamines, calcium channel blockers, diuretics, iron supplements, opioids, and pseudoephedrine (found in many cough and cold preparations).

Try to go half an hour after eating The gastrocolic reflex—a wave of muscle activity along the intestines that leads to a bowel movement—usually happens within half an hour after a meal. Digestion experts often recommend that people prone to constipation make a point of spending some time on the toilet after meals as a form of bowel retraining—getting your body on a schedule that can lead to better regularity. If nothing happens, don't linger, as sitting for a long time won't help.

▶ WHAT CAUSES IT
Slow movement of waste material along the intestinal tract due to a lack of fibre and fluids, ageing, lack of a regular bathroom routine, taking medications or having a health condition (such as diabetes) that slows bowel speed.

▶ SYMPTOMS TO WATCH FOR
Bloating, abdominal discomfort, having two or fewer bowel movements per week (with hard stools), straining and pushing when you have a bowel movement, and feeling that your bowel movement was incomplete.

▶ LATEST THINKING
People with chronic constipation are twice as likely to have frequent headaches as people with regular bowel movements, report researchers from the Norwegian University of Science and Technology. The more frequent the headaches, the worse the constipation. Experts aren't sure why the two are connected, but they warn that prescription painkillers such as morphine, codeine and oxycodone could make constipation worse.

Coronary artery disease

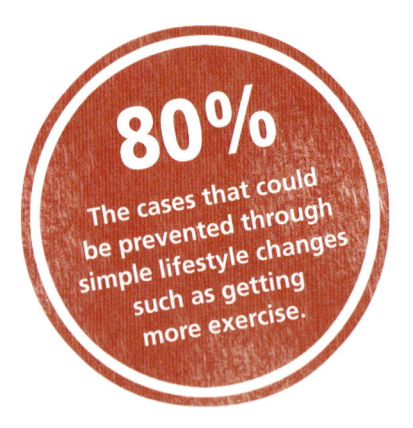

80% The cases that could be prevented through simple lifestyle changes such as getting more exercise.

The stage is set for getting heart disease as early as your teens, or even preteens. Getting too little exercise and eating too much saturated fat pads artery walls with plaque. Fast forward 20, 30 or 40 years, and you may have chest pain as narrowed arteries can't deliver enough blood to heart muscle—or worse, a heart attack. While genes play a role, your heart's fate is mostly in your hands. Even if your arteries are slightly blocked, changing your ways can change your future.

Key prevention strategies

Walk for 30 minutes five times a week Getting out for a walk at a moderate pace, brisk enough to quicken your breathing a little, five days a week can cut heart disease risk in half, according to one large study of middle-aged and older women. Researchers looking at men found that those who rarely if ever exercised were three times more likely to die from heart disease than men who exercised at least five days a week.

Exercise helps your heart in many ways. It raises HDL ('good') cholesterol, lowers LDL ('bad') cholesterol and triglycerides, puts a damper on high blood pressure and heart-threatening inflammation, and can even improve the circulation of anti-oxidants that protect the cells of the heart and the cells lining blood vessels from injury.

One particular study demonstrated the heart-friendly powers of exercise. Researchers looked at 101 men who had surgery to open blocked arteries in their hearts: half of them received stents to keep the arteries open; the other half didn't. Instead, they rode exercise bikes for 20 minutes a day to achieve the same effect. The result? The bike riders had fewer heart attacks, strokes and serious chest pain, which is reason enough to invest in an exercise bike.

Quit smoking Cigarette smoking doubles, triples or even quadruples your risk of developing heart disease, and once you have it, smoking doubles your risk of sudden cardiac death. Smoke damages arteries, giving plaque an easier foothold, and nicotine constricts blood vessels, while the carbon monoxide in cigarette smoke displaces oxygen in the bloodstream, forcing your heart to pump harder to oxygenate cells.

Quit smoking, and you'll begin to lower your risk almost immediately. Within two years after your last cigarette, risk drops by more than 30 per cent, and it drops to normal within 10 to 14 years. (Turn to page 62 for some top strategies for kicking the habit.)

Eat more oily fish If you eat more fish rich in omega-3s, you'll eat fewer kilojoules than you would if steak were on your plate, and you'll not only avoid unhealthy saturated fats that raise cholesterol levels but also get 'good' fats that are heart-healthy. In one study of nearly 85,000 women, those who ate fatty fish just one to three times a month cut their risk of developing coronary heart disease by 21 per cent; eating fish five times a week or more lowered it by 34 per cent. Fish fat helps prevent blood clots and inflammation of the arteries, and it protects against irregular heart rhythms, or arrhythmias, that can lead to heart attacks.

Aim to eat at least 300 g of fatty fish such as salmon, trout, sardines, mackerel or canned light tuna each week. And don't worry too much if the salmon is farmed or wild; unless you're pregnant, the benefits of eating it outweigh any risks.

Consider fish-oil capsules The Australian Heart Foundation recommends that people with heart disease eat about 1 g of omega-3 fatty acids from marine sources every day. People with high triglycerides should start with 1.2 g per day and check their response three to four weeks later. It is also recommended that all Australians and New Zealanders eat at least 2 g of omega-3s from plant sources every day, by eating two slices of soy and linseed bread with a canola-based margarine spread, or 30 g of walnuts (about a small handful), for example.

In one study, people who got 1.5 g of omega-3 fatty acids a day from fish-oil capsules saw plaque regress after two years. Even if you don't have heart disease, ask your doctor about taking 1 g of fish oil daily. Vegetarians can look for omega-3 capsules that provide DHA from algae instead of fish.

Eat nuts and heart-healthy oils Walnuts, canola oil, ground linseeds (they must be refrigerated), tofu and soybeans are all good sources of alpha linolenic acid (ALA), a type of omega-3 fatty acid that your body converts into DHA and EPA. These foods are not a replacement for fish and fish oil—your body gets only a small amount of DHA and EPA from them—but they're a good add-on.

'Getting out for a walk five days a week can cut heart disease risk in half.'

Eat foods that 'offer best protection' It's a mnemonic device for remembering the foods richest in soluble fibre—oats and oranges; beans, barley and berries; and pears and peas. Soluble fibre forms a gel in your intestines that actually reduces the absorption of the fat you eat, which, in turn, lowers cholesterol. In one study that followed 9776 women and men for 19 years, those who got about 6 g of soluble fibre a day (about the amount in a bowl of porridge, $1/2$ cup of barley and a whole pear) had a 15 per cent lower risk of heart disease than those who got less than a gram a day.

Choose smarter carbs The key here is whole grains. Studies show that people who eat more of them (think 100 per cent wholegrain bread, wholegrain breakfast cereal and whole grains such as brown rice and burghul) are less likely to have heart disease, whereas people who eat a lot of refined grains (think white bread, white rice and snack foods such as crackers, biscuits and doughnuts) have more heart attacks. Chalk up the difference largely to the effects of refined grains on insulin; generally speaking, they raise insulin more than whole grains do, and high insulin levels have a domino effect that raises heart disease risk. A diet that keeps insulin low also helps lower levels of potentially harmful blood fats called triglycerides.

Go low salt A recent US study from Harvard Medical School shows that cutting back on salt cuts your risk of heart disease by 25 per cent, even if you don't have high blood pressure. Taking the saltshaker off your table is just the first step. Infinitely more important is completely avoiding processed foods, from which we get 70 to 80 per cent of the salt we eat. That means everything from ham, salami and canned soups to microwave meals and salad dressings (make your own or look for low-sodium versions).

Ask your doctor about wine Drinking any form of alcohol in moderation (for healthy men and women, no more than two standard drinks, with meals, on any day) can lower your risk of heart disease as much as 30 per cent by improving cholesterol ratios and helping to prevent blood clots. But if your triglycerides are high, consume wine only in moderation or not at all. While some studies suggest that just one glass a day may lower triglycerides, this strategy doesn't work for everyone. (If you have trouble keeping your alcohol intake in check, consume in moderation. Binge drinking even once a month increases your heart attack risk.)

Lower your blood pressure High blood pressure puts added stress on your heart, making the heart muscle thicker and stiffer. This extra pressure damages artery walls, speeding up the accumulation of plaque. It can also diminish your sensitivity to chest pain to the point that you don't even notice the warning signs of heart disease, and could even suffer a 'silent' heart attack, according to Canadian researchers who studied 900 people with hypertension. Lowering your blood pressure can cut heart disease risk by up to 30 per cent, according to current research.

Watch your cholesterol levels If you don't know your cholesterol levels—LDL, HDL and total cholesterol—see your doctor to have them tested. You should have your cholesterol checked every two years after the age of 45, or every year if you already have chronic disease. While many people who have heart attacks don't have elevated blood cholesterol, having high cholesterol does increase risk. If your cholesterol levels are less than ideal, take steps to improve them (see 'High cholesterol', starting on page 214).

Prevention boosters

Brush and floss regularly Using a toothbrush and dental floss are two very basic ways to protect your heart. When used daily (brush at least twice and floss once), they can cut your risk of gum disease, which recent studies suggest doubles your odds for heart disease. The link is thought to be inflammation caused by bacteria. People with severe gum disease have four times higher levels of bacterial by-products, called endotoxins, in their bloodstream than people with healthy gums. Battling these toxins involves an immune system response that triggers inflammation, and chronic inflammation contributes to the formation of plaque in artery walls.

Have a guilt-free treat Thirty grams of dark chocolate a day—that's just a small piece—helps arteries stay flexible and can help nudge your blood pressure lower, some studies show. For the most anti-oxidants it has to be dark chocolate, so look for a minimum of 60 per cent cocoa solids.

Avoid secondhand smoke Being exposed to smoke from someone else's cigarette, cigar or pipe raises your own risk of developing heart disease by a significant 25 to 30 per cent.

▶ WHAT CAUSES IT

Damage to the inner layers of arteries in your heart due to high blood pressure, smoking and high blood sugar. As your heart tries to heal itself, fatty plaque accumulates in artery walls, especially if you have high levels of 'bad' LDL cholesterol. This buildup narrows arteries and can lead to the formation of heart-threatening blood clots. Infections (e.g. gum disease) and excess belly fat fuel the process by releasing inflammatory compounds into the bloodstream that spur the growth of plaque.

▶ SYMPTOMS TO WATCH FOR

Chest pain, or angina, which occurs when the heart muscle can't get enough oxygen-rich blood. Angina can feel like pressure or squeezing in your chest, but you may also feel it in your back, jaw, shoulders, neck or arms. It usually gets worse during activity and improves at rest.

▶ LATEST THINKING

Marital stress can harm the heart. In a US study of 150 couples, those who unleashed angry, mean-spirited verbal assaults during a 6-minute conversation about a 'touchy' subject had more atherosclerosis (caused by severe plaque buildup). Husbands had a 30 per cent higher risk of atherosclerosis when either spouse was dominant or controlling; wives' risk rose by 30 per cent when either partner was hostile.

Depression

61% The amount by which learning to problem solve could reduce your risk of depression.

When we asked more than 100 doctors which health conditions are most likely to cause chronic disease, depression ranked surprisingly high—not far below high blood pressure. Depression is linked with a higher risk of nearly every major health issue, from diabetes to heart disease, and is the leading cause of physical disability in the world. And it's hardly the type of thing you just 'snap out of'. The best way forward is to prevent depression in the first place or, failing that, prevent a recurrence (up to 60 per cent of people who have had one major depressive episode go on to have another). Here are strategies that the research finds helpful.

Key prevention strategies

Learn to solve problems Quite often, depression starts with a particular challenge in life that you just don't know how to cope with. Finding ways to manage the issues you're facing now may well help you avoid depression further down the track—think of it as preventive maintenance for your mind.

One study looked at older adults who were recently diagnosed with macular degeneration, a leading cause of vision loss. Those who were taught to solve many of the problems they would encounter as their sight failed were 61 per cent less likely to be depressed two months after their diagnoses than those who didn't receive such coaching. They were also less likely to have to give up an activity they enjoyed—the very types of activities that help prevent depression.

Learning to solve problems can be as simple as sitting down with pen and paper, listing the issues that are making you unhappy, and identifying three concrete steps you can take to improve things. Other options include brainstorming solutions with close friends or family,

DRUGS THAT PREVENT DISEASE

If you've had at least two episodes of major depression, or you have a chronic illness such as diabetes, heart disease or cancer, talk to your doctor about continuing your antidepressant medication for longer than the recommended 12 months after the depression recedes. A review of several studies found that about 60 per cent of people are at risk of having another depressive episode within a year of ending treatment, but just 10 to 30 per cent of people who continue their medication will have a recurrence. Another study found that people with a form of depression called seasonal affective disorder (SAD), which occurs in some climates during winter, can prevent an episode by starting antidepressants early on, while they still feel well.

or scheduling as many sessions as you need with a therapist who is trained in cognitive behavioural therapy.

Try to view the glass as half full Numerous studies find that optimistic people are less likely to develop depression than pessimistic people. In fact, in one study of 71 older adults, researchers found that people who expected bad things to happen in the coming month experienced more depressive symptoms at the end of the month than those who didn't have negative expectations, regardless of what actually happened.

Not everyone is a born optimist, but anyone can work on adopting a more positive attitude. Being an optimist begins with the belief that bad events are temporary and changeable. For instance, rather than complaining about a bad boss and assuming nothing will change, an optimist would identify opportunities for growth elsewhere in the company, update his or her CV and apply for a new—possibly better—job. It also involves looking on the bright side. If a pessimist were diagnosed with breast cancer, she might immediately assume she's going to become sick from chemotherapy, lose her hair and eventually die from the disease. An optimist might count herself lucky that women today are much less likely to die from breast cancer and that new treatments address many of the negative effects of chemotherapy.

'Anyone can work on adopting a more positive attitude.'

See a therapist once a month If you've ever been diagnosed with major depression, a once-a-month psychotherapy session may be all that's required to prevent a recurrence. Researchers randomly assigned 99 previously depressed women to interpersonal psychotherapy (a short-term form of counselling that focuses on resolving issues related to grief, role transitions or problems interacting with others) weekly, twice a month or once a month for two years or until they had another depressive episode. The result was that just 26 per cent of the women who completed the maintenance phase saw their depression recur (versus an average 60 per cent recurrence rate), no matter how often they had therapy.

Stay connected Join a bowling team, a knitting or sewing club, or a committee at your child's school or your local church—anything to bring you into regular contact with others and enhance your social network. According to research, these sorts of connections do a great job of guarding against depression.

Ten instant mood boosters

Snapping at your children, spouse or the supermarket check-out person? Feeling out of sorts or just sad for no reason? Here are 10 quick ways to raise your spirits.

1. **Call a friend and chat about anything** Staying in touch and laughing is a great stress buster.
2. **Take a walk in the sunshine** Sunlight has proven mood-boosting properties, as does exercise.
3. **Meet someone for coffee** Good conversation coupled with an energy burst from the caffeine is a quick way to lighten things up.
4. **Give thanks for something** You'll remember how much you have to be grateful for and stop dwelling on your problems for a while.
5. **Plant some brightly coloured flowers** The physical activity of gardening and the bright colours of the flowers might raise your spirits.
6. **Bake a loaf of bread** Nothing spells contentment like the scent of freshly baked bread filling the house. Even instant-mix bread can do the trick.
7. **Clean out a cupboard** You'll get an instant sense of accomplishment. Donate old clothes and get the added mood benefit of helping someone else.
8. **Soak in a hot bath** Light some candles (try lavender or vanilla scents, which studies find can relieve anxiety and boost mood), listen to music or just drift for 20 minutes. Relaxing helps to improve mood.
9. **Pat a puppy** Actually, even a fully grown dog will work. Studies find that patting animals reduces stress and boosts mood.
10. **Enjoy a small piece of dark chocolate** It contains compounds that influence levels of serotonin, a feelgood brain chemical.

Prevention boosters

Seek treatment for anxiety If you find that you're worrying beyond reason, obsessing over events in your life or pathologically afraid of certain things such as going outside or being around other people, you may have an anxiety disorder and thus an increased risk of depression. The more severe your anxiety, the more likely you are to become depressed. Researchers think the anxiety disorder may alter the way the brain releases and takes up serotonin, a chemical important to mood. Or the anxiety may change your normal interactions and lifestyle so much that it triggers depression. Regardless, your best option is to seek out a therapist trained in cognitive behavioural therapy, which studies find is the best way to treat most anxiety disorders.

Get moving regularly Countless studies underscore the emotional boost that exercise provides and its ability to help relieve symptoms of depression. But a pile of research also suggests that people who get regular exercise are less likely to become depressed in the first place. A recent UK study showed that, at least in middle-aged men, more intense exercise (think running or playing soccer or basketball) was most effective. But in another study of older adults with arthritis, taking aerobics classes led to fewer depression symptoms. It may be key to get your heart rate up; slow walking may not do the trick.

Grill some salmon for dinner Can twice-weekly meals of salmon, trout or tuna help keep depression at bay? It's entirely possible. Fatty fish such as these are excellent sources of omega-3 fatty acids. In countries where people consume a lot of these healthy fats, depression rates tend to be low. In fact, women who eat fatty fish regularly often have half the risk of developing depression than those who don't eat fish often. If you don't eat fish, ask your doctor about taking a daily fish-oil supplement containing at least 2 g of omega-3 fatty acids.

And also try to cut back on corn, safflower and sunflower oils as well as processed foods such as chips and biscuits. These are high in omega-6 fatty acids, which counteract the beneficial effects of heart-healthy omega-3s.

Get a good night's sleep Researchers used to think that insomnia was a symptom of depression. Now they're finding that it typically precedes depression, with up to 50 per cent of people with insomnia that lasts two weeks or longer later developing a major depressive episode. Of course, the insomnia may be a sign of an underlying problem in your life that may lead to depression, but good evidence shows that poor sleep by itself can lead to symptoms of depression. (See 'Insomnia', starting on page 228, for more information.)

Include more folate-rich foods in your diet Just a cup of cooked green soybeans contains about 200 mcg of folate, a B vitamin in which many people who are depressed are deficient. Many wholegrain breakfast cereals are fortified with folate. Studies find that men who get 234 mcg of folate for every 4200 kilojoules they eat are half as likely to become depressed as men who get 119 mcg. Other great sources of folate include spinach (150 mcg in 1 cup of cooked spinach), chickpeas (100 mcg in 1 cup) and lentils (40 mcg in 1 cup of cooked lentils).

▶ WHAT CAUSES IT

Usually a mix of factors that results in an imbalance in mood-regulating chemicals called neurotransmitters (such as serotonin and dopamine). These factors may include a genetic predisposition, a single traumatic event and stress, particularly the kind of stress that comes from feeling a loss of control over your life. Other triggers include specific situations, like the death of a loved one.

▶ SYMPTOMS TO WATCH FOR

Changes in your sleeping and/or eating habits; loss of pleasure in things that you used to enjoy; thoughts of hurting yourself; lack of interest in sex; feeling hopeless or worthless; crying for no apparent reason; trouble concentrating and making decisions; irritability or restlessness; feeling fatigued or weak; unexplained physical problems such as back pain or headaches.

▶ LATEST THINKING

People who have had depression are more likely to develop Alzheimer's disease than those who were never depressed. Researchers don't know yet whether the depression contributes to the development of Alzheimer's or whether something else is at work to cause both the depression and the Alzheimer's.

Diabetes

58% The drop in your risk of developing Type 2 diabetes if you lose just 7 per cent of your body weight.

Genes play a role in getting diabetes, but the less exercise you get and the more you weigh, the greater your risk. If you aren't part of the 'diabetes epidemic' yet, congratulations. But watch out for prediabetes—elevated blood sugar that's not yet high enough to trigger alarms—in case you need to address that issue now. Doctors don't always check for prediabetes (a fasting blood test can indicate if you have it), so now's the time to prevent it from turning into diabetes.

Key prevention strategies

Drop just a few kilos Excess weight is the number one reason adults and children are at higher risk for Type 2 diabetes now than ever before. Gaining weight can pack excess fat around internal organs at your midsection—especially if you're stressed out on a regular basis (stress hormones can send extra fat to the belly). New research shows that this dangerous abdominal fat sends out chemical signals that desensitise cells throughout your body to insulin, the hormone that persuades cells to absorb blood sugar. Insulin resistance is the first step on the path to Type 2 diabetes.

In a landmark clinical trial that followed 3234 people with prediabetes for three years, those who lost just 7 per cent of their body weight (5 kg if you now weigh 70 kg) lowered their diabetes risk by 58 per cent. In fact, weight loss worked better than insulin-sensitising diabetes medications at cutting the odds of diabetes.

A brisk cardio work-out three to five times a week can get rid of belly fat better than dieting, say US researchers at Syracuse University. Brisk walking for 30 minutes each day also works.

Aim for at least seven serves of fruit and vegetables daily
And factor in three servings of whole grains, too. Following a low-glycaemic diet packed with fresh fruit and vegetables and whole grains—and cutting back on white bread, white rice, foods made with white flour, and sweets—helps keeps blood sugar low and steady. Research shows it also redresses chronic low-grade inflammation in the body, which interferes with the action of insulin and the absorption of blood sugar by cells.

In a recent study of 486 women, Harvard School of Public Health researchers found that those who ate the most fruit were 34 per cent less likely to have metabolic syndrome, a cluster of risk factors, including insulin resistance, that predispose a person to diabetes. Women who ate the most vegetables cut their risk of metabolic syndrome by 30 per cent. Meanwhile, German researchers who followed 25,067 women and men for seven years recently found that those who got the most fibre from whole grains were 27 per cent less likely to develop diabetes than those who got the least.

Give up the 'lolly water' Start quenching your thirst with water, soda water (with a squeeze of lemon or lime), unsweetened tea or skim milk instead of soft drinks, fruit juice drinks, coffee or sweetened iced-tea drinks.

A single daily serving of soft drink raised the risk of metabolic syndrome (described above) by a staggering 44 per cent in a headline-grabbing study from Boston University School of Medicine in the US. Experts have many theories as to why this is. It could simply be all those extra kilojoules in soft drinks and other sugary drinks or in the high-fat, high-kilojoule foods we tend to pair them with (hot chips and pizza). Experts are also finding that drinking even a single soft drink a day is associated with being overweight—perhaps because the kilojoules in drinks don't register in our brains, so we don't compensate for them by eating less food.

Another possible culprit is high-fructose corn syrup. It's essentially sugar in liquid form, except that for technical chemical reasons, some experts believe it's more likely to lead to insulin resistance.

For a healthier thirst quencher, drop several tea bags (black, green or herbal) into a jug filled with water and refrigerate overnight before drinking. And don't rule out a glass of skim milk. The calcium,

Ten low-glycaemic snacks

Low-glycaemic foods are those that have a slower effect on blood sugar. Studies show that people who eat more of these foods and fewer high-glycaemic foods are less likely to develop insulin resistance, a core problem underlying Type 2 diabetes. Low-glycaemic foods are often rich in fibre, protein or fat, though it's not a good idea to eat fatty foods just for the sake of your blood sugar unless they're healthy (unsaturated) fats.

1. **An apple with skin**
2. **Wholegrain bread with peanut butter**
3. **Baby carrots dipped in low-fat sour cream**
4. **A small handful of walnuts or almonds**
5. **Low-fat yogurt sprinkled with fresh fruit or untoasted muesli**
6. **Toasted wholemeal pita with white bean dip**
7. **Edamame (fresh soybeans)**
8. **Lentil soup (with no added salt)**
9. **A small handful of dried apricots**
10. **A hard-boiled egg**

vitamin D and other minerals in dairy foods may be the reason that getting at least one serve of low-fat or skim milk (or yogurt or cheese) a day lowered metabolic syndrome risk by up to 62 per cent in one particular UK study.

Turn off the TV and go for a walk Exercise helps protect against diabetes by transporting blood sugar into fuel-hungry muscle cells and making cells more sensitive to insulin. A Harvard study of 40,000 women found that 30 minutes a day of brisk walking, plus a TV limit of 10 hours per week, cut diabetes risk by 43 per cent. If you get bored walking, sign up for an aerobics class, take up bowling, gather your children or grandchildren for a bushwalk, or just put on some music and dance.

Eat less fast food Does regular drive-through dining lead to diabetes? When US researchers at the University of Minnesota tracked the eating habits and health of 9514 people aged between 45 and 64 for up to 10 years, they discovered that those who ate two serves of red meat (beef patties in hamburgers) a week were 26 per cent more likely to wind up with metabolic syndrome. A daily helping of fried foods raised it another 10 to 25 per cent. These foods are high in saturated and trans fats, which have been linked to diabetes.

Swap burgers and butter for fish and olive oil Each bite of a burger and each smear of butter you consume is full of saturated fat. These fats not only clog arteries, they also increase insulin resistance, which propels you down the path to genuine diabetes. Saturated fats also trigger inflammation, which is toxic to cells, including those that handle blood sugar. Fish and olive oil have the exact opposite effect and could actually lower your diabetes risk. The same goes for nuts (including peanuts) and canola oil.

Of course, you don't want to overdo even these good fats, which are high in kilojoules. Cutting total fat intake as well as saturated fat helped participants in the US Diabetes Prevention Program study cut their diabetes risk. Participants limited

Get out the tape measure

Women whose waists measure 88 cm or more and men whose waists measure 102 cm or more are more likely to have fat deep in their abdomens, which can triple the risk of diabetes. While you're probably overweight if your waist is big, researchers report that they're seeing more people at a normal weight who also have larger waistline measurements, so don't think it's enough to simply watch the numbers on the scale.

their intake of saturated fat to 7 per cent of total kilojoules a day, which is about the amount in 60 g of cheese plus 5 g of butter if you eat 8400 kilojoules a day.

Prevention boosters

Eat breakfast In one study, people who ate breakfast were 35 to 50 per cent less likely to be overweight or have insulin resistance than breakfast skippers. What's going on? An overnight fast puts your body into 'starvation mode'. If you don't eat breakfast, your liver churns out stored glucose to keep your blood sugar levels up. At the same time, skipping breakfast flips biochemical switches that reduce the body's response to insulin. And it raises levels of an appetite-stimulating hormone called ghrelin so you want to eat more all day long. Do this often enough, and you gain weight, say scientists from Children's Hospital Boston in the US.

Avoid eating bagels (too many carbohydrates) or a shop-bought muffin (too many kilojoules and hydrogenated oils) for breakfast. Instead, pour yourself a bowl of muesli or high-fibre cereal with skim milk and add some berries on top for good measure. One Canadian study from the University of Toronto looked at people with prediabetes and found that high-fibre cereals made their cells 'listen' better to insulin than lower-fibre ones. Yogurt with fresh berries is also a good breakfast choice.

If you're depressed, get help If you're depressed, you're much less likely to exercise and eat well. But the health dangers don't end there. US scientists from Stanford University think that depression itself alters body chemistry in profound ways that spell trouble for anyone at risk for diabetes. Rates of insulin resistance were 23 per cent higher among depressed women than among women who weren't depressed, regardless of body weight, exercise habits or age. (See 'Depression', starting on page 160, for more advice.)

Get better sleep A chronic lack of sleep leads to weight gain and reduces your body's sensitivity to insulin. In one US study of 1709 men, those who averaged 5 to 6 hours of sleep per night doubled their risk of diabetes. Studies of women have found similar results.

▶ WHAT CAUSES IT

Heredity definitely plays a role, but it usually takes extra kilos and a sedentary lifestyle to develop Type 2 diabetes. Excess body fat (especially visceral fat deep in the belly) and inactivity conspire to make cells stop obeying signals from insulin to absorb blood sugar. Your body compensates by pumping out more insulin, but if it can't keep pace, you've got high blood sugar.

▶ SYMPTOMS TO WATCH FOR

Often, there are none. You can have Type 2 diabetes for years without noticing anything's amiss. But as it progresses, symptoms include thirst, frequent urination, intense hunger, weight loss, tiredness, blurry vision, sores that are slow to heal and more frequent bladder and vaginal infections for women.

▶ LATEST THINKING

Diet soft drinks aren't safe, either. Sipping just one can of diet soft drink per day raised the risk of metabolic syndrome by 34 per cent in one recent study and 48 per cent in another, although experts aren't sure why.

Diverticular disease

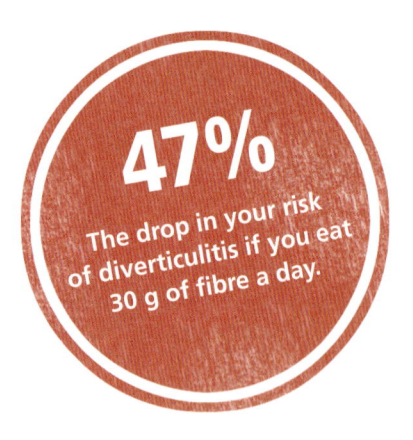

47% The drop in your risk of diverticulitis if you eat 30 g of fibre a day.

Years of constipation, straining during bowel movements and eating a low-fibre diet can take an invisible toll on the walls of your intestinal tract. Hard stools and repeated high-pressure 'pushing' can create tiny, pea-sized pouches that balloon outward. These sacs, called diverticula, can number in the hundreds—and usually don't cause any trouble. But if stool gets trapped in a pouch, the sac can become inflamed and even infected, and you have diverticulitis, which can cause intense abdominal pain, fever, nausea and constipation or diarrhoea, putting you at risk for intestinal blockages or tears, and bleeding if a blood vessel bursts.

Key prevention strategies

Eat more fibre Packing about 30 g of fibre into your diet each day could cut your risk of developing diverticulitis by 47 per cent, say Harvard School of Public Health researchers who tracked the health and diets of nearly 44,000 men for four years. And if you've already had a painful episode, boosting the fibre in your meals could help prevent a repeat attack. In one UK study of people who had been hospitalised once for diverticulitis, 90 per cent of those who switched to a high-fibre diet were symptom free and stayed that way when researchers checked up on them seven years later.

Provided you drink plenty of fluids along with the fibre you eat, fibre protects intestinal walls by making stools soft and fluffy, which makes them easier to pass, and by decreasing tension within the walls. Researchers now suspect that it also promotes a healthier environment in the intestines by providing a haven for beneficial bacteria and by maintaining the layer of protective mucus that lines the inner walls. This healthy 'inner landscape' seems to prevent the immune system from overreacting and causing inflammation in diverticula.

If you're planning to increase your fibre intake, go slowly. Add a few higher-fibre foods to your diet each week over the course of a month or two so you and your body grow accustomed to the changes. And be sure to drink several large glasses of water a day to avoid discomfort.

Add a fibre supplement If you can't get 30 g of fibre from food every day, experts say it's OK to use a fibre supplement to close the gap. (However, you should avoid taking supplements during flare-ups of diverticulitis as they can cause discomfort.)

Snack on fruit instead of chips, biscuits and fries Eating french fries, biscuits or a small bag of chips five or six times a week raised the risk of diverticular disease by as much as 69 per cent in one study of 48,000 men. In contrast, those who snacked regularly on peaches, blueberries, apricots, apples or oranges lowered their risk by as much as 80 per cent. The trick is to avoid those fruits that give you diarrhoea.

Have chicken or fish instead of fatty or processed red meat
Greek researchers have found that a diet loaded with red meat can raise your odds for diverticulitis an incredible 50 times more than a vegetarian diet can. Eating even a medium (110- to 170-g) serve of beef, pork or lamb five or six nights a week tripled the risk of diverticular disease in the Harvard study noted earlier. Having a weekly hot dog raised the odds by 86 per cent; a serve of processed meat (such as salami or ham) five or six times a week nearly doubled the risk. In contrast, fish and chicken eaters barely increased their risk at all. Some experts speculate that red meat may prompt bacteria in your colon to produce substances that weaken the intestinal wall, so it's easier for pouches to form.

Don't worry about coffee or tea
In the past, people at risk for diverticulitis have been warned to avoid these popular drinks. But newer research suggests that they actually have little effect on

Eating the right foods

Fruit, vegetables and whole grains packed with a type of insoluble fibre called cellulose seem to have a special talent for protecting intestinal walls from damage that leads to bowel problems. The foods listed below contain the most.

FOOD	SERVING	TOTAL FIBRE	CELLULOSE
Legumes (cooked or canned)	½ cup	6.7 g	2.8 g
Peas	½ cup	4.4 g	2.1 g
Tomato pasta sauce	½ cup	4.2 g	2.0 g
Potato, with skin	1 medium	4.2 g	1.6 g
Apple	1 medium	3.7 g	1.0 g
Carrots	½ cup	2.6 g	1.0 g
Wholegrain cereal	1 cup	6.0 g	0.7 g
Banana	1 medium	2.7 g	0.5 g
Wholegrain bread	1 slice	1.1 g	0.3 g
Orange	1 medium	3.0 g	0.3 g

diverticulitis. (Of course, if a food or drink makes your symptoms worse, you should eliminate it from your daily diet.)

Start exercising Perhaps because it can prompt stools to move more swiftly through the intestinal tract, physical activity lowered the risk of diverticular disease by as much as 48 per cent in one study. People who jogged got the most benefit, but any kind of exercise may help, especially if you also eat a high-fibre diet.

Schedule in some 'toilet time' Straining to have a bowel movement puts extra pressure on the intestinal walls, setting the stage for the formation of pouches. If you're prone to constipation, be sure to take advantage of a key, after-meal opportunity for a bowel movement. During the half hour or so after eating, your gastrointestinal system makes room for the new food by moving everything else further down the line. This wave of muscle activity, called the gastrocolic reflex, often results in a bowel movement if you give it a chance by spending a few minutes on the toilet about 30 minutes after a meal.

Ask about your medications Ask your doctor if constipation is a common side effect of any prescription or over-the-counter medication you're taking. Culprits include antacids that contain aluminium or calcium, antidepressants, antihistamines, calcium channel blockers, diuretics, iron supplements, opioid painkillers, and pseudoephedrine (found in many cough and cold preparations). You may be able to substitute a different medication.

Prevention boosters

Consume more healthy fats Getting plenty of omega-3 fatty acids from fish, linseeds (which also act as a laxative) and linseed oil, walnuts, or fish-oil capsules may nudge down levels of inflammation in your colon—a big plus because inflammation can trigger serious diverticulitis symptoms. Taking 1 g of fish oil once or twice a day could help, according to digestive disease experts from the University of Maryland in the US. However, you should always check with your doctor before taking any supplement.

Take probiotics Diverticular disease can decimate beneficial bacteria in the gut. These 'good' bacteria, available in supplements known as probiotics, play a role in the speedy movement of stools, in protecting the lining of intestinal walls and even in reducing inflammation. Studies from Italy and Germany are beginning to suggest that bolstering their levels may cut the risk of repeat attacks of diverticulitis. Look for *Lactobacillus acidophilus*, *L. gasseri* and *Bifidobacterium bifidum*. Many probiotic products include a combination of these. And the yeast *Saccharomyces boulardii* may help to prevent diarrhoea caused by infections.

If you've had an attack of diverticulitis, probiotic supplements alone may not be enough to prevent a repeat. Make an appointment to see your doctor and follow his or her advice about medication and lifestyle steps you can take.

Lose weight Traditionally, diverticular disease has been a problem for people over the age of 50, brought on by decades of low-fibre eating and constipation, but that may be changing. Because of the obesity epidemic, doctors are beginning to notice that people as young as 20 have the thin-walled, bulging pouches along their intestines—yet another good reason to keep your weight in check.

People who snacked regularly on peaches, blueberries, apricots, apples or oranges lowered their risk by as much as 80 per cent.

▶ WHAT CAUSES IT

Increased intestinal wall tension from hard stools plus straining to have a bowel movement can make tiny sections of the wall bulge outwards. If these pouches become infected or inflamed, you may experience pain, bleeding or even perforations in the intestinal wall.

▶ SYMPTOMS TO WATCH FOR

You may have severe, sharp pain in your abdomen (often on the lower left side) or milder pain that lasts for several days and may occasionally get worse. Other symptoms include fever, nausea, bouts of diarrhoea or constipation, and bloating. If you have severe pain or bleeding, call your doctor immediately.

▶ LATEST THINKING

Nuts, seeds and popcorn are fine. In the past, doctors have told people with diverticular disease to avoid these foods, fearing that they could get stuck in the intestinal pouches. But when researchers tracked more than 47,000 men for 18 years, they found that those who ate these healthy, high-fibre foods had no extra risk of problems. In fact, those who ate popcorn twice a week had a 28 per cent lower risk of flare-ups than those who indulged less than once a month, possibly because popcorn is a good source of fibre.

Dry eyes

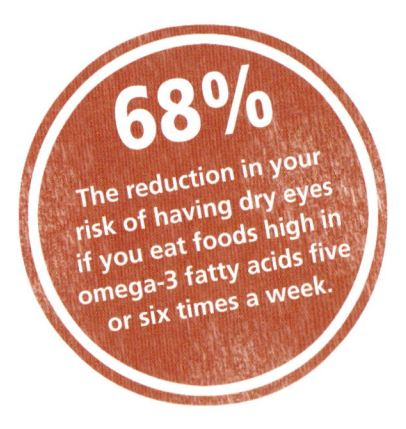

68% The reduction in your risk of having dry eyes if you eat foods high in omega-3 fatty acids five or six times a week.

Tears are your eyes' first line of defence against infection and damage from dust and airborne debris. Each time you blink, a new layer of moisture rolls across the surface of your eyes. Or at least it should. If tears evaporate too quickly (due to age-related changes in tear production) or aren't renewed often enough (because you're staring at the TV or computer for too long), your eyes begin to dry out. Try the following steps to keep your eyes comfortably moist.

Key prevention strategies

Remind yourself to blink Your 'blink rate' drops from a normal 17 to 22 blinks per minute to as few as four when you're doing anything that requires intense visual focus. In one study, people playing computer games blinked just once every 2 to 3 minutes! Keeping your eyes wide open allows the protective film of tears to evaporate. To protect your eyes, remember to blink whenever you turn the page of a book or check your rear-vision mirror while driving (which should be several times each minute). If you're working at a computer, try the 20–20 rule: give your eyes a 20-second rest every 20 minutes. Look out a window or at something across the room and be sure to blink.

Lower your computer monitor Shifting your eyes upwards to read the top lines on your screen could double your odds for dry eyes. The reason is that looking up exposes more of the surface of your eyes to the air. (This is one reason computer use dries out eyes more than reading a book does—when you read, you tend to look down, which partially closes your eyes.) Raise your chair or lower your monitor so you can see the top third of the screen while looking straight ahead.

Medical help for dry eyes

If self-care steps aren't keeping your eyes moist, see an eye doctor. He or she may suggest one of these treatments:

Ocular lubricants Artificial tears, gels and lubricating ointments are the mainstay of treatment for dry eyes. Two things to note are that they may need to be applied as often as every 2 hours and that it's important to use preservative-free formulations if you are doing this frequently (frequent exposure to preservatives can damage the surface of the eye). Examples include Bion Tears, Polygel and Lacrilube.

Punctal plugs for more tears These tiny silicone stoppers, installed in an opthalmologist's office, close off your eyes' drain holes for tears. Some doctors use temporary plugs first so you can see if they'll help. They are usually recommended for people with moderate to severe dry eyes who haven't been helped by other treatments.

Eat healthy fats When researchers from Brigham and Women's Hospital in the US checked the diets and eye health of nearly 32,500 women, they found that those who ate the most omega-3 fats had the lowest risk of dry eyes. In fact, those who ate five or six serves of fatty fish a week were 68 per cent less likely to have dry eyes than those who had less than one. Try to get your omega-3s from a variety of sources, including herring, sardines, salmon and trout, as well as linseed oil, walnuts, freshly ground linseeds (ground in a spice grinder, not a coffee grinder that may have coffee grounds still in it), canola oil, walnut oil and pumpkin seeds.

Eye experts think fish-oil or linseed-oil capsules may also promote eye health, but they're still debating the best dosage. Follow the package directions on one of the dry eye-prevention supplements available in pharmacies, such as TheraTears Nutrition, or take fish-oil capsules with a total of 1 g of DHA and EPA per day. It may take up to three months to notice a difference, so stick with this treatment to see some results.

Stop smoking Research that checked lifestyle habits against the eye health of several thousand people, found that smokers had an 82 per cent higher risk of dry eyes than nonsmokers.

Prevention boosters

Take care of rosacea, blepharitis and eyelid problems All can cause dry eyes. People with rosacea have a 50 per cent chance of developing ocular rosacea, which can cause dry eyes, frequent sties and the feeling that there's something in your eyes. Tell your eye doctor that you have rosacea and ask about a check for this type, too. Your doctor can also help treat blepharitis, or inflammation of the eyelids, as well as eyelids that curl outwards or inwards with age. Both conditions can change the way you blink, resulting in tears not spreading across the entire eye.

Use artificial tears Keep artificial tears, also called lubricating drops, on hand for times when you'll be in airconditioned or heated buildings, or in a car, aeroplane, desert or any other place with extremely dry air. Eye experts recommend choosing preservative-free drops if you'll be using them more than four to six times a day for more than two or three days; otherwise, your eyes may become sensitised to preservatives and become inflamed.

▶ WHAT CAUSES IT

Ageing; for women, hormonal changes at menopause; eye problems that interfere with blinking or tear production; medications such as antihistamines, diuretics, sleeping pills, contraceptive pills and tricyclic antidepressants; exposure to dry air; and medical conditions such as diabetes, rheumatoid arthritis, lupus, scleroderma and Sjögren's syndrome.

▶ SYMPTOMS TO WATCH FOR

A stinging, burning or scratchy sensation in your eyes; sensitivity to light, wind and/or smoke; stringy mucus in or around your eyes; and blurry vision at the end of the day or after focusing intently on a close-range task.

▶ LATEST THINKING

Before having LASIK surgery, have a dry-eye check-up. In the US, 50 per cent of people who opt for laser surgery to improve their vision wind up with dry eyes for at least a few months after surgery—and 10 per cent develop ongoing, severe problems. If your eyes are dry, ask your doctor about starting treatment with artificial tears and/or tear duct plugs before considering surgery.

Eczema

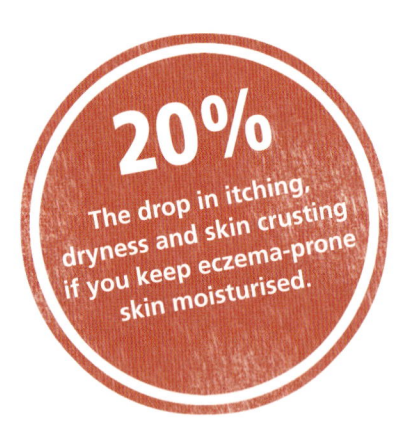

20%
The drop in itching, dryness and skin crusting if you keep eczema-prone skin moisturised.

Could itchy skin be worse than a life-threatening health condition such as diabetes or high blood pressure? When scientists asked 92 adults with severe eczema about the quality of their daily lives, they reported that having a serious medical problem might be easier than dealing with itchy, bumpy, scaly skin all the time. Half said they would trade up to 2 hours a day of their lives for normal skin, and 74 vowed they'd spend whatever it took for a cure. The following strategies may help avoid flare-ups, and beat the 'itch, scratch, itch' cycle that makes skin so much worse.

Key prevention strategies

Avoid hidden triggers Among the everyday things that can cause an outbreak are: perfumes and dyes in laundry and personal-care products, dust, cigarette smoke, walking barefoot on sand (or letting it rub the creases of your legs or arms at the beach), and chlorine or bromine left on the skin after swimming in a pool or soaking in a hot bath. Avoid them or get them off your skin as soon as possible. Sunburn is another trigger.

Bathe less often Long hot baths or showers can take the natural oils out of skin, making it drier and more easily irritated. While some experts recommend a long soak in a tepid bath to soothe skin, many others say it's better to go a day or two between washing. When you do bathe, keep it short and use warm—not hot—water. Avoid soaps, including antibacterial or deodorant soaps, which may strip more moisture from your skin. In fact, use a mild soap only where you really need it: on your underarms, genitals, hands and feet. Try using just water, or sorbolene cream and water, everywhere else. When you're done, pat yourself dry, then slather on moisturiser.

Keep your skin super-moist If you have eczema, you know first-hand how dry, itchy and sensitive your skin is, and that dryness makes itching and rashes even worse. That's why it's important to apply a thick layer of moisturiser once or twice a day to seal the water in the top layer of skin. Keeping your skin moist may mean you'll need less steroid cream to control rashes. In a Spanish study of 173 children with eczema, those who were slathered daily with moisturisers needed 42 per cent less high-potency steroid cream.

Always apply moisturiser generously. In one German study of 30 adults with eczema, those who applied the amount their doctors recommended saw their itching, dryness and skin crusting improve about 20 per cent more than those who skimped. If you're using moisturiser and a steroid cream, apply the steroid first.

Keep a steroid cream handy just in case Steroid creams, ointments, gels and lotions can't cure eczema, but when it flares up, they're the number-one choice for controlling it. The catch is that overuse (more than four continuous weeks) can lead to thinning of the skin, reduced bone density in adults and growth problems in kids—but these side effects are rare. In fact, some researchers say fear of steroid creams can have worse side effects than the creams themselves. In one UK study of 200 people with eczema, 73 per cent admitted to being worried about using a steroid cream, and 24 per cent admitted to skimping on or skipping the treatment as a result. But studies show that sensible use brings relief, usually without adverse effects.

If you're worried about stronger creams recommended by your doctor, remember that they're safe and very effective when used as directed. When UK researchers followed 174 children and teenagers with mild to moderate eczema for 18 weeks, they found that when treating flare-ups, three days of a high-dose cream worked as well as seven days of a low-dose cream. Both groups had the same number of itch-free days and neither showed signs of skin thinning.

Get tested for allergies Pet dander, pollen and dust mites can all trigger eczema flare-ups. In fact, one Scandinavian study of 45 people with eczema found that everyone with severe skin problems was allergic to at least one of these airborne allergens. But get an allergy test. It makes sense to know who (or what) the enemy is before you launch an all-out battle.

Sunlight or a sunlamp?

Go the sunlamp. Stubborn, severe eczema that isn't healed by creams or even steroid medication may respond to exposure to ultraviolet (UV) light. In one study of 73 people with moderate to severe eczema, those who got twice-weekly narrow-band UVB treatments with sunlamps for 12 weeks saw a 28 per cent reduction in itching, oozing and crusting of their skin rashes. In contrast, those who were exposed to regular sunlight saw a 1.3 per cent improvement. See a dermatologist about UV therapy—and don't go to a tanning salon; any potential benefit has to be balanced against the risk of skin cancer.

Experts have conflicting opinions about the effectiveness of strategies for avoiding allergens at home (such as removing carpets, keeping pets out of the bedroom and covering mattresses and pillows with allergen-proof covers). While some recommend it, studies tend to show that these steps often don't reduce eczema flare-ups, simply because it's tough to keep the air completely allergen free. Allergy injections may help. In one German study of 89 people with eczema who were allergic to dust mites, those who got immunotherapy had an easier time keeping their eczema under control than those who didn't have the injections.

Consider food allergies Intolerance to milk, wheat and other foods can cause flare-ups in children with eczema. While food allergies are usually rare among adults with eczema, don't rule them out. In one Danish study, 25 per cent of adults with severe eczema were allergic to at least one food. Before you start cutting whole food groups out of your diet on your own, though, talk to an allergy specialist or a registered dietitian about the best way to test yourself. Often this involves keeping a detailed food diary, removing one suspect food from your diet for several weeks and then reintroducing it again to see what happens.

Try an immunomodulator cream For severe eczema, an immunomodulator cream may help. Pimecrolimus (Elidel) reduces eczema symptoms by 50 per cent or more, according to UK researchers who reviewed 31 well-designed studies.

Pimecrolimus cream doesn't have the skin thinning and other side effects of steroid creams, so it is often used for sensitive areas such as the face or body folds. It can also be used for long-term control of eczema. Talk to your doctor about reports of increased risk of skin cancer and lymphoma. Major medical organisations say that the evidence for a connection is extremely weak and that these warnings may keep people from getting the eczema relief they need.

Cut the odds for eczema

Most eczema begins in early childhood. Now it appears that what the mother eats during pregnancy can lower her child's risk for the condition. Scientists from the University of Aberdeen in Scotland tracked the eating habits of mothers as well as allergies and asthma in 1212 kids from birth to the age of five and found that the babies of women who ate fish once a week or more often during pregnancy were significantly less likely to develop eczema. They also concluded that a woman's diet during gestation may have a bigger impact on a child's risk of developing eczema than the child's own diet in the first few years of life. Fish is a rich source of inflammation-soothing omega-3 fatty acids, but scientists aren't yet sure how this healthy food may bolster protection in a child. For toddlers who are eating solid foods and can have dairy products, adding probiotic-rich foods such as yogurt with live, active cultures may help, too.

Prevention boosters

Soothe your emotions Several studies have linked stress and anxiety with eczema outbreaks. If anger, frustration or stress seems to trigger a rash, consider adding a little 'emotional therapy' to your skin-care routine. Studies show that relaxation therapy, cognitive behavioural therapy and biofeedback can all help. For best results, ask your doctor for a referral to a psychologist or a program specifically designed for people with skin conditions.

Dress for comfort Rough, scratchy fabrics and clothing that's too tight can irritate sensitive skin. Instead, choose smooth cotton weaves and knits to avoid irritation and allow skin to breathe. And avoid itchy wool and synthetic fabrics that trap sweat.

Wash all new clothes before you wear them to remove irritating chemicals used to make them look smooth and wrinkle free in the shop. If you suspect that your laundry detergent or fabric softener is irritating your skin, switch to products without perfumes or dyes and rinse clothes twice in the washing machine.

Keep the temperature and humidity levels comfortable Too much humidity in the air can make you sweat; too little can leave skin parched and flaky. Both situations can prompt an eczema flare-up. Keep your home's humidity level comfortable by using an airconditioner in summer and a humidifier in winter if your heating system dries out the air too much. Research suggests that big temperature swings can also trigger flare-ups, so try to keep the room temperature on an even keel.

Keep using your medications A recent study showed that people's use of medication recommended for eczema dropped by 60 per cent within three days of starting treatment—perhaps because their skin improved quickly or because they were afraid of side effects. Discuss with your doctor any concerns you may have about your treatment, and how often you really use the medication so he or she can plan the treatment that's best for you.

▶ WHAT CAUSES IT

Experts are still trying to identify the culprits behind eczema. While the causes aren't fully understood, allergies, dry skin and low levels of a skin-protecting protein may play a role.

▶ SYMPTOMS TO WATCH FOR

Small, itchy bumps that may leak fluid when scratched; dry, itchy, red to brownish grey skin patches or areas of thick, scaly skin, especially on the hands, feet, arms, neck, face and chest, and behind the knees.

▶ LATEST THINKING

While many experts have traditionally believed that allergies trigger eczema, there's evidence that a genetic quirk that makes skin fragile could be behind many eczema cases. Researchers in Ireland and Scotland have found a lack of filaggrin, a compound that normally makes the skin's outer layer watertight, in up to half of adults and children with eczema. The result is that the skin dries out, and particles of dust, pollen—virtually anything—from the outside can creep in, causing irritation. While experts continue investigating this intriguing clue, researchers say it underscores the importance of protecting eczema-prone skin by slathering on moisturisers.

Emphysema and chronic bronchitis

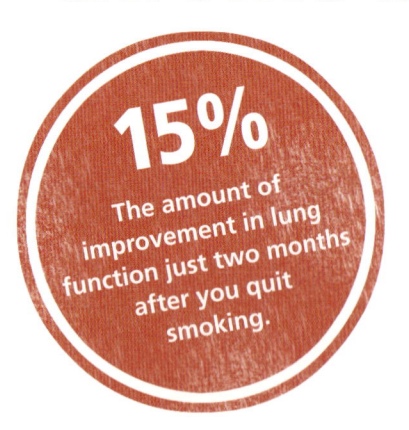

15% The amount of improvement in lung function just two months after you quit smoking.

The best thing you can do to avoid emphysema and chronic bronchitis—two types of chronic obstructive pulmonary disease (COPD)—is avoid tobacco smoke, dust and fumes. Although it sounds rare and obscure, COPD is shockingly common. In some nations, it's the fourth leading cause of death, right behind heart disease, cancer and stroke. Emphysema weakens the air sacs in your lungs so that they can't force out stale air, leaving little room for your next fresh, oxygen-rich inhalation. Chronic bronchitis occurs when damaged bronchial linings produce excess mucus and can't remove it. COPD makes you cough, wheeze and feel incredibly tired; it also raises your risk of lung infections.

How to prevent flare-ups

If you already have emphysema, try these strategies to help you avoid wheezing episodes.

Get a yearly flu vaccination Viral and bacterial infections can make breathing problems worse. This vaccine can cut the risk of influenza among people with COPD by up to 81 per cent.

Get a pneumonia vaccine at least once COPD raises your risk of life-threatening forms of pneumonia.

Use an over-the-counter mucus thinner Medications such as guaifenesin and acetylcysteine dilute mucus and make it easier to cough up, cutting flare-ups by 20 per cent.

Use an inhaler with one or two medications A long-acting bronchodilator or an inhaled corticosteroid can each cut flare-ups by 20 per cent. Combining the two cuts your odds by 25 per cent.

Follow an exercise routine Work with your doctor or physiotherapist. Half an hour of exercise most days of the week can ease breathlessness significantly.

Key prevention strategies

Quit smoking Smoking cigarettes, cigars and pipes causes an estimated 85 per cent of COPD cases. Over a lifetime, half of all smokers will develop this debilitating lung disease. Quitting is the most effective way for smokers to reduce their risk. But to be honest, if you already have COPD quitting won't reverse lung damage that's already been done, but experts say it's still crucial. By kicking the habit, you may cut future declines in lung function by half.

Avoid second-hand smoke Passive smoking exposes you to chemicals and particles that irritate your lungs. Living with a smoker raises your own odds of developing COPD by 55 per cent. Working in a smoky environment, such as a bar, raised risk 36 per cent in one study. New legislation in Australia now prevents people from smoking in pubs and bars, but it's essential that you also insist on smoke-free air in your home and car.

Bad air at work? Ask for a respirator Chemical fumes as well as dust from grain, cotton, wood or mining products can raise your risk for lung damage whether or not you smoke. A face mask fitted with special air filters could save your lungs.

Keep the air at home clean If you already have COPD, you can cut your risk of an attack by avoiding fumes from paint as well as perfumes and the smell of burning candles and incense. Even cooking odours can make you cough or wheeze. Keep the humidity in your home between 40 and 50 per cent (you can buy a device that measures humidity from most hardware shops) and check air filters on your heating and airconditioning systems regularly—as often as monthly—and clean or change them when they look dirty so that the air stays irritant free.

Prevention boosters

Skip bacon, frankfurters, salami and other cured meats
Eating cured meats at least once a day raised smokers' risk of emphysema and other progressive lung problems 2.64 times higher than that of those who ate these foods only a few times a year, according to a Harvard School of Public Health study of nearly 43,000 men. Nitrites in these meats generate cell-damaging particles, called free radicals, in the body. People with higher levels of free radicals are more susceptible to lung damage.

Eat more fibre Getting about 27 g of fibre a day translated into a 15 per cent drop in risk for emphysema and other lung problems compared to eating just 9.5 g a day, according to a study of nearly 12,000 people. Those who got a lot of their fibre from fruit cut their risk further—by 27 per cent. The reason may be that fibre simply acts as a marker for a diet that includes more fruit and vegetables. It's possible that the real protectors are the anti-oxidants in fresh fruit and vegetables, which protect lungs from free-radical damage.

▶ **WHAT CAUSES IT**
Smoking and chronic exposure to fumes and dust. Occasionally, genes play a role.

▶ **SYMPTOMS TO WATCH FOR**
A cough that brings up yellowish, grey or green mucus; chest soreness or tightness, or a tickling feeling when you breathe; infections, chills and a low fever; tiredness; wheezing; sore throat; and sinus congestion.

▶ **LATEST THINKING**
A new twist on standard breathing exercises makes exhaling even easier for people with emphysema. US researchers at the University of Michigan have found that people with emphysema who learned to play the mouth organ improved their breathing significantly.

Erectile dysfunction

70% The amount by which you can reduce your risk if you stay physically active in middle age and beyond.

Before 1998, it was quite rare to hear anyone speak openly about erectile dysfunction (ED) or impotence. Then Viagra arrived on the scene, and suddenly everything changed. Overnight, conversations about the ability to have and maintain an erection became commonplace. Although there are now five medications approved to treat ED, including two injectable agents, simple lifestyle changes are still the best way to try to prevent it occurring in the first place.

Key prevention strategies

Eat like the ancients The Mediterranean diet is rich in healthy monounsaturated fats from foods such as olive oil. It's also loaded with fruit, vegetables, nuts, legumes, whole grains and fish and is relatively low in red meat. When Italian researchers compared 100 men with ED to 100 men without it, they found that those whose diets closely matched a Mediterranean diet were significantly less likely to be impotent. The reason, researchers speculate, is probably the anti-inflammatory effect of the diet. Inflammation contributes to plaque buildup, narrowing blood vessels, and narrow vessels mean less blood gets through to the penis, making an erection less likely.

Get into sport Exercise isn't just good for your muscles; it's also good for an erection. Men who become more physically active in middle age drastically reduce their risk of impotence by 70 per cent compared with men who stay on the couch. In fact, physical activity—no matter what kind—reduced the risk of impotence even more than quitting smoking, losing weight or drinking less alcohol.

Stop smoking If the idea of protecting your heart and lungs isn't enough to make you stop smoking, perhaps the threat of

DRUGS THAT PREVENT DISEASE

Although medications such as sildenafil (Viagra) are designed to be used on an as-needed basis, preliminary studies suggest that taking them every night for a year could actually prevent impotence once you stop using the medication. German researchers had 112 impotent men take either 50 mg of sildenafil every night or 50–100 mg as needed for a year. After six months with no treatment, 58.3 per cent of the men who took nightly sildenafil had normal erections without any medication, compared to only 8.2 per cent of those who used the tablet as needed. One medication, tadalafil (Cialis), is already approved for daily use in the US, but not as yet in Australia, New Zealand or South Africa.

sexual embarrassment is. One study of 7684 Chinese men found that smoking probably accounted for about one in five cases of ED. The more you smoke, the more likely you are to have problems. The study found that smoking 20 cigarettes a day increased the risk by 60 per cent compared to not smoking at all. The reason could be that smoking constricts blood vessels and contributes to the buildup of plaque, both of which reduce blood flow—which obviously results in trouble getting and maintaining an erection. Smoking also reduces levels of nitric oxide, a chemical compound that keeps blood vessels, including those in the penis, dilated. Even one day without a cigarette can improve erections.

Prevention boosters

Maintain normal blood sugar levels Half of all men with diabetes have erection problems—twice the rate of men without the disease. (See 'Diabetes', starting on page 164, to find out how to prevent Type 2 diabetes.)

Take medication The three most popular choices include: sildenafil (Viagra), tadalafil (Cialis) and vardenafil (Levitra). All work by increasing levels of nitric oxide, the chemical that helps dilate blood vessels in the penis and keep them dilated so you can have and maintain an erection. The major difference between the three is how long they take to begin working. Vardenafil works the fastest, with one study finding it began working in as few as 10 minutes and remained effective for up to 12 hours. However, if you're away for a romantic weekend, consider tadalafil: studies find that one dose continues working for up to 36 hours.

▶ WHAT CAUSES IT

Anything that affects the health of blood vessels—heart disease, diabetes, high blood pressure or smoking—can affect a man's ability to have an erection. Stress and relationship problems are other causes.

▶ SYMPTOMS TO WATCH FOR

The inability to have or maintain an erection.

▶ LATEST THINKING

Men with impotence have a greater risk of developing Parkinson's disease. Researchers evaluating the medical records of 32,616 medical professionals found those with a history of ED were nearly three times more likely to develop Parkinson's than those who didn't have erection problems. The link seems to be related to damage in the autonomic nervous system, which regulates functions such as breathing and digestion. Identifying the underlying reasons for the link could theoretically lead to ways to prevent Parkinson's disease.

Even one day without a cigarette can improve erections.

Fatigue

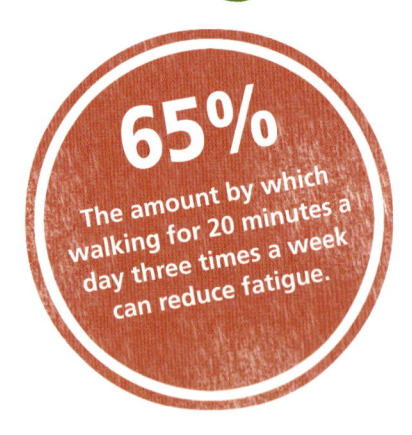

65% The amount by which walking for 20 minutes a day three times a week can reduce fatigue.

Fatigue is classically characterised by a chronic lack of energy. When you're fatigued, you may not need to sleep, but you don't feel like doing much else. Your brain feels muddy, and your muscles feel like lead. Fatigue can be the result of a condition such as depression, cancer, diabetes, fibromyalgia or congestive heart failure, but about one in four people experience fatigue that's not related to any medical problem.

Key prevention strategies

Get a good night's sleep It's the most obvious way to keep your natural energy up. If you're tossing and turning, waking up in the middle of the night or waking up too early, see 'Insomnia', starting on page 228. If you snore, also read 'Snoring', starting on page 292. Obstructive sleep apnoea, which is associated with severe snoring, is a common cause of daytime tiredness.

Hit the walking trail As little as 10 minutes of brisk walking helps power up energy levels more effectively—and for much longer—than eating a chocolate bar. Just 20 minutes of walking three times a week can increase energy levels by 20 per cent and reduce fatigue by 65 per cent.

Eat a high-fibre breakfast One study found that people who started their mornings with a high-fibre meal, such as muesli or baked beans on wholegrain toast, were more alert throughout the morning, probably because these meals take longer to digest than, say, a bowl of cornflakes or a muffin, so blood sugar levels remain steadier. It also helps to include some protein with breakfast—and every other meal, too.

Good breakfast options, then, are wholegrain toast with a slice of cheese or a teaspoon of peanut butter and a piece of fruit, a bowl of high-fibre cereal (aim for at least 5 g of fibre per serve) with skim milk, or a bowl of porridge sprinkled with freshly ground linseeds. For an afternoon snack, instead of a chocolate bar or chips from a vending machine, choose a small handful of almonds, trail mix or wholegrain crackers with peanut butter.

Get your blood tested Common causes of fatigue that a blood test can reveal are low iron levels (you don't have to be anaemic to be low on iron) and hypothyroidism, which occurs when the thyroid gland doesn't make enough thyroid hormone. Both are common in women and often go undetected. One US study found that about 16 per cent of women had low iron levels.

Prevention boosters

Tip your head up to the sun Bright light—whether from the sun or a full-spectrum fluorescent light designed to mimic the sun's rays—pumps up alertness levels like a shot of adrenaline. You don't have to sunbathe; in one Japanese study, women who sat near a sunny window for 30 minutes reported feeling more alert than when they sat in a darkened room for the same time period. Sunlight boosts activity in brain regions associated with alertness and dampens levels of the so-called 'sleep hormone', melatonin.

Sip small coffees Too much caffeine can backfire by keeping you up at night, but sipping just 60 ml of coffee every hour from about 10 am to 2 pm boosts alertness levels, thanks to caffeine's ability to block a sleep-inducing brain chemical called adenosine.

Use the power of peppermint If you need a quick pick-me-up, the smell of peppermint may do the trick. Purchase peppermint essential oil from a health food shop or pharmacy and rub a drop between your hands once every hour, or place a few drops on a tissue and breathe in the scent.

Find a new hobby Boredom and loneliness are twin contributors to depression, which is a major cause of fatigue. Join a book club, a bowling team, a knitting or sewing club—anything that gets you out of the house, helps you meet new people and gives you something interesting to do.

▶ WHAT CAUSES IT

The most common reason for fatigue is lack of sleep, but it can also be a side effect of illness, cancer treatment or medical conditions such as fibromyalgia, chronic fatigue syndrome, diabetes, lupus, multiple sclerosis, low iron levels or hypothyroidism. Depression and boredom may also contribute. Certain medications, either prescription or over-the-counter, can have fatigue as a side effect as well.

▶ SYMPTOMS TO WATCH FOR

Lack of energy and the inability to concentrate.

▶ LATEST THINKING

In women with breast cancer, fatigue from chemotherapy can last up to six months or more after the treatment ends. But a recent review of studies shows that good old exercise is effective at relieving even cancer-related fatigue.

Flatulence

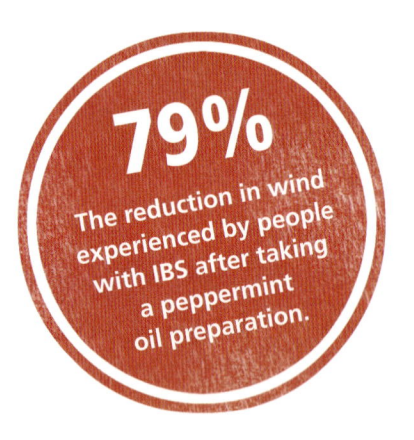

79% The reduction in wind experienced by people with IBS after taking a peppermint oil preparation.

Flatulence is hardly a disease. In fact, everyone passes wind from 14 to 23 times a day (women emit as much as men), but most of the time it's odourless. However, knowing that doesn't make passing wind in company any less embarrassing. If smelly emissions are giving you grief, follow our advice.

Key prevention strategies

Go easy on beans and 'windy' vegetables Dried beans are very good for you, but wind is often part of the deal. The culprit is an indigestible sugar called raffinose, also found in cabbage, brussels sprouts, broccoli and asparagus. Humans lack an enzyme needed to break down raffinose, so beneficial bacteria in the intestinal tract do the work of consuming this sugar. The bacteria emit gas, so within a few hours, you do the same. US experts say that by gradually increasing the amount of beans and similar foods in your diet, you can minimise this side effect.

Minimise bean gas Draining and rinsing canned beans before use gets rid of some of the gas-causing raffinose. If you're cooking dried beans, always soak them first. Add $1/8$ teaspoon of bicarbonate of soda to the soaking water to leach out more raffinose, and rinse soaked beans well. Never cook beans in their rinse water.

Eat slowly It's normal to swallow some air when you're eating—accounting for half the wind you pass—but gulping down food or drinking through a straw adds to this considerably. So slow down and cut back on chewing gum and hard lollies, which also increase the amount of air you swallow.

When wind is a symptom

Sometimes intestinal gas is a sign of a food intolerance or digestive condition. Among the most common are:

Lactose intolerance If you have wind and abdominal pain after eating dairy products or drinking milk, you may lack the enzyme lactase, needed to break down the sugar, called lactose, in these foods. A simple breath test can diagnose this problem. The solution is lactase supplements, lactase drops to add to milk and lactose-reduced dairy products.

Gluten intolerance If your body can't digest gluten, a protein found in wheat and some other grains, you may experience gas, bloating, weight loss, oily and foul-smelling stools, and other symptoms. The only solution is to avoid gluten, but see your doctor first for a diagnosis.

Irritable bowel syndrome (IBS) If you emit normal amounts of wind but feel extremely bloated on a regular basis and have bouts of diarrhoea and/or constipation, you may have IBS. Dietary changes, stress reduction and medications may help; discuss options with your doctor.

Check your reaction to these major wind producers Other foods contain tough-to-digest sugars that often become food for gassy bacteria in your gut. Everyone reacts differently, so don't write off a nutritious fruit or vegetable unless you're sure it's causing a reaction. Prime culprits include foods high in the sugar fructose, such as dates, grapes, apples and pears, as well as foods that contain sorbitol, such as apples, pears, peaches and plums.

Prevention boosters

Opt for still water over soda water All those bubbles in soda water and soft drinks contain gas, and you swallow a lot of it when you sip a carbonated drink. Switching from the fizzy stuff to still water helps. (This tip includes beer and champagne, too.)

Have rice instead Starchy side dishes such as potatoes, noodles made from wheat flour (that's most pasta) and corn produce wind when they're digested in your large intestine. Rice won't—it's just about the only starch that is completely absorbed in the small intestine, making it a more comfortable choice if you're bothered by excessive wind.

Skip low-carbohydrate sweets Many 'sugar-free' and low-carb chewing gums, lollies, chocolates, biscuits, cake mixes and even pancake syrups are sweetened with sugar alcohols such as sorbitol and mannitol. When bacteria in your intestinal tract break them down, the result can be tummy rumbling and windy emissions.

Switch antacids Using bicarbonate of soda or an antacid containing sodium bicarbonate to ease heartburn and acid indigestion could backfire, loudly. Experts caution that while it's busy neutralising stomach acid, it produces plenty of carbon dioxide—some of which may exit through your intestinal tract. As little as $1/2$ teaspoon of bicarb could produce enough gas to give you wind. Look for another type of antacid, such as one that contains calcium carbonate, which neutralises acid, or ask your doctor or pharmacist about H2 blockers, which reduce acid production.

Season beans to get rid of gas Researchers from India report that adding garlic and ginger (either fresh or dried) to beans while they cook can reduce gas when you eat them.

▶ WHAT CAUSES IT

Gas is produced when bacteria in your colon ferment indigestible carbohydrates in high-fibre foods and fibre supplements. Lactose intolerance, gluten intolerance, irritable bowel syndrome, ulcerative colitis and Crohn's disease can also cause wind. So can antibiotics, some diabetes medications, laxatives, weight-loss drugs, medications to help you stop smoking and gastric bypass surgery. Eating foods sweetened with sugar alcohols such as sorbitol and mannitol can also cause cramps and excess wind.

▶ SYMPTOMS TO WATCH FOR

Passing wind, sharp abdominal cramps and bloating.

▶ LATEST THINKING

If you have irritable bowel syndrome (IBS) and flatulence, meditation may help. In a small study of 16 people, twice-daily relaxation-response meditation for 15 minutes improved flatulence and belching over a two-week period.

Flu

75% The drop in your risk if you take Tamiflu as soon as someone in your household shows signs of the flu.

The odds of catching the flu range from 5 to 20 per cent each winter, depending on the virulence of the circulating virus. That sounds low, but once you've had a miserable case of the flu, you'll be motivated to tilt those odds a little more in your favour. Start by doing all you can to keep your immunity strong: eat a healthy diet and get plenty of sleep and physical activity. Beyond that, the following suggestions may help to stack the deck in your favour.

Key prevention strategies

Get vaccinated The flu isn't just miserable; it can be dangerous, especially in older people. In a 10-year study of thousands of elderly men and women, having a flu vaccine cut the risk of being hospitalised with flu-like illnesses by 27 per cent and reduced the risk of dying from the flu by 48 per cent. This is not a perfect vaccine, and it works better some years than others. At best, it protects against 70 to 90 per cent of the flu viruses being passed around. But at worst, it may provide only 40 to 50 per cent immunity. However, those are still far better odds than you'd have with no flu shot.

Definitely get vaccinated if you're over the age of 65, if you have a medical condition that lowers your immunity or affects your lung function, or if you live in a household with anyone on that list (to protect yourself and them).

Take an antiviral drug asap People who took the prescription drug oseltamivir (Tamiflu) or zanamivir (Relenza) after someone in their household caught the flu significantly reduced their risk of getting it themselves in one major study. Among

Vaccination know-how

The flu vaccine works by introducing a tiny dose of several dead flu viruses into your body. The antibodies you develop to fight them help to protect you if you're exposed to the real thing. The more antibodies, the better the protection. The following four factors can affect the flu vaccine's effectiveness:

Stress Feeling stressed-out 8 to 10 days after having a flu injection could suppress your immune response to the vaccine by 12 to 17 per cent.

A fever If you have a fever on the day of your injection, reschedule. Fever is a sign that your immune system is already fighting an infection, so don't overload it.

Sleep Getting a few good nights' sleep before the vaccine could boost your antibody production by 50 per cent.

Tai chi or qigong US researchers found that people who performed one of these two activities for an hour three times a week for 20 weeks produced significantly more antibodies after getting a flu vaccine.

people who took oseltamivir, 81 per cent didn't get sick; among those who took zanamivir, 75 per cent stayed well. People who got a placebo were five to seven times more likely to develop flu symptoms than those who took the antiviral drugs. The potential downside is an upset stomach and a depleted wallet—the Australian Government doesn't pay for the treatment, though it may be cheaper than losing time off work due to sickness.

Wash your hands often The flu virus can survive for hours on hard surfaces such as metal, glass and plastic—and even on cloth, paper and tissues. Your best defence is washing your hands, and the more you do it the better. Lather vigorously for at least 20 seconds to get rid of all the germs. Choose hand washing over antibacterial hand wipes and gels when you have the option; relying on rubs and wipes could allow bugs to build up on your hands if you use them too many times in a row without washing.

Carry the right alcohol-based hand sanitiser Viruses are hard to kill; even some alcohol-based hand sanitisers won't kill them if the alcohol concentration isn't high enough. (Hand washing doesn't kill viruses; it simply washes them away. That's why you don't need antibacterial soap.) Buy a sanitiser that contains 60 to 95 per cent ethyl alcohol. Rub the gel or foam on all sides of your hands, then rub your hands together vigorously until they're dry.

Prevention boosters

Sneeze smart Wipes impregnated with anti-viral agents aren't a substitute for hand washing, but they could cut the number of virus particles on your children's hands and may even reduce the number lurking on surfaces in your home. Also, teach your children to sneeze into the crook of their elbow, not their hand.

Move your exercise routine indoors In a small Canadian study, people who exercised most days of the week for three months had fewer flu symptoms and higher levels of flu-fighting immunoglobulin A in their bloodstreams compared to people who didn't exercise. We know that exercising can be a challenge when the weather is cold and wet. If that's the case, try following an exercise DVD at home, or do old-fashioned calisthenics such as sit-ups and jumping jacks, or get that exercise bike back into action.

▶ WHAT CAUSES IT

Dozens of strains of the influenza virus. These viruses are extremely infectious because they're always mutating. This means that even though you develop antibodies to the flu if you're infected, your immune system won't recognise and fight off a new strain.

▶ SYMPTOMS TO WATCH FOR

A sudden high fever, severe headache, aches and pains, fatigue, chest discomfort, coughing and sometimes a sore throat, stuffy nose, and sneezing.

▶ LATEST THINKING

To avoid flu over the holidays, don't fly. In 2002, the flu season started several weeks later than usual and peaked in March instead of January or February. US researchers at Harvard University suspect the cause was the 27 per cent drop in air travel after the terrorist attacks of 11 September. Exposure to airport crowds and germs on aeroplane surfaces plus hours spent in close quarters can increase your risk of catching the flu virus.

Gallstones

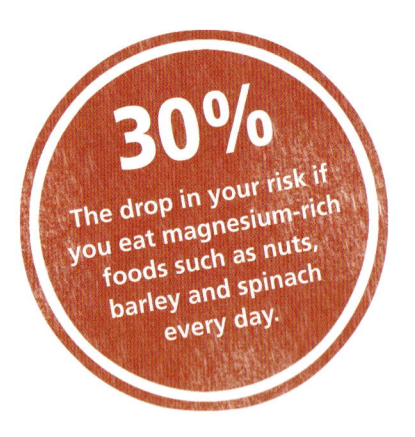

30% The drop in your risk if you eat magnesium-rich foods such as nuts, barley and spinach every day.

Built from layers of cholesterol or calcium salts, gallstones grow slowly and silently in your gall bladder or bile ducts the way a pearl grows inside an oyster. While most gallstones never cause a problem, some trigger incredibly painful attacks and ultimately have to be treated with surgery or medication. Fortunately, there's a lot you can do to lower your chances of developing these painful stones and to prevent their return if you've already had them.

Key prevention strategies

Aim for a healthy weight and a trim waist Being overweight or obese more than triples your odds for gallstones; carrying extra kilos around your middle is especially dangerous. In a Harvard School of Public Health study of more than 42,000 women, those whose waistlines measured 92 cm or more were twice as likely to have gallstones that required surgery compared to women whose waists measured less than 66 cm. If you're not within your healthy weight range now, losing extra kilos slowly and steadily is the best way to protect yourself. Don't crash diet; losing more than 1.5 kg a week raises gallstone risk, while losing 0.5–0.75 kg a week doesn't seem to.

Avoid yo-yo dieting at all costs The more weight you gain and lose repeatedly, the higher your risk of gallstones becomes. US researchers found that men who lost and regained as few as 2–4 kg in five years had a 21 per cent higher risk of gallstones compared to those who maintained the same weight. Men whose weight fluctuated by 5–8 kg raised their odds by 38 per cent. Weight-cycling 9 kg or more increased risk by 78 per cent.

Foods that fight gallstones

A diet rich in magnesium can lower gallstone risk by 30 per cent, according to a US study from the University of Kentucky. Men with the lowest risk got an average of 454 mg a day from supplements plus food. A standard multivitamin has about 100 mg. The following nine foods deliver a healthy dose of magnesium:

Almonds, unblanched	1 cup	370 mg
Buckwheat flour, wholemeal	1 cup	265 mg
Oat bran, raw	1 cup	220 mg
Tahini (sesame paste)	¼ cup	200 mg
Pumpkin seeds	¼ cup	180 mg
Pearled barley, raw	1 cup	180 mg
Brazil nuts	10 nuts	175 mg
Spinach, cooked	1 cup	150 mg
Burghul, soaked	1 cup	100 mg

Why is yo-yo dieting so risky? While dieting, you may not be eating enough fat to keep your gall bladder active; this may allow cholesterol to sit long enough to begin forming stones. Meanwhile, when you regain weight, you may develop insulin resistance because most of the kilos you put back on after a diet are body fat (not muscle), and body fat increases the risk of this condition. Changes in body chemistry that lead to insulin resistance also increase gallstone risk, according to researchers.

Exercise more Getting 2 to 3 hours of physical activity per week can lower your risk of gallstones by 20 per cent.

Focus on good fats Cutting out too much fat could cause problems, but regularly eating a little fat helps prevent gallstones by prompting the gall bladder to empty, pumping bile acids into your digestive system to help digest your meal. It's the type of fat that matters. In studies from Denmark and France, people who ate more saturated fat were more likely to develop gallstones, so opt for 'healthy' fats, found in olive and canola oils, nuts, and fatty fish.

Cut back on sugar and add fibre Eating 40 g of sugar a day, the amount in 8 teaspoons of sugar or a serve of sweetened breakfast cereal plus a couple of biscuits after lunch, doubles gallstone risk, according to research. Experts think this is because of an increase in cholesterol in the bloodstream, which is triggered by the surge of insulin that occurs when blood sugar rises. Eat a high-fibre diet, on the other hand, and you'll protect against gallstones by whisking cholesterol (found in bile acids) out of your body.

Prevention boosters

Enjoy coffee A cup or two of coffee in the morning could cut your risk of gallstones by 40 per cent, according to researchers who tracked the gall bladder health of more than 46,000 men for a decade. Components in coffee stimulate the release of bile acids, and lower levels of stone-forming cholesterol in bile fluid.

Toast your gall bladder's health One drink a day can lower gallstone risk by 27 per cent. Alcohol may help by raising 'good' HDL cholesterol, which removes 'bad' LDL (found in gallstones) out of your body. Beer, wine and spirits are equally protective.

▶ WHAT CAUSES IT

An imbalance of the 'ingredients' in bile acids, the digestive juices that break down dietary fat, or incomplete emptying of your gall bladder. Either problem can allow cholesterol particles from bile acids to group together, forming stones.

▶ SYMPTOMS TO WATCH FOR

Indigestion, which may be worse after you eat a high-fat meal. Also wind, bloating, sudden steady pain in your right upper abdomen, nausea and vomiting.

▶ LATEST THINKING

Research suggests that people of European ancestry have a 10 per cent chance of having a gene variation that increases gallstone risk. Carrying the gene doubles or even triples the risk by causing the liver to pump extra cholesterol (a major component of gallstones) into the gall bladder. But experts say that eating well and exercising can prevent gallstones from ever causing trouble.

Glaucoma

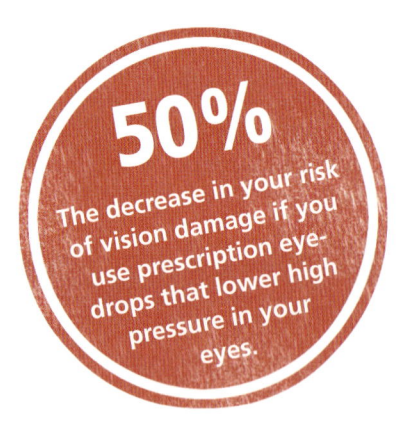

50%
The decrease in your risk of vision damage if you use prescription eye-drops that lower high pressure in your eyes.

Glaucoma slowly destroys the delicate fibres of the optic nerve, making it impossible for your eyes to tell your brain what they're seeing. The result is a loss of sight. The damage usually begins decades before you realise something's wrong, as pressure within your eyes builds and begins erasing peripheral vision. Untreated, glaucoma leaves you with tunnel vision—and then darkness. Regular vision checks can pick up dangerously high eye pressure early, and prescription eye-drops and surgery can help bring it under control.

Key prevention strategies

Make sure you get your eyes tested regularly Everyone should have comprehensive eye exams every two to four years from the age of 40, and every one to two years after 65. Your optometrist or eye doctor will dilate your pupils to look for signs of optic nerve damage, measure pressure levels in your eyes and check the thickness of your cornea (a thin cornea is associated with higher glaucoma risk). You should also have a visual field test to check for tiny blind spots in your vision.

Know your risk While anyone can develop glaucoma, your risk is significantly higher if other people in your family have it, if you're over the age of 60 or if you're of African or Asian descent and over the age of forty. Diabetes, high blood pressure, nearsightedness, severe eye injuries and long-term use of steroid medications may also increase your risk.

If you're at increased risk, catching problems early should be a top priority. You may need more frequent eye examinations as recommended by your doctor.

Use prescription eye-drops If the pressure inside your eyes is elevated, using

The coffee controversy

Glaucoma specialists don't all agree, but several studies suggest that a serious coffee habit could raise eye pressure and your risk of optic nerve damage. Harvard researchers found that drinking five cups a day increased glaucoma risk by 61 per cent in a long-term study of more than 76,000 women. Meanwhile, Australian researchers who studied the eye health of more than 3600 people found that the more coffee they drank, the higher their eye pressure. Some studies suggest that caffeine is the culprit, but in other research, tea and caffeinated soft drinks seemed to have little effect—whereas coffee did.

pressure-lowering eye-drops every day could save your vision. In a landmark study of 1686 people with high eye pressure but no signs of optic nerve damage, those who used drops cut their risk of damage over the next five years in half. If eye-drops don't work, or if your optic nerve loss is progressing despite the use of drops, your doctor may suggest surgery to help lower your eye pressure.

Control diabetes Researchers from the Harvard School of Public Health found that having Type 2 diabetes raises your risk of developing glaucoma by 70 per cent. Experts suspect that diabetes may somehow raise eye pressure or make the optic nerve more vulnerable to damage. If you have diabetes, keep your blood sugar under control and have your eyes checked once a year for glaucoma and other diabetes-related vision problems.

Prevention boosters

Move it! It's no substitute for eye exams and eye-drops, but physical activity is a great add-on strategy for lowering glaucoma risk. Studies show that exercise that raises your heart rate—walking, swimming or even vigorous housework—for about 20 minutes can lower your eye pressure by four points immediately afterwards. Exercising four times a week can keep your pressure lower throughout the day. (If you use eye-drops, keep using them unless your doctor advises otherwise.) Avoid moves that involve lowering your head below heart level (such as the downward-facing dog position in yoga or any exercise involving bending over); they can raise pressure.

Quit smoking When Greek researchers reviewed seven glaucoma studies, they found that smokers were 37 per cent more likely to develop glaucoma than nonsmokers. Not all studies have found an association, but if you've been told you're at risk for glaucoma or already have it, it's just another good reason to kick the habit.

Relax and refresh There's some evidence that emotional stress raises fluid pressure inside the eyes and that relaxation techniques can reverse that trend. In one German study of people with glaucoma, those who did guided imagery exercises to relax reduced their eye pressure significantly. Again, it's no substitute for drops if you need them, but it could help.

WHAT CAUSES IT
Untreated elevation of intra-ocular pressure. Pressure can build if your eyes' drainage system doesn't work efficiently. Some people with apparently normal pressure also develop glaucoma.

SYMPTOMS TO WATCH FOR
Usually, none. In advanced glaucoma, you will develop tunnel vision. A less common form of glaucoma, called acute angle-closure glaucoma, causes very sudden blurred vision, halos around lights, red eyes, severe eye pain and nausea and vomiting, all due to a rapid, dramatic increase in eye pressure. This is a medical emergency.

LATEST THINKING
Glaucoma is a warning sign of heart trouble. When researchers followed the health of 4092 Barbados residents for five years, they found that those with glaucoma were 38 per cent more likely to have fatal heart disease. The connection could be underlying health problems that lead to both. If you have glaucoma, keep tabs on your blood pressure and cholesterol levels, too.

Gout

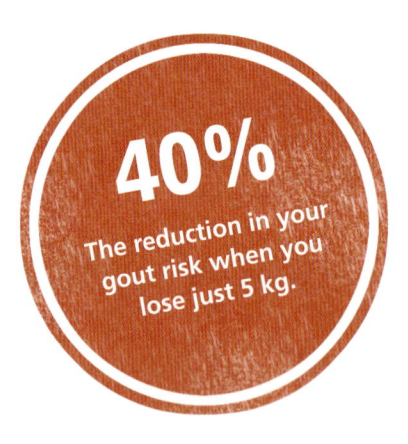

40%
The reduction in your gout risk when you lose just 5 kg.

Gout is part of a growing epidemic involving excruciating joint pain in an ever-increasing number of men and women, thanks to the developed world's obesity problem—and to the fact that more people are ingesting food, drinks and medications that raise levels of uric acid in the blood. Too much leads to the development of crystals that collect in joints. Here's how to cope with gout, or to simply avoid it.

Key prevention strategies

Maintain a healthy weight Gaining 15 kg could more than double your risk of developing gout, according to researchers from Massachusetts General Hospital in the US. Losing just 5 kg lowered the odds by 40 per cent.

Sweat a little In a California study of 228 men, those who were leaner and fitter were less likely to develop gout than men who had only one of those healthy attributes. In the study, men who ran around 6 km a day lowered their risk by 50 per cent, but doing any form of aerobic exercise—such as brisk walking, swimming or cycling—for any amount of time will help to some extent.

Limit red meat or seafood A daily serving of red meat raised the likelihood of developing gout by 45 per cent in a study of 228 men conducted by US researchers. Meanwhile, men who ate the most seafood (including fatty fish) increased their risk by 51 per cent in another study. Why? Purines, found in foods (game and organ meats, and seafood, including anchovies, sardines and scallops, have especially high levels) and in our body tissues. When purines break down, blood levels of uric acid rise.

Instead, try chicken or legumes, and limit meat and seafood to less than three 100-g serves a week. (If you don't have problems with gout, it's a good idea to keep eating oily fish.)

Eat dark red cherries Cherries are a traditional remedy for gout, and now science reveals why they work. When 10 volunteers breakfasted on 45 dark red cherries for two days, researchers at the University of California discovered that levels of uric acid in their blood fell by an impressive 30 points. Black, yellow and red sour cherries are effective, too. Just 1½ cups a day is all you need.

Include soy foods in your daily diet Based on current research, people with gout may benefit from limiting animal protein in their diet, because it contains purines, but soy foods are a different story altogether. Several studies show that soy reduces uric acid, making it a great way to include healthy protein in your daily diet and combat gout at the same time. Try to eat soy foods such as tofu or soy milk at least twice a week, in place of meat.

Check your hypertension medication Studies suggest that blood pressure-lowering diuretics can push gout risk three and a half times higher than normal. Older, 'thiazide' diuretics may raise risk the most. If your gout is a problem and you already take one of these medications, ask your doctor about an alternative.

Drink wine instead of beer A little alcohol may protect your heart, but it also raises gout risk. In one study, men who drank two or more 375-ml beers a day increased their odds 2.6 times more than those who abstained. But two small glasses of wine did not raise risk. Beer contains higher levels of purines than most wines.

Skip sweetened soft drinks Sugary soft drinks, iced teas and fruit punches raise gout risk just as much as alcohol does. Fructose seems to increase uric acid levels, so opt for water or herbal tea.

Prevention boosters

Enjoy your coffee Four or five small cups of coffee a day cut gout risk by 40 per cent compared to not drinking it at all, according to a US study of 228 men. Decaffeinated coffee lowered risk, too, but tea had no effect, suggesting that a strong anti-oxidant in coffee, called chlorogenic acid, is the ingredient at work.

Have low-fat milk and yogurt Two daily serves of dairy can lower gout risk by about 45 per cent—as long as it's low fat. Proteins in dairy called casein and lactalbumin may protect against gout by promoting the excretion of uric acid in urine. Low-fat dairy foods also help with weight loss, which may help you avoid getting gout.

▶ WHAT CAUSES IT

High blood levels of uric acid, which crystallises in joints, causing inflammation and pain. Certain foods and beverages raise uric acid levels, and some medications may make it more difficult for your body to excrete it or may increase production.

▶ SYMPTOMS TO WATCH FOR

Sudden, severe pain; redness and tenderness in joints. Gout often begins in a big toe or knee.

▶ LATEST THINKING

People with gout have a 20 per cent higher risk for heart attack than people who don't have it, according to new research. The connection may be inflammation: gout can trigger ongoing inflammation in the body, and inflammatory compounds may also trigger blood clots that can lead to a heart attack. If you have gout, be extra vigilant about your cholesterol, blood pressure and blood sugar to help protect your heart. People with gout also have an increased risk of kidney failure.

Gum disease

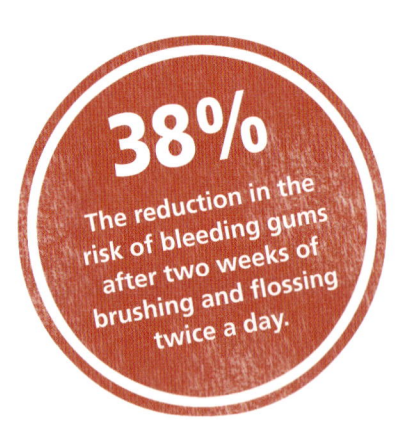

38% The reduction in the risk of bleeding gums after two weeks of brushing and flossing twice a day.

Gum disease can affect more than just your mouth. Heart disease, diabetes, pneumonia and chronic obstructive pulmonary disease are all linked to gum disease, probably because of the low-level inflammation created as bacteria from your gums travel throughout your bloodstream.

Key prevention strategies

Floss frequently Flossing takes less than a minute, and it's one of the best ways to prevent bad breath. Here's how to make flossing easier.

- **Buy non-shredding monofilament floss** The only thing worse than food stuck between your teeth is floss stuck between your teeth.
- **Keep floss everywhere** At your desk, in your purse, in the bathroom (of course) and in the car glove box.
- **Buy minty floss** The fresh taste in your mouth is a bonus.
- **Use a battery-operated flosser** A 10-week study found that these flossers (available online) got rid of more plaque on molars, premolars and hard-to-reach back teeth than regular floss.
- **Ask for a demonstration** Although the process may seem obvious, there is a right and wrong way to floss. Ask your dentist or dental hygienist for a demonstration.

Rinse with an antibacterial mouthwash daily A study of 156 healthy volunteers found those who brushed their teeth and used either mouthwash containing antimicrobial chlorhexidine or cetylpyridinium chloride had lower scores on a test that measures plaque levels than those who brushed and flossed or only brushed.

Try a battery-powered toothbrush After six months of brushing—but not flossing—with an automated toothbrush, people who already had gum disease showed significantly less plaque in the morning and immediately after brushing than those using a regular toothbrush.

Quit smoking Not only is cigarette smoking a major risk factor for gum disease, but exposure to second-hand smoke can also increase your risk by up to 70 per cent.

Prevention boosters

Watch your blood sugar If you have diabetes, your risk of gum disease is already higher than it is for someone who doesn't have it. But if your diabetes isn't well controlled, you're in the danger zone: researchers find that people with poorly controlled diabetes have more inflammatory chemicals such as cytokines in their gums, which contribute to the formation of gum disease.

Eat foods high in vitamin C When researchers evaluated the link between diet and gum disease in 12,400 adults, they found that those who didn't get the recommended daily amount of vitamin C (45 mg, or about the amount in one orange) were nearly 20 per cent more likely to have gum disease than those who got more. Aim to include more vitamin C-rich foods, such as citrus fruit, red capsicum and broccoli, in your daily diet.

Up your calcium intake People who get less than 500 mg of calcium a day (1 cup of low-fat milk has about 350 mg) are nearly twice as likely to have gum disease as those who get at least three serves a day of calcium-rich foods (a serve is 1 cup of milk or a 200-g tub of yogurt, 100 g of sardines with bones or 50 g of cheddar cheese). Aim to get around 1000 mg of calcium a day from food. Calcium helps build density in the jaw bone, which supports the teeth, enabling it to withstand the bacterial attack from plaque.

Don't overdo the alcohol Researchers have found a direct correlation between the amount of alcohol people drink and their risk of gum disease. Ten drinks a week increased the risk by 10 per cent, 20 drinks increased it by 20 per cent, and so on. Heavy drinking may influence gum disease by affecting the immune system's ability to fight infection, interfering with blood clotting and leading to vitamin and protein deficiencies that impair healing.

If you have a dry mouth, see your doctor Dozens of medications, including some antidepressants and cold remedies, contain ingredients that dry up saliva production. Saliva helps clean teeth and hinders the growth of bacteria, so if your mouth is dry, you may be courting gum disease.

▶ WHAT CAUSES IT
Bacteria in plaque (a sticky, colourless film that forms on teeth) inflames gums. Over time, the inflammation can spread beneath the gumline.

▶ SYMPTOMS TO WATCH FOR
Gums that become reddish, swell or bleed easily; later, you may have loose teeth, bad breath and visibly receding gums.

▶ LATEST THINKING
New research suggests that obesity and gum disease may be related. When you're very overweight, fat cells release inflammatory chemicals that can contribute to numerous diseases, including gum disease.

Haemorrhoids

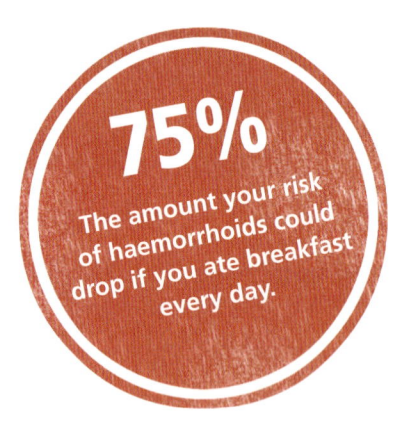

75% The amount your risk of haemorrhoids could drop if you ate breakfast every day.

Haemorrhoids are very common in middle age, and also in pregnancy. Over-the-counter treatments can help some people, but if the problem gets bad enough, you may need more serious help. In fact, haemorrhoids—marked by swollen and inflamed veins around the lower rectum—form a large portion of any colorectal surgeon's workload. They're also probably much more common than we know, since many people are, understandably, too embarrassed to admit they have them. Try to avoid the pain, itching and operating table by following the suggestions outlined below.

Key prevention strategies

Don't strain If you have to bear down to have a bowel movement, something's wrong. And if you've been sitting on the toilet for more than 5 minutes, get off. Straining is the primary cause of haemorrhoids, and a longer time spent on the toilet doesn't guarantee success. Instead, try again an hour or so later.

Soften your stool If you're straining, the problem could well be constipation. Keep things moving along by eating a high-fibre diet, and drink plenty of clear fluids to help the fibre move through the bowel. It's a good idea to slowly increase your daily fibre intake to avoid further constipation.

Focus on fibre When we asked a leading gastroenterologist what he recommends to his patients to prevent haemorrhoids, he answered with one word: linseed. It's one of the best sources of fibre you'll find, with nearly 3 g in 1 tablespoon. Add a couple of teaspoons of ground linseeds to muffin or pancake batter and sprinkle it over yogurt or breakfast cereal. Add freshly ground seeds to salads for added crunch, to pasta

Stop the burning

Once you have haemorrhoids, it can make going to the toilet difficult: you're afraid something might burst, not to mention the burning. Try these suggestions:

- **Avoid dry, scratchy toilet paper** Instead, try using moist towelettes to wipe after a bowel motion.
- **Use over-the-counter haemorrhoid cream or pads** They usually contain topical anti-inflammatories to decrease inflammation and anaesthetics to reduce pain.
- **Try a sitz bath** A sitz bath is a salt bath. Sit in about 15 cm of warm water for about 20 minutes. Or you can hold a cloth washer soaked in warm water over the sore area. Do this several times a day.

sauce for added bulk and even to a bowl of ice-cream. Fibre acts like a sponge in your intestinal tract, soaking up liquid and creating bulkier stools that are easier to move out of your body.

Get out of the chair A good way to get your bowels moving is to get yourself moving with regular exercise. It can be dancing, swimming, walking, golf—anything that gets the blood flowing. One study of 43 people with constipation found that those who walked every day for 30 minutes and did 11 minutes a day of weight-based exercises at home improved their rankings by nearly 35 per cent on a scale designed to evaluate constipation.

Drink up A major reason people get constipated and have a hard time moving their bowels is that their stools don't absorb enough water. Often it's because they're not drinking enough fluids, so make sure you always have water on hand throughout the day.

Go on a schedule Believe it or not, there's actually an ideal time for a bowel movement: about 30 minutes after you wake up, just after a cup of hot coffee or tea, and about 30 to 60 minutes after meals. So factor in bathroom time, even if nothing happens. What you're doing is training your bowels to 'let go' on time.

Prevention boosters

Change your position Modern toilets work against you when it comes to haemorrhoids, since they require you to sit instead of squat (squatting facilitates bowel movements). To get around this, try propping up your feet on a small footstool and pulling your knees up towards your chest.

Load up on berries Not only will the extra fibre help with constipation, but these fruits are also high in flavonoids, natural plant compounds that help reduce inflammation and strengthen blood vessel walls. In some countries, prescription medications containing highly purified flavonoids are used to treat haemorrhoids. In certain studies, the medications significantly reduced the risk of bleeding, pain and itching and also lowered the risk of recurrence by 47 per cent. Ask your doctor about taking one, or simply try to eat $3/4$ cup of your favourite berries every day.

▶ WHAT CAUSES IT
Haemorrhoids occur in pregnancy because of changing hormones and abdominal pressure, straining during bowel movements due to constipation, obesity, and sitting for prolonged periods.

▶ SYMPTOMS TO WATCH FOR
Bright red blood covering the stool, on toilet paper or in the toilet bowl. An internal haemorrhoid may protrude through the anus outside the body, becoming irritated and painful. Other symptoms include painful swelling or a hard lump around the anus.

▶ LATEST THINKING
To treat bad haemorrhoids, instead of surgery or cutting off the blood supply to haemorrhoids with a tight band, doctors can now zap them with infrared light to cut off the blood flow.

Headaches

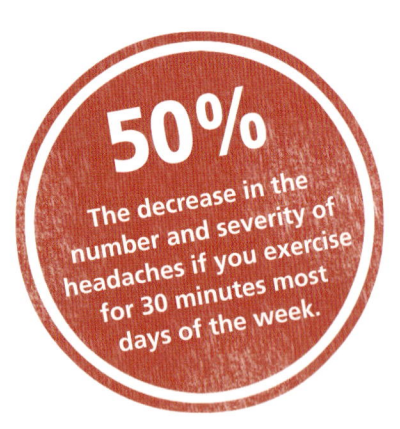

50% The decrease in the number and severity of headaches if you exercise for 30 minutes most days of the week.

Whether you get a tension headache once in a while or experience fiercely excruciating 'cluster' headaches, the best headache is the one you don't get at all. Experts say most headaches can be avoided with the following steps, but if you get a sudden intense headache that's unlike any previous headache, call your doctor immediately.

Key prevention strategies

Stick to your schedule Sleeping-in on weekends or not drinking tea or coffee could trigger a headache. One survey found that 79 per cent of headache sufferers have a headache if they sleep longer than 8 hours. And if you're used to a cup of coffee at 7 am, delaying it could make blood vessels clench, leaving you with a pounding head.

Show up for breakfast, lunch and dinner If you get 'hunger headaches', the culprit could be low blood sugar. Keeping your blood sugar on an even keel with low GI foods could help. Try to include whole grains, fruit and vegetables, and protein to keep levels steadier for longer. Avoid loading up on white rice, white bread, white potatoes and processed sugary snacks and desserts, which make blood sugar spike and then crash again.

Move your muscles Getting half an hour of exercise on most days of the week can cut headache pain and frequency by an impressive 50 per cent, according to research. Physical activity fights headaches in two ways: by boosting feelgood brain chemicals called endorphins and by easing stress.

Practise relaxation You don't have to meditate—any kind of relaxation that eases stress could help you escape from frequent tension headaches. Italian office workers who took brief relaxation breaks every 2 to 3 hours cut their monthly headaches by 41 per cent, report researchers from the

DRUGS THAT PREVENT DISEASE

Cluster headaches are excruciating and can be a major problem for weeks, months or years on end. The most popular preventive medication, verapamil, is effective but carries risks. In one study of 30 people, 12 of 15 participants who got the medication had fewer attacks in just two weeks. But other research shows that it significantly raises the risk of irregular heart rhythm. If you take verapamil, have your heart monitored regularly.

University of Turin. And when US researchers from Ohio University tracked 203 adults with chronic daily tension headaches, 35 per cent of those who got five sessions of stress management advice saw headache frequency fall by more than 50 per cent. Ask your doctor about mindfulness-based stress-reduction training. Meanwhile, try a few minutes of slow, deep breathing on a regular basis.

Check the ergonomics of your workstation Reposition your chair, desk and computer screen so you can sit up straight with your feet on the floor. The centre of your monitor should be just below your gaze when you look straight ahead. Make sure your glasses prescription is current (if you need a new pair, it's worth paying extra for the anti-glare coating). Finally, get up and take frequent breaks from the screen.

Quit your pain reliever If you take medicine for headache more than 15 times each month, you may have 'medication overuse headaches' or 'rebound headaches'. These happen when painkillers wear off and blood vessels swell, then pain returns, you take something to relieve it and the cycle begins again.

Studies show that rebound headaches can happen with over-the-counter remedies such as ibuprofen and aspirin, and with stronger prescription drugs for headaches and migraines, such as opioids, triptans and ergots. The best remedy is to stop taking your pain reliever (and understand that it'll hurt). But once the rebound effect wears off, your doctor will be able to treat the underlying cause of your headaches.

Prevention boosters

Stay hydrated That nagging pain could be your brain's way of asking for a glass of water. Mild headaches can be a sign of mild dehydration, so drink up.

Let go of tension in your jaw, face, shoulders and/or neck
It's easy to unconsciously clench muscles in these areas when you're tense, boosting your odds for a headache. Studies confirm that this is a frequent cause of chronic tension headaches. So if these muscles are tight, take a few slow, deep breaths and imagine the stress flowing out until you feel relaxed. Repeat several times a day.

▶ WHAT CAUSES IT

We don't know exactly what causes tension headaches, but researchers now suspect that fluctuating levels of serotonin—feelgood endorphins—and other brain chemicals play an important role. Anaemia, anxiety, arthritis of the neck or spine, depression, menopause, muscle tension, severe high blood pressure and sinus infections can cause headaches. So can prescription and over-the-counter medications, including oral contraceptives, some antihistamines and decongestants, and oral contraceptives.

▶ SYMPTOMS TO WATCH FOR

Head pain, of course, as well as trouble sleeping, tiredness, irritability, loss of appetite and difficulty concentrating. If you have cluster headaches, you will have intense pain plus teary swollen eyes, a stuffy nose and sweaty skin.

▶ LATEST THINKING

Chronic headaches and depression are linked. In a study, one in four women and men with chronic headaches also had major depression, report researchers from the University of Tsukuba in Japan. The researchers suggest that if you have had chronic headaches for longer than six months, it's a good reason to see your doctor for an evaluation for depression.

Hearing loss

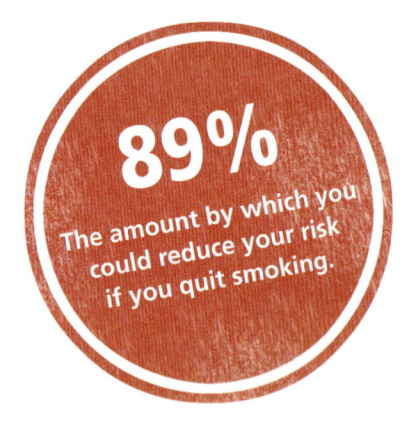

89% The amount by which you could reduce your risk if you quit smoking.

Hearing tends to worsen with age, partially due to some health conditions, smoking and years of noise. But thanks to rock bands, MP3 players, leaf blowers and electronic kids' toys, noise-related hearing loss is now turning up in younger adults and in children as young as six.

Key prevention strategies

Protect yourself against major disease Diabetes, heart disease and high blood pressure can increase the risk of age-related hearing loss, probably by impeding blood flow to the inner ear. Find tips for preventing them in each respective entry in this book.

Use the lawnmower test If something sounds as loud as a lawnmower (about 90 decibels), it's too loud. You need to cover your ears with earmuffs or at least use earplugs from a pharmacy. Here's another way to gauge whether your tasks or hobbies are hurting your hearing: before mowing the lawn or listening to the stereo, turn on the television and set the volume on low. Notice how well you hear what's said. Afterwards, try the test again. If you don't hear as well, you're experiencing some temporary hearing loss. With continued exposure, it could become permanent.

Turn down the volume on your MP3 player When you're plugged into your MP3 player, you may not realise how loud the sound really is. When in doubt, turn down the volume. If you keep the volume control no higher than 50 per cent of maximum, you can listen as long as you like, but if you're used to turning up the sound loud enough so that someone standing next to you could identify the song, limit yourself to 5 minutes if you're using an iPod with earbuds that sit inside your ear and 18 minutes if you use earphones that rest on top of your ears. Any longer and you're putting your hearing at risk, according to current research findings.

Quit smoking Add hearing to the list of body functions damaged by cigarette smoke. After analysing eight major studies, researchers concluded that smoking increases your risk of hearing loss by 33 to

Got the gene?

While most hearing loss results from noise, everyone's hearing reacts differently. Two people exposed to the same noise level could experience it differently in each ear, even at different times of the day. That makes researchers suspect there's some genetic component to hearing loss. Another clue to your risk may come from your blood type. In one study, researchers found noise-induced hearing loss much more common among people with blood group O. So if your parents or grandparents wear hearing aids, or you have type O blood, you may have a higher risk of noise-related hearing loss, so should be extra careful about prevention.

89 per cent. It reduces the flow of blood and oxygen to your inner ear, weakening the hair cells that transmit sound to your brain.

Get plenty of B vitamins A growing body of evidence suggests that people with low levels of the B vitamins folic acid and B_{12} tend to have poorer hearing. When Dutch researchers gave 728 older men and women 800 mcg of folic acid or a placebo daily for three years, those who got this vitamin had less hearing loss than those who took the placebo. In another study, researchers injected 20 young volunteers daily with either a placebo or vitamin B_{12} for seven days, then exposed each group to a loud noise. The vitamin group's hearing recovered better from the noise than the placebo group's did.

The B vitamins reduce levels of the amino acid homocysteine, which damages blood vessels. When homocysteine is cleared out blood flow is improved, leading to healthier inner-ear hair cells. That's important, given that loud noises can reduce blood flow to the cochlea, or inner ear, by up to 70 per cent. Good sources of B vitamins include soybeans, leafy green vegetables, lentils, beans, mussels (for vitamin B_{12}) and fortified cereals.

Prevention boosters

Hop on a bike, go jogging or walk After cycling twice a week for 30 minutes a day over two months, 17 moderately fit young adults suffered less hearing loss after a loud noise than before they started cycling. It was as if the exercise 'inoculated' them against noise-related hearing loss. Researchers suspect this is related to the cyclists' stronger hearts. The stronger the heart and the better the circulation, which exercise improves, the more oxygenated blood gets to those fragile inner-ear hair cells, helping them resist noise-related damage.

Snack on unblanched almonds They're packed with magnesium, which studies find can help prevent hearing-related damage. When researchers had 20 men drink juice containing 122 mg of magnesium or take a placebo for 10 days, then exposed them to white noise designed to exhaust the cochlear hair cells, they found the men recovered more hearing more rapidly after the magnesium-laced juice than after the placebo drink. Researchers think it's because magnesium helps cells use energy better, the kind of energy you need to repair noise-induced damage. Raw oat bran, pumpkin seeds, barley and spinach are also good sources.

▶ WHAT CAUSES IT
Noise damages minuscule hair cells in your inner ear that transmit sounds to your brain. When these cells die, they can't be replaced. You're born with about 16,000 hair cells, and you can lose between one-third and one-half of them before you notice yourself saying 'what?' all the time.

▶ SYMPTOMS TO WATCH FOR
Ringing in the ears, dizziness, difficulty perceiving and differentiating consonants, feeling that words often 'run together', and the inability to hear high-pitched sounds like a ringing phone or a crying baby.

▶ LATEST THINKING
One reason why noise damages ears may be that it stimulates the production of free radicals, dangerous molecules that can damage cells. Anti-oxidants in your body neutralise free radicals, but if you're exposed to too much noise, those anti-oxidants can't keep up. In animals, certain anti-oxidants such as n-acetyl-l-cysteine and acetyl-l-carnitine reduce the risk of that damage.

Heartburn and GORD

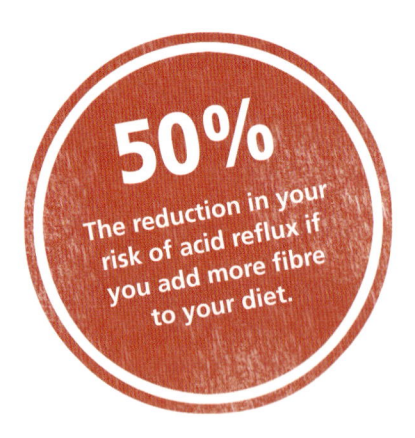

50% The reduction in your risk of acid reflux if you add more fibre to your diet.

A muscular valve at the bottom of your oesophagus normally keeps corrosive digestive juices in your stomach. But if you have heartburn, this valve sneaks open at inopportune times, such as after a big meal, allowing acid to rise up, causing pain that can be mild or so strong you could mistake it for a heart attack. Over time, heartburn becomes gastro-oesophageal reflux disease (GORD), a more serious condition that may raise your risk of oesophageal cancer. Take it seriously—and try to discourage acid backwash.

Key prevention strategies

If you're overweight, shed some kilos Losing 12 kg cut reflux episodes 40 per cent in one study reviewed by researchers from Stanford University in the US. It helps because losing weight may lower pressure at the valve that keeps stomach acid in its place, known as the lower oesophageal sphincter (LOS). It also reduces the body's output of acidic digestive enzymes.

Catch the early-bird special When Japanese researchers tracked the bedtimes and GORD symptoms of 441 women and men, they found that those who went to bed within 3 hours of finishing dinner were seven and a half times more likely to have acid indigestion than those who turned in four or more hours later. If you go to bed at 10 pm, aim to finish dinner no later than 6 pm.

Prop up the head of your bed Raising the head of your bed about 30 cm with bricks or old telephone directories could cut reflux episodes dramatically and make the ones you do have shorter.

Favour your left side In one study, people who slept on their left sides had only half as much reflux as right-side sleepers. Due to the location of your stomach and oesophagus, lying on your right side puts more pressure on the LOS.

Take the pepperoni pizza test There's plenty of controversy about which foods trigger heartburn. The truth is, what bothers you may be no problem at all for the person sitting next to you. (They, on the other hand, may be in agony after eating a few chocolate-covered after-dinner mints.)

When US researchers from Stanford University reviewed more than 100 studies of lifestyle remedies for acid reflux, they found that avoiding chocolate, mint, spices, greasy foods and late-night eating doesn't help most people. But plenty of other research, and the experience of digestive disease specialists, suggests that, for some people, these are exactly the things they should avoid.

The take-home lesson is to figure out what your personal trigger foods are, then steer clear of them. Possibilities include citrus fruits, chocolate, coffee and tea, alcohol, fatty and fried foods, garlic and onions, mint flavourings, spicy foods, and tomato-based foods such as pasta sauce, hot curries, chilli dishes and some pizza.

Avoid sleeping pills According to a large health survey, people who took benzodiazepines such as alprazolam (Xanax), diazepam (Valium) and triazolam (Halcion) in order to fall asleep were 50 per cent more likely to have GORD at night than those who didn't take them. Other research has shown that these medications loosen the LOS, lowering your chances of a comfortable night's sleep.

Quit smoking A Swedish study of more than 43,300 people found that long-time smokers had a 70 per cent higher risk of heartburn and GORD than nonsmokers. Smoking raises risk four ways: it may make you cough more, which puts pressure on the LOS; it can weaken the LOS; it reduces production of saliva, which normally neutralises stomach acids that find their way into your oesophagus; and it boosts production of corrosive digestive acids.

Prevention boosters

Try chewing gum For times when you don't have any antacid on hand, you might be able to head off heartburn with some chewing gum. A small UK study found that chewing gum for 30 minutes after a large fatty meal doubled saliva production and saliva swallowing. Researchers estimate that 10 extra swallows could cool mild

When to call the doctor

Chronic or severe heartburn can be a sign of more serious reflux disease or other digestive problems. Call your doctor if you have heartburn for more than two weeks or if it's making you wheeze or giving you a sore throat; preventing you from sleeping; interfering with daytime activities; causing pain in your neck, chest or back; creating discomfort or difficulty when you swallow; making you vomit or have black stools (from digested blood); or resulting in weight loss.

heartburn by pushing acids back where they belong. Other research shows that gum chewing neutralises the acids in stomach backwash for up to 3 hours after a meal.

Take a relaxation break Science has yet to uncover the link between stress and acid indigestion, but plenty of heartburn sufferers know it exists. In one survey conducted by the US National Heartburn Alliance, 58 per cent of people who had frequent heartburn said hectic lifestyles made their pain worse. Stress may prompt you to smoke more, drink more alcohol, eat the foods that trigger acid backwash or simply to feel discomfort more intensely. Pay attention to your own stress levels, and when they get too high, look for ways to relax, such as deep breathing.

Control asthma Three out of every four people with asthma also have acid reflux. Coughing and difficulty exhaling may trigger the backwash of stomach acid into the oesophagus. Asthma medications that widen airways in the lungs may also relax the LOS. Keeping your asthma under control can help, but if you still have acid reflux, tell your doctor.

Keep blood sugar at healthy levels
Over time, the high blood sugar levels that inevitably come with Type 1 and Type 2 diabetes can damage nerves throughout your body, including those that regulate the emptying of your stomach. If food sits in your stomach, it can be regurgitated more readily into your oesophagus. Some research studies suggest that better blood sugar control can help this problem, but it's still important to use the other lifestyle strategies mentioned here.

> **DRUGS THAT PREVENT DISEASE**
>
> If you already have GORD, acid-stopping medications known as H2 blockers and proton-pump inhibitors (PPIs) can help you accomplish two important health goals: halting the searing pain of heartburn and healing damaged tissue in your oesophagus. (It's important to note that there is also non-acid reflux that does not respond to PPIs.)
>
> **H2 blockers** Drugs such as cimetidine (Tagamet), famotidine (Pepcid), nizatidine (Tazac) and ranitidine (Zantac) reduce acid levels in your stomach. Your doctor may suggest over-the-counter H2 blockers for two weeks to relieve symptoms or prescription-strength forms for long-term relief. Studies show that H2 blockers work best for people with mild to moderate reflux problems but are less effective if your oesophagus is inflamed or has already been damaged by exposure to stomach acids. If you know which foods or situations are more likely to make heartburn flare up, taking an H2 blocker in advance may help you avoid discomfort better than taking an antacid afterwards.
>
> **Proton-pump inhibitors (PPIs)** Medications such as esomeprazole (Nexium), lansoprazole (Zoton), omeprazole (Losec), pantoprazole (Somac) and rabeprazole (Pariet) work by blocking production of about 90 per cent of stomach acids. Doctors often prescribe PPIs if H2 blockers don't bring relief or if you have severe heartburn or oesophageal damage. In one study of people with GORD, 78 per cent of those who took a PPI saw damaged oesophageal tissue heal in four to eight weeks. After about eight weeks, your doctor should check to see if your oesophagus is healing and may cut back on your dosage.

Find out if any medications are the culprits Many prescription and over-the-counter medications and supplements can keep the LOS from staying tightly shut. These include some antibiotics, antidepressants, calcium channel blockers, opioid pain relievers such as codeine and oxycodone, osteoporosis medications, sedatives, and tranquillisers, as well as over-the-counter pain relievers and supplements such as iron, potassium and vitamin C. If you have heartburn or GORD, ask your doctor if any of these could be contributing to your discomfort, and whether you should switch to another medication or remedy.

Up your fibre intake People who ate high-fibre breads (wholegrain and multigrain) had half the risk of GORD compared to people who ate low-fibre breads (white) in one large Scandinavian study. Fibre may help by soaking up excess nitric oxide, a compound that relaxes muscles in the digestive system. When US researchers scanned the oesophaguses of 164 people, they found that those who ate more fruit, vegetables, whole grains and legumes were 20 per cent less likely to have signs of erosion of delicate oesophageal tissue caused by reflux. People who took in more fat, protein and kilojoules were at higher risk.

Avoid cola drinks When US researchers from the University of Arizona College of Medicine polled more than 15,000 people about their lifestyle habits and history of GORD, they found that those who drank more than one carbonated, caffeinated drink per day were 24 per cent more likely to have sleep-disturbing night-time reflux than those who drank fewer soft drinks. Many carbonated drinks have a high acid level, which may explain the connection.

Try acupuncture if prescription medication isn't working
When 30 people with persistent heartburn received either a double dose of proton-pump inhibitors or twice-weekly acupuncture plus their regular dose for four weeks, the acupuncture group enjoyed a significant decrease in GORD symptoms. The group that simply got more medications didn't see much improvement at all, according to researchers at the University of Arizona.

WHAT CAUSES IT
Weakening or relaxation of the lower oesophageal sphincter, the muscular valve at the bottom of your oesophagus. Normally, the LOS keeps digestive juices and food in your stomach. But smoking, alcohol, lying down too soon after a meal, some foods and medications can weaken or partially open the LOS, letting stomach acids backwash into the oesophagus.

SYMPTOMS TO WATCH FOR
A burning pain in your throat or chest, under your breastbone. It may become worse after a meal, at night or when you lie down. Less obvious symptoms include a persistent cough and chronic laryngitis.

LATEST THINKING
New research shows that nearly 40 per cent of heartburn/GORD sufferers who use an acid-stopping PPI medication once a day still get heartburn symptoms two to four times a week. Many wind up taking antacids, which can stop pain but may not protect the oesophagus from damage. If you're taking medication for heartburn or GORD and are still in pain, ask your doctor about upgrading your treatment plan.

Hepatitis

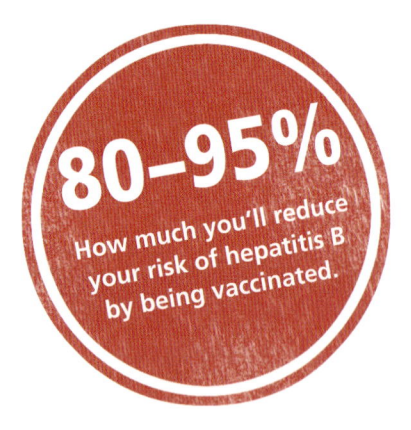

80–95% How much you'll reduce your risk of hepatitis B by being vaccinated.

Hepatitis is inflammation of the liver. There are five types of viral hepatitis: A, B, C, D and E. If hepatitis A, B or C gains control, liver cells are infiltrated and turned into virus-producing factories. Sometimes hepatitis heals on its own or it can last a lifetime. Cirrhosis, liver failure and liver cancer may result from years of infection.

Key prevention strategies

Get vaccinated The number-one way to prevent hepatitis A, B and D is with a vaccine. Unfortunately, there are no vaccines yet for hepatitis C or E, though researchers are working on them.

- **Hepatitis A vaccine** Recommended for all Aboriginal and Torres Strait Islander children outside of NSW and Tasmania, people with intellectual disabilities, travellers to countries where the virus is prevalent (for a complete list, visit www.cdc.gov/ncidod/diseases/hepatitis/b/country_listing.htm or consult your doctor or local travel clinic), men who have sex with men, users of IV and injectable drugs, people with blood disorders (such as haemophilia) who often require transfusions, those with chronic liver disease and those who work with the virus in lab settings. The vaccine requires three doses given over 12 to 18 months, depending on your age and the vaccine type. Studies suggest it could last up to 25 years or more.
- **Hepatitis B vaccine** Recommended for all children and anyone who works in the healthcare field. If you're under 19 years of age and have never been vaccinated, do it now. The vaccine is also recommended for men who have sex with men, heterosexual people who have had a sexually transmissible infection or more than one partner in the previous six months, and those travelling to areas of the world with high rates of infection (for a list, see the website above). It's typically given in three doses over six months, though a few studies find that a shorter dosing schedule is also effective—perhaps

DRUGS THAT PREVENT DISEASE
If you may have been exposed to the hepatitis A or B virus, see your doctor as soon as possible. He or she may give you a shot of immune globulin, which contains antibodies that destroy the virus. The sooner you receive this injection after being exposed to the virus—within two weeks for hepatitis A and 72 hours for hepatitis B—the more likely it is to work.

more effective. In one study, participants who received the second dose two weeks after the first showed protective antibody levels much higher than in those receiving the vaccine according to the traditional schedule. The protection lasts for at least 15 years but in most cases is believed to be lifelong. However, if you're over the age of 40 or obese, have kidney failure, are on dialysis, or have a suppressed immune system, it's not quite as effective. This vaccine also protects against hepatitis D.

- **Combined vaccine** Three combination vaccines protect against both hepatitis A and B. Some are formulated for infants and young children; others are for adults. The vaccine is given either three times in six months or three times in 30 days, followed by a fourth at one year.

Prevention boosters

Wash your hands regularly Not everyone washes their hands properly, so when you shake a person's hand and then touch your mouth, eyes or nose, you could easily end up with a hepatitis A infection. Always wash with soap and water whenever you can (especially when travelling), and for times when you can't, carry hand wipes or hand-sanitising gel. Always wash thoroughly after using the toilet or changing a nappy, and before preparing food.

Use condoms Safer sex is one of the best ways to prevent transmission of the hepatitis B virus.

Stay away from injectable drugs We're talking about recreational drug use, not insulin. The most common cause of infection with hepatitis B and C viruses is from use of injectable drugs.

Don't share personal items Using razors, toothbrushes or any other personal item that could have come in contact with an infected person's blood can lead to hepatitis B or C infection.

Choose your tattoo parlour carefully It's possible, though unlikely, that you could get hepatitis C when you get a tattoo. Make sure the tattoo parlour you choose complies with health regulations, looks clean and tidy, and uses an autoclave to sterilise all equipment properly. The tattoo artist should remove the needles and tubes from a sealed package and wear gloves while working.

▶ WHAT CAUSES IT

Hepatitis A and E Ingesting food or water contaminated by stools from an infected person or through some other contact with an infected person's stool, such as nappy changing or shaking hands with someone who hasn't washed after using the toilet.

Hepatitis B and D Unprotected sexual contact with an infected person, sharing needles or drugs, or a needle-stick injury from an infected person. These viruses can also be passed from mother to infant during childbirth.

Hepatitis C Exposure to infected blood products or sharing needles. It can also be passed from mother to infant during childbirth.

▶ SYMPTOMS TO WATCH FOR

Infection may initially go unnoticed or feel like a mild case of the flu. With serious infection, you may experience jaundice, fatigue, abdominal pain, loss of appetite, nausea, diarrhoea, fever and dark urine. Hepatitis B infection may also cause skin rashes, joint pain and arthritis.

▶ LATEST THINKING

People infected with hepatitis B should be started on treatment as early as possible, even before they show signs of liver damage. This may help prevent harm.

Herpes simplex

71%
The percentage of genital herpes outbreaks that can be prevented if you take an antiviral medication daily.

Herpes—whether it's cold sores on your lips or blisters on your genitals—is painful in many ways. The blisters sting and burn for days. And while an attack is under way, herpes can be both embarrassing and risky because it's so contagious. Once you've been infected by the herpes virus, it lives in your skin cells or nerve cells, dormant until it's reactivated by stress, sun exposure, trauma, surgery, illness or even menstrual cycles. The following strategies can keep it under control and help you to stay safe.

Key prevention strategies

Not infected? Practise safe sex—and safe kissing If your partner has herpes blisters around the mouth or genitals, you should avoid skin-to-skin contact. An estimated 60 per cent of adults harbour the herpes virus—and at least one in five never has symptoms, but could be contagious anyway. The reason for this is that tiny viral particles can migrate to the skin's surface without causing an outbreak. This is known as viral shedding, and it's dangerous because it makes it possible to pass the virus around even when no one can see it.

That's why it's so important to practise safer sex. This includes using a condom during intercourse, though condoms won't always prevent spread of the virus simply because they don't cover all the areas that are infected or could become infected. The surest way to avoid genital herpes is to abstain from sexual contact or to stay in a mutually monogamous relationship with a partner who has been tested (testing for herpes antibodies is available, although the results may be difficult to interpret) and is known to be uninfected.

Keep antiviral drugs on hand These prescription medications can short-circuit a cold sore and dramatically reduce genital herpes outbreaks and viral shedding. The specific medications are aciclovir (Zovirax), famciclovir (Famvir) and valaciclovir (Valtrex). In one international study of 384 women and men with genital herpes, 71 per cent of those who took valaciclovir every day for six months had no more outbreaks, compared to just 43 per cent of those who took a placebo. Daily use can also reduce viral shedding by 94 per cent, helping to keep partners infection free.

In cold-sore studies, antivirals healed outbreaks in three days, compared to just over four days for placebos, and reduced the number of blisters by 50 per cent. You can take these medications in advance to prevent cold sores, too, such as when you'll be outdoors in bright sunlight all day. Your doctor will tell you what dosing schedule to use, and talk to your pharmacist about the costs involved (the Pharmaceutical Benefits Scheme [PBS] in Australia covers only genital herpes).

What about antiviral creams? The truth is, many doctors don't even recommend them anymore. In some studies, they've proven no more effective than a placebo cream for clearing up blisters. And they're expensive. Having a supply of antiviral medication on hand, and even carrying some for sudden outbreaks away from home, is a much better herpes-control strategy.

Always wear sunscreen The sun's ultraviolet rays may reactivate the herpes virus. In one US National Institutes of Health study of 38 people prone to cold sores, 71 per cent developed blisters after exposure to UV rays. The number dropped to zero when they all wore lip balm with built-in sunblock.

Prevention boosters

Breathe, and try to release the tension In one survey of nearly 500 Canadian doctors, dentists and pharmacists, 60 per cent said their patients and customers complained that emotional upheaval was certain to bring on unwanted blisters. The best possible fix for this is using your favourite stress-reduction technique. In one study, men who made time for daily relaxation had lower levels of antibodies associated with herpes.

Eat well, sleep well Experts aren't sure why, but letting yourself become run down increases blister risk, perhaps due to stress, lowered immunity or both. When your life is tense, make an extra effort to go to bed earlier and to opt for healthier food choices— simply to pamper yourself so you don't feel worn out.

WHAT CAUSES IT

The herpes simplex virus. Type 1 usually causes oral herpes and Type 2, genital herpes. But either type can show up in either area.

SYMPTOMS TO WATCH FOR

Open sores or small, painful blisters surrounded by swollen, painful skin. Often there's pain or tingling for a day or two before the blisters appear. They typically occur around the lips or on the genitals, but they can also show up in your nose, mouth or eyes; on your chin or fingers; or on your buttocks or the upper part of your inner thighs. Outbreaks may be accompanied by flu-like symptoms.

LATEST THINKING

Your doctor's not talking—or you're not listening. A Canadian survey found that 75 per cent of people with herpes say they were never told about antiviral medications that can control this virus, but doctors say they're telling 60 per cent of their patients about them. So if you haven't heard, ask.

High blood pressure

11.5 points
The likely reduction in blood pressure if you eat the right diet.

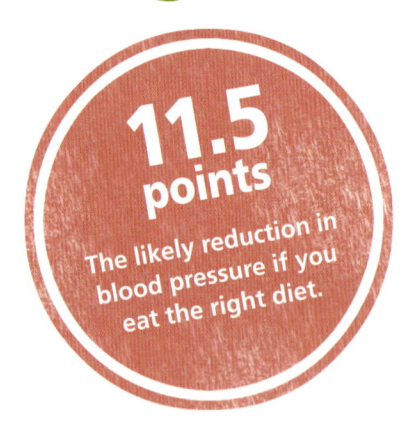

If avoiding a single health problem could cut your odds of having a stroke by 30 per cent, reduce your chance of a heart attack by 23 per cent and cut your heart failure and dementia risk by half, you'd start now, right? These health dividends—and more—all involve keeping blood pressure at a healthy level. After the age of 55, your odds of developing high blood pressure jump to 90 per cent—unless you take action. So if it's creeping over 120/80 mmHg, start now.

Key prevention strategies

Drop excess weight Carrying extra weight, especially around your waist, raises your odds for high blood pressure by an incredible 60 per cent. The reason is that fat around the waistline pumps inflammatory compounds into your bloodstream where they, in turn, stiffen artery walls. Stiff arteries mean higher blood pressure. Excess fat can also interfere with your kidneys' ability to filter pressure-raising sodium out of your bloodstream.

Being overweight seems to be the cause of half of all cases of high blood pressure, according to research. Losing a modest amount can protect you from this silent killer. When researchers followed 1191 overweight women and men with high to normal blood pressure for more than two years, 65 per cent of those who lost 5 kg and kept it off nudged their blood pressure down to healthy levels.

The lesson is to start sooner rather than later. Researchers suspect that, over time, chemicals churned out by body fat can make artery stiffness hard to reverse.

Cut back on sodium A little sodium—a component of salt—is essential for human survival; too much is a problem. When sodium levels in your blood rise, your body pumps more water into your bloodstream to dilute it. This results in a growth in blood volume, and the speed of the blood pumping through your body increases. Too much sodium, research suggests, can also stiffen arteries, further raising your blood pressure.

If you make just one dietary change to lower blood pressure, eat less sodium. In one US study from Duke University, 71 per cent of people with high blood pressure who cut back on salt but made no other menu changes brought their readings down to normal. If your blood pressure is optimal, the Heart Foundation of Australia recommends getting less than 2300 mg of sodium a day—that's about a teaspoon of salt. But, better still, aim for about two-thirds of that amount, closer to 1500 mg. If your pressure is beginning to rise, you'll need to seriously cut back and eat less than that—500 mg or about one-quarter of a teaspoon. And don't believe the hype that only an unlucky few are 'salt-sensitive'; this may still be true if your blood pressure has only crept up just a little over the years. And remember that most of the salt we eat is found in foods that may not even taste salty, such as packaged and processed foods, some cereals, and processed meats such as ham and salami.

When you cook, add salt at the end (if at all); long cooking dulls salt's flavour, so you're more likely to add more at the table.

Eat plenty of fresh fruit and vegetables A low-fat diet packed with fruit and vegetables can work wonders for your blood pressure. In one remarkable study, people with high blood pressure who followed a low-fat diet rich in fruit and vegetables and low-fat dairy foods for just eight weeks lowered their systolic pressure (the top number) by 11.4 points and their diastolic pressure (the bottom number) by 5.5 points—an improvement on par with some blood pressure medications. Blood pressure began to fall after just two weeks. Other studies show that eating this way daily can lower your odds of developing high blood pressure in the first place.

The star performers here are calcium, magnesium and potassium. These three minerals help lower pressure in several ways; for example, potassium helps the body excrete excess sodium, while calcium and magnesium work together to keep artery walls flexible.

The landmark US study of nutrition and blood pressure known as Dietary Approaches to Stop Hypertension, or DASH, found that people who increased their fruit and vegetable intake were able to lower their blood pressure, which lowers your risk for heart attack and stroke. The recommendation is 7 to 10 serves of fruit and vegetables daily,

Is your diet too salty?

Most people eat double or even triple the amount of salt recommended by blood-pressure experts. You could be one of them if you answer yes to one or more of these questions.

1. Do you often use processed foods, such as frozen dinners; packet or canned goods (including soups and vegetables); processed meats such as ham, sausages and salami; cheeses; or bottled salad dressings?
2. Do you often eat salty snack foods, such as potato chips, salted nuts, cheese snacks or pretzels?
3. Do you often eat in restaurants or fast-food places?
4. Do you often add salt during cooking and/or at the table?

which is easier to achieve than you might think. Here are the best food sources of the three essential minerals:

- **Calcium** Low-fat dairy foods, sardines (with bones), tofu (firm), canned salmon (with bones and liquid), almonds, cooked soybeans and cooked spinach.
- **Magnesium** Almonds (unblanched), buckwheat flour, oat bran, tahini, pumpkin seeds, pearled barley, brazil nuts, cooked spinach, burghul, tofu and kidney beans.
- **Potassium** Raisins, cooked spinach, potatoes (baked, with skin on), avocados, cooked pumpkin, baked beans in tomato sauce, broccoli, canned tomatoes (crushed or pureed) and bananas.

Have milk or low-fat dairy foods two or three times a day

Treats such as a low-fat cheese sandwich, a low-fat yogurt and fruit smoothie, and hot chocolate made with low-fat milk and dark chocolate are more than delicious, they're an essential part of a strategy to keep your blood pressure normal. Low-fat dairy foods are a top source of calcium, which helps prevent artery walls from stiffening. Low-fat or skim versions will help to keep the saturated fat in your diet low. If dairy products are problematic for you, get 600–900 mg of calcium a day in supplement form.

Keep walking shoes handy Half an hour of brisk walking three to five days a week can keep your blood pressure five to six points lower than if you didn't exercise. And when UK researchers checked the blood pressures of 106 government workers on a walking program, they found that those who got their exercise in short bursts enjoyed the same blood pressure-lowering benefits as colleagues who preferred one longer exercise session a day.

Other research suggests that exercising in short bursts is actually better. In one study, people who used this strategy saw their blood pressure stay lower for longer during the day compared to people who got all their activity in one hit.

Kick the habit Puffing on just one cigarette makes arteries less elastic, allowing blood pressure to rise even if you're young, slim and fit. Smoking 15 cigarettes a day raises your risk of high blood pressure by 11 per cent; smoking 25 cigarettes raises it 21 per cent.

Snorers, ask your bedmate a question 'Do I seem to stop breathing, then catch my breath, during the night?' If the answer is yes, or if you wake up tired despite a full night of rest, you may have obstructive sleep apnoea, which makes your high blood pressure risk up to seven times higher than normal. Mild sleep apnoea raised risk 2.5 times, and even snoring, without apnoea, doubled it. Disturbed sleep raises levels of artery-tightening stress hormones in your body.

Prevention boosters

Drink coffee instead of diet cola Drinking just one diet cola a day raised the risk of high blood pressure by 5 per cent, and four a day increased the odds by 19 per cent in a landmark US study. Risks were even higher for women who drank regular colas. Experts can't explain the association, but suggest that coffee might be a better alternative; women who drank coffee every day had no added risk for hypertension. Coffee triggers a temporary rise in blood pressure, but it doesn't persist in regular coffee drinkers.

Try to relax Regularly practising meditation, yoga or another relaxation technique can help pressure-proof your blood vessels. When US scientists analysed 107 studies of the effect of meditation on blood pressure, they concluded that it produces significant drops (one of the studies found a 10-point drop in systolic pressure and a 6-point drop in diastolic pressure). When other researchers tested the blood pressure of 33 people taking a yoga class that met three times a week, they found improvements after just six weeks. Average blood pressure fell from 130/79 to 125/74 mmHg. Tai chi has also been shown to be effective.

Sip beetroot juice UK researchers report that drinking 2 cups of beetroot juice a day can lower your blood pressure by 8 to 10 points, fast. Volunteers who sipped 2 cups a day saw their pressure drop significantly after 3 hours, and stay lower for up to a day. Emerging research suggests that nitrates in beetroots (and in green leafy vegetables) keep the lining of your arteries (endothelium) supple.

Have a piece of dark chocolate When people with slightly elevated blood pressure ate 125 kilojoules of dark chocolate each night after dinner for 18 weeks, their blood pressure fell by two to three points. Artery-friendly compounds called flavonols may be responsible for the improvement. And dark chocolate is also a source of magnesium.

▶ WHAT CAUSES IT
Stiff arteries and excess salt play a role. Eating too much salt prompts your body to pump extra water into your bloodstream in an effort to dilute high sodium levels. Meanwhile, everything from smoking to being overweight to eating a diet low in fruit and vegetables, dairy, and whole grains can stiffen arteries, leaving them unable to flex, stretch and make room for fast-moving blood.

▶ SYMPTOMS TO WATCH FOR
Usually, none. To keep tabs on your pressure, have it checked at least every two years and ask your doctor for your reading. If it's 120/80 mmHg or higher, it's time to take action—even if your doctor doesn't suggest it first. Studies show that many physicians aren't aggressive enough about putting a lid on pressure that's inching higher, especially in people over sixty.

▶ LATEST THINKING
There's nothing normal about 'high normal' blood pressure. Until recently, experts thought blood pressure readings between 120/80 and 140/90 mmHg were perfectly healthy. Now those levels are considered 'prehypertensive' or 'high normal'—and they can raise your risk of dying from heart disease by 58 per cent, making this problem more deadly than smoking.

High cholesterol

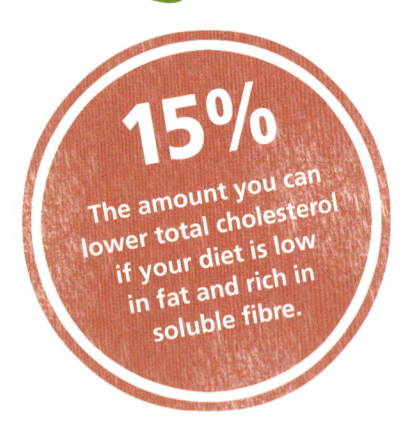

15% The amount you can lower total cholesterol if your diet is low in fat and rich in soluble fibre.

Cholesterol is necessary to make cell membranes as well as hormones, and your body produces this cholesterol. What you eat also contributes to blood cholesterol levels, but it's not so much this as the saturated fat in your diet that raises your cholesterol. Some cholesterol is 'bad' (LDL attacks arteries and contributes to plaque buildup), while some is 'good' (HDL escorts the bad cholesterol out of the body). Only about half of people who have heart attacks have high cholesterol, but it's still important to keep your levels healthy.

Key prevention strategies

Eat less saturated fat This is the fat found in hamburgers, steaks, butter, cheese and ice-cream. To lower your risk of heart attack, switch to skinless chicken breasts, oily fish, olive or canola oil, and low-fat dairy foods. Experts estimate that every 5 per cent increase in saturated fat intake bumps up your risk of heart disease by 17 per cent. And one US study found that eating just one meal high in saturated fat had an adverse effect on the elasticity of arteries. Keep your daily intake of saturated fat to less than 7 per cent of daily kilojoules—about 1 tablespoon of butter or a slice of cheddar cheese plus 1/2 cup of ice-cream if you eat 8500 kilojoules a day—and you could lower your LDL by 9 to 11 per cent.

Avoid foods with 'hydrogenated' on the label Read the back of a bag of chips or biscuits, crackers or baked goods, and you may well see 'partially hydrogenated oil' on the list. These oils, also known as trans fats, extend the shelf life of a product, but they can spell disaster by raising LDL and triglycerides, reducing HDL, and increasing your odds of having a heart attack. In one study of 50 men with healthy cholesterol levels, eating trans fats for five weeks raised LDL 5 per cent and lowered HDL a heart-damaging 11 per cent.

Cholesterol targets

Total cholesterol Under 4.0 mmol/L.

LDL ('bad' cholesterol) Under 2.5 mmol/L for people at higher risk, and under 3.0 mmol/L for those at lower risk.

HDL ('good' cholesterol) Over 1.0 mmol/L.

Triglycerides Like cholesterol, these blood fats are dangerous to the heart. Ideal levels are below 2.0 mmol/L.

Note: Any lowering of total or LDL cholesterol, or raising of HDL cholesterol, is likely to be of benefit, even if the desired targets aren't reached.

Food served in restaurants and at fast-food chains—especially fried food—can also be high in trans fats; ask how food is cooked before you order it, and find out what oils are used and how often they're replenished. Even if they have made the switch to healthier oils, fried food is still generally too high in fat and kilojoules to eat safely except on the odd occasion.

Stop smoking Smoking depresses levels of HDL cholesterol by 7 to 20 per cent and at the same time can raise your LDL cholesterol 70 per cent, according to one analysis of several studies. It also unleashes toxic chemicals that make LDL more dangerous to your arteries. By quitting smoking, you'll see benefits incredibly quickly: blood levels of heart-protecting HDL bounce back within a month or two of making this one change.

Eat oats, barley and legumes every day These three 'superfoods' are packed with a type of soluble fibre called beta-glucan. It acts like a sponge, trapping cholesterol-rich bile acids in your intestines so they can be eliminated before they have the chance to raise your cholesterol. Whole grains such as wholemeal bread and brown rice, which are rich in insoluble fibre, just can't perform that trick. In one study of 36 overweight men, those who ate two large serves of foods rich in soluble fibre a day lowered their LDL by 17 per cent. Here are three great ways to include more fibre into your diet:

- Enjoy grated apples over porridge at breakfast; oats contain more soluble fibre than any other grain. Having just two serves of porridge a day can lower your cholesterol by 2 to 3 per cent.
- Cook up barley and serve it instead of rice. In a US study from the Beltsville Human Nutrition Research Center, 25 people with slightly high cholesterol who ate barley daily for several weeks saw their LDL drop significantly.
- Try to eat a combination of soy protein, almonds, oats, barley and plant sterols at the same meal. Studies show that this can reduce LDL by 28 per cent in people with high cholesterol who also have a diet low in saturated fats.

The heart-friendly fruit

If you haven't yet discovered the rich, creamy flavour of avocados, it's time you did. Slice one up and enjoy a few pieces as a snack, add it to a salad or use it in sandwiches and in nachos, or to make fresh guacamole. In a study from Mexico's Instituto Mexicano del Seguro Social, women and men who ate one avocado a day for a week saw total cholesterol drop by 17 per cent. 'Bad' LDL cholesterol fell, and 'good' HDL rose. The reason? Avocados are incredibly rich in heart-healthy monounsaturated fat and contain respectable levels of beta-sitosterol, the same stuff found in some cholesterol-lowering margarines.

Snack on nuts It may seem odd, since nuts are fatty, but they really are excellent for your cholesterol, thanks in part to the cholesterol-lowering monounsaturated fats they contain. Choosing almonds instead of a doughnut, chips or biscuits for your afternoon snack every day could cut LDL cholesterol by nearly 10 per cent. A bonus is that vitamin E in the almond's 'meat' plus flavonoids in its papery skin protect LDL from oxidation, which is the first step in the development of artery-clogging plaque.

If you want to raise your HDL at the same time, choose walnuts. Bad cholesterol fell 10 per cent and good cholesterol rose 18 per cent when 58 women and men in one study snacked on about 14 walnut halves a day for six months.

Nuts are high in kilojoules, so control the portions. A 15-g, 375-kilojoule serve is about 12 almonds, 8 whole cashews, 8 pecans, 26 pistachios or 7 walnut halves. Double that for a 750-kilojoule serve. Eating a small handful of any type of nut is a good rule of thumb when it comes to portion control.

Feast on fruit, double your vegetables Eating nine serves of fruit and vegetables a day can reduce your LDL by as much as 7 per cent. Researchers aren't sure why, but it could be because of soluble fibre, which blocks the reabsorption of cholesterol found in the bile acids (digestive juices) that make their way into your intestines. This effectively lowers your LDL levels. Apples, pears and prunes are all good sources of soluble fibre. Or it could just be that people who tend to eat more fresh fruit and vegetables probably eat fewer fatty meats, snacks and desserts.

Get moving to boost good cholesterol Recently, doctors have discovered that having high levels of good cholesterol is every bit as important as having low levels of bad. Unfortunately, there aren't a lot of effective ways to increase your HDL—but exercise is one of them. Aerobic exercise, whether it's walking, swimming, cycling or even working hard in your garden, can raise HDL by 5 to 10 per cent. If you're also following a healthy diet, adding exercise can nudge LDL down 0.075 to 0.4 points, other studies suggest. A recent Japanese

Mind over cholesterol?

Stress can raise levels of 'bad' LDL cholesterol—and relaxation exercises such as yoga and tai chi can lower them, studies suggest. In one study of 113 people with heart disease, researchers from India report that those who added regular yoga sessions to a healthy diet lowered their LDL by 26 per cent after one year. If yoga isn't your thing, try to find another soothing activity.

study of 1400 people found that those who took a 40-minute brisk walk four times a week raised their HDL by about 0.05 points—enough to lower heart disease risk by about 6 per cent. For raising HDL, longer work-outs are better than several short ones.

Prevention boosters

Have up to two glasses of alcohol a day, with food Studies suggest that people who drink alcohol in moderation (no more than two standard drinks a day, for both men and women, with food) get a double cholesterol benefit. In one study, one drink a day lowered LDL nearly 0.2 points. Drinking moderately also increases HDL; in one Dutch study, HDL rose by a respectable 7 per cent.

Trim your personal fat zones Losing about 6 per cent of your body weight (about 4 kg if you now weigh 70 kg) could lower your LDL by 12 per cent and raise your HDL by 18 per cent, researchers say. The best weight-loss strategy for making your cholesterol levels healthier is a moderate-fat diet with lots of fresh fruit, vegetables and unsaturated fat from fish, nuts and olive and canola oils. Skip extremely low-fat diets: while research shows that they can make plaque in arteries shrink, they're impossibly difficult for most people to follow. And plenty of studies show that a moderate-fat diet not only protects your heart well, but is also much more pleasurable.

Lower your LDL with plant sterols and stanols These natural compounds, found in cholesterol-lowering margarine spreads, block the absorption of some cholesterol in your intestines. In one study, people with normal cholesterol levels who used margarine spreads fortified with sterols, such as Flora pro-activ or Logicol, saw their LDL cholesterol decrease 7 to 11 per cent after three months. Experts recommend getting up to 2 g of sterols and stanols a day, about the amount in 2 tablespoons of fortified margarine. Eat an extra serve of red, yellow or orange fruit or vegetables a day if you use these cholesterol-lowering spreads, as they can reduce absorption of heart-friendly compounds called carotenoids from foods you eat.

▶ WHAT CAUSES IT

For most people, a high-fat diet and a sedentary lifestyle combine to raise levels of LDL and decrease HDL. Cholesterol levels also rise with age. Your genes play a role, too: a few people inherit a genetic mutation that raises total cholesterol sky-high.

▶ SYMPTOMS TO WATCH FOR

Usually none. If you have familial hypercholesterolaemia, you may develop small, bumpy cholesterol deposits on your elbows, knees and buttocks. If you have them, have your cholesterol checked immediately; diet and exercise can help, but it's likely you'll need medication to bring levels back down to normal.

▶ LATEST THINKING

Don't worry (too much) about cholesterol in food. Studies show that for most people, foods such as whole eggs, and even prawns, won't raise LDL cholesterol. US researchers have found, for example, that eating up to seven eggs a week doesn't raise LDL levels. And despite the fact that 12 large prawns deliver 200 mg of cholesterol, a US study found that people who ate prawns did raise their LDL slightly, but their cholesterol ratios improved because HDL rose even higher and triglycerides fell.

Hot flushes

90% The amount by which supplemental oestrogen therapy can reduce hot flushes.

A hot flush usually begins as warmth in the chest region, then slowly rises up into your neck and face like mercury rising in a thermometer. And just a few minutes later, you're chilled and shivering. Mimicking a fever, hot flushes are a symptom that some 80 per cent of women experience as they transition through menopause. Most women aren't overly bothered by them, but for some, hot flushes and their nocturnal counterparts—night sweats—can make life miserable and difficult. Here's how you can try to keep hot flushes to a minimum.

Key prevention strategies

Take hormone replacement therapy (HRT) Nothing works as well as supplemental oestrogen to cool hot flushes, with studies finding it reduces episodes by up to 90 per cent. The key is to take the lowest possible dose for the shortest possible time. Although a major study found higher rates of breast cancer, heart disease and stroke in women who took an oestrogen-plus-progestin medication (progestin is included with oestrogen therapy to lower the risk of uterine cancer) and higher rates of stroke in women who took an oestrogen-only medication, major medical organisations say it's safe to use HRT in the short term (up to five years) to get you through the worst of the menopausal transition. The risks of any associated health problems are low if you're under sixty.

Take a supplement Many supplements have been investigated for possible hot flush-fighting activity, but few have come up to the mark, despite promising initial results. Options include herbs such as black cohosh, dong quai and chasteberry, and supplements containing phyto-oestrogens, such as those based on soy products, which contain isoflavones or aglycones, or those containing red clover extracts. Phyto-oestrogens are similar in some ways to natural oestrogens and, like them, may increase breast cancer risk. Of all the supplements investigated to date, black cohosh has the best evidence to support its use, but even here the evidence is weak and there is a small risk of serious liver damage.

Try antidepressants Researchers trying to find non-oestrogen options to relieve hot flushes in women with breast cancer stumbled onto the cooling benefits of certain antidepressants prescribed in lower-than-normal doses. These include fluoxetine (Prozac), paroxetine (Aropax) and venlafaxine (Effexor). Studies find they can reduce the number of hot flushes by up to 63 per cent compared to a placebo.

Prevention boosters

Drop a dress size Researchers used to think that having a bit of extra padding would actually reduce hot flushes because hormones in body fat called androgens are converted to oestrogen, which helps prevent hot flushes. It turns out they were wrong. A study of women aged 47 to 59 found that those with the highest percentages of body fat were about 27 per cent more likely to have hot flushes than those with lower percentages. Ideally, aim for body fat levels below 33 per cent (but above 5 per cent). There are devices you can buy to measure your body fat percentage; your gym may have one. Your doctor can also perform a more accurate test. In this study, the average body fat percentage was thirty-seven point nine.

While losing weight will certainly reduce your overall body fat, strength training is your best option for converting fat into muscle (and losing the aforementioned dress size, even if your weight remains the same). Consider a couple of sessions with a personal trainer to get you started.

Take up yoga Australian research suggests yoga may be an effective and inexpensive way to control hot flushes. But don't forget to tell your instructor about any pre-existing injuries you may have.

Consider vitamin E Studies on its benefits for preventing hot flushes are mixed, but one recent study in which 51 women received either 400 IU of vitamin E or a placebo found that those taking vitamin E had about two fewer hot flushes a day compared to when they took a placebo, and the flushes they did have were less severe. High doses may increase stroke risk, so talk with your doctor before supplementing with vitamin E, and don't take more than 400 IU daily.

▶ WHAT CAUSES IT

Fluctuating levels of oestrogen. These fluctuations affect the temperature-control system in the brain so that it overreacts to tiny changes in temperature by dilating blood vessels in a mistaken attempt to cool down.

▶ SYMPTOMS TO WATCH FOR

A feeling of warmth, flushing, heavy perspiration. When hot flushes occur at night, they can disrupt sleep and leave you lying in a muddle of wet sheets.

▶ LATEST THINKING

Ultra-low doses of oestrogen—as little as 25 per cent of previously used conventional doses—can still significantly improve a woman's hot flushes.

Incontinence

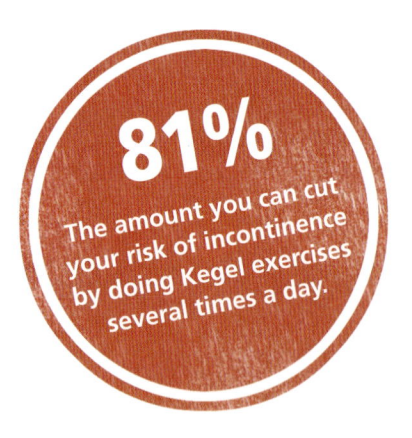

81% The amount you can cut your risk of incontinence by doing Kegel exercises several times a day.

The term 'overactive bladder' may have been dreamed up by marketing gurus at some pharmaceutical company, but the reality is that up to 25 per cent of women and 5 per cent of men under 65—and much higher numbers of those who are older—experience some form of urinary incontinence at some point. It's embarrassing, smelly and one of the major reasons older people end up in nursing homes. Follow these recommendations to stay dry.

Key prevention strategies

Do Kegel exercises every day These exercises strengthen the pelvic floor muscles, which help control the release of urine. The stronger the muscles are, the less likely you are to have an accident. In fact, Kegels are even better than medication at improving existing incontinence. They are particularly effective in pregnant women and in men who have undergone surgery for prostate cancer.

You can do them anytime, anywhere because no one knows you're doing them. First, figure out which muscles to target by stopping in midstream when you're urinating. The muscles you use to do this are your pelvic floor muscles. To perform Kegels, squeeze those muscles and hold for a count of ten. Relax, then repeat. Perform at least three sets of 10 contractions a day. If you're unsure whether you're doing them properly, check with your doctor or a physiotherapist —doing them incorrectly can worsen any existing problems.

Eat smaller portions Studies find that losing weight is one of the most effective ways, next to pelvic floor exercises, to prevent incontinence. Always dole out appropriate-sized portions onto your dinner plate and leave the platter on the stove or elsewhere in the kitchen—not on the dinner table, where you may be tempted to have seconds. Another trick is to use the smallest dinner plates you own. The plate will be fuller, so it will look like you're eating more.

Put your bladder on a schedule Doctors think one reason for incontinence is that some people tend to urinate too often. This can reduce the amount your bladder is able to hold and teaches your bladder muscles to send 'must go' signals even when the bladder is barely half full. If you find yourself going every hour or two, try bladder training. Numerous studies find that this approach, which strengthens bladder muscles, improves incontinence, so there's good reason to think it could help prevent it in the first place.

One way to train your bladder is to start out by going to the toilet every hour whether you have to or not. The next day, go every hour and a half. Continue to increase the time between toilet visits by 30 minutes a day until you're going every few hours, or whatever time frame works best for you to prevent incontinence.

Prevention boosters

Avoid caffeine If you're a tea drinker, you're more likely to develop incontinence, according to a large Norwegian study. It may or may not be due to the caffeine; researchers suspect that tea contains other chemicals that contribute to incontinence, although they don't yet know what they are. However, there is a link between caffeine and incontinence if you drink more than 4 cups a day.

Avoid a hysterectomy Studies suggest that women who have hysterectomies, the most common of gynaecological surgeries in the world, are twice as likely to later require surgery for urinary incontinence than women who don't have them. Some hysterectomies are medically unnecessary; if your doctor recommends one, ask about other options and get a second opinion.

▶ WHAT CAUSES IT

There are numerous causes, ranging from urinary tract infections and pregnancy to being overweight. Over time, particularly after menopause, bladder muscles can thin and weaken. In men, removing the prostate can lead to incontinence. And in both men and women, weak pelvic floor muscles often play a role.

▶ SYMPTOMS TO WATCH FOR

Releasing small amounts of urine when you laugh, sneeze, cough or otherwise exert yourself and/or a sudden urge to urinate that you may or may not be able to control until you get to the toilet.

▶ LATEST THINKING

An injection of botulinum A (Botox) into the bladder muscle can improve incontinence even in people who haven't responded to medication or other treatments.

Weight loss is one of the most effective ways to prevent incontinence.

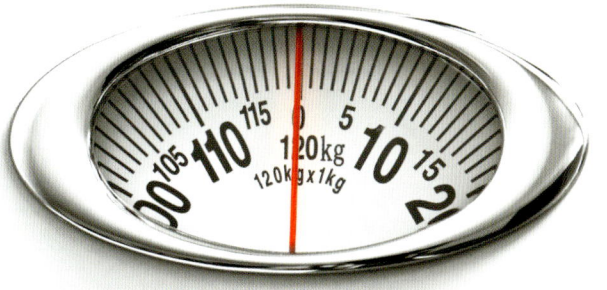

Infertility

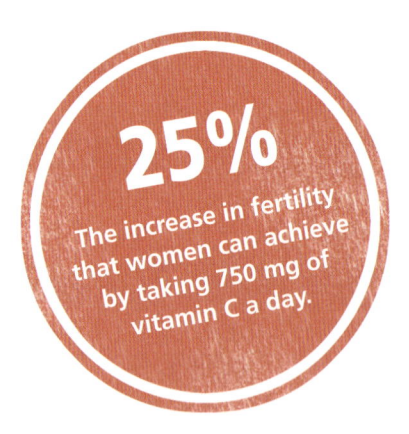

25%
The increase in fertility that women can achieve by taking 750 mg of vitamin C a day.

Within a year of trying, nine out of ten healthy young couples will find themselves pregnant. The others, however, face the possibility of needing medical help for one or both partners. Infertility may be due to a combination of factors unique to a couple, but our advice for reducing the risk of infertility includes options for both men and women.

Key prevention strategies

Start trying to conceive early The odds of getting pregnant plummet with age. In men, the drop usually begins in the early forties thanks to sperm that tend to move more slowly with age. Women are most fertile between 19 and 26, when they have a one-in-two chance of getting pregnant if they have sex when they're most fertile (typically, two days after ovulating). A woman aged 35 to 39 has only about a one-third chance of getting pregnant during that time, and less if her partner is at least five years older.

Maintain a healthy weight In women, obesity plays havoc with reproductive hormones, more than doubling the risk of infertility and increasing by tenfold the likelihood that it will take longer than usual to get pregnant. In men, a 10-kg weight gain increases the risk of infertility by about 10 per cent. If you decide to lose weight by dieting, consider a high-protein, low-carbohydrate approach, which several studies suggest works best to return reproductive hormones to their normal levels.

Quit smoking Smoking is definitely out for women trying to conceive, but a man's smoking habit also lessens the chances of his wife becoming pregnant. Because smoking creates free radicals—molecules that damage healthy cells—the number of sperm that are made and how fast they swim is affected. Free radicals are also triggered by an unhealthy diet.

Boxers or briefs?

As it turns out, it probably doesn't matter. For a long time, experts advised men to switch to boxers since briefs, which are tighter, trap more heat in the groin area. This heat was thought to cause a drop in sperm count, but recent studies discount this theory. Researchers measured scrotal temperatures among 97 men who wore either boxers or briefs and found that those who wore boxers were just as heated as those who wore briefs.

Prevention boosters

Chill out It's not clear whether stress contributes to infertility or vice versa, but studies find that infertile women who seek help from assisted reproductive techniques such as in-vitro fertilisation (IVF) have much higher levels of stress hormones than women who aren't infertile. Studies also find higher levels of stress hormones in women with disturbances in their menstrual cycles that could affect fertility, such as endometriosis. One study also found lower rates of pregnancy associated with higher stress levels in couples undergoing IVF.

Switch from wine to water Women trying to become pregnant shouldn't wait until they conceive to stop drinking alcohol. One study of healthy women who were not alcoholics found that those who had more than three drinks a day had disrupted menstrual cycles and temporary infertility.

Consider some supplements A German study of 7900 women found that taking a daily multivitamin for a month before trying to fall pregnant increased women's fertility rate by 5 per cent compared to taking a placebo containing trace elements.

Studies also find improved fertility in men and women who take vitamin C supplements. In men, supplementing daily with 200–1000 mg of vitamin C increases sperm production. Buy a vitamin C supplement that contains flavonoids; the two together may work better than either alone to reduce oxidative damage to sperm. In women, the dose required was 750 mg a day. But don't take more than 500 mg at once, as your body can't absorb more than that.

Men should also consider selenium and vitamin E. A study of 54 infertile men found that those who supplemented with 400 IU of vitamin E and 225 mcg of selenium for three months had healthier, faster sperm. Talk to your GP before taking any supplements.

Get regular screenings Women who have mulitple sexual partners should be screened at least annually for sexually transmissible infections (STIs), which can result in pelvic inflammatory disease, in which bacteria move up through the cervix into the uterus and fallopian tubes, creating scarring that can prevent a normal pregnancy from developing. In addition to STIs, men should be checked regularly for inflammation of the prostate gland as this can also lead to damaged sperm.

▶ WHAT CAUSES IT

In women, common causes include problems with ovulation, such as polycystic ovary syndrome (PCOS), blocked fallopian tubes and endometriosis, in which uterine tissue grows outside the uterus. In men, the most common causes are slow sperm, low sperm count and malformed sperm.

▶ SYMPTOMS TO WATCH FOR

If you are under 35 and have been trying to get pregnant for a year or more with no success, or if you're 35 or older and have been trying for at least six months, you should see a doctor. Also see a doctor if you or your partner has any known fertility issues (such as previous cancer treatment, endometriosis, blocked fallopian tubes, etc.) or other reproductive problems (uterine fibroids or ovarian cysts, or testicular problems in men).

▶ LATEST THINKING

Chlamydia reproduces inside the early bundle of cells that forms after conception and replicates, which hinders the cells' production of oestrogen and progesterone, hormones needed to keep the embryo growing. This can lead to early miscarriage.

Inflammatory bowel disease

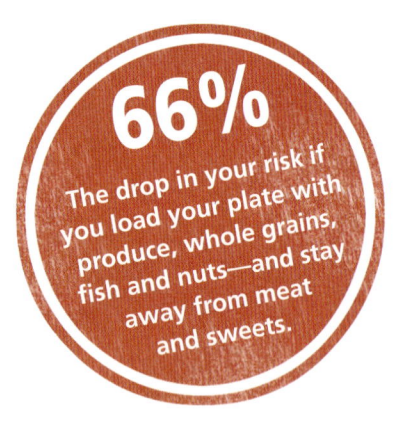

66% The drop in your risk if you load your plate with produce, whole grains, fish and nuts—and stay away from meat and sweets.

Inflammatory bowel disease (IBD) encompasses two painful and sometimes life-threatening conditions: ulcerative colitis and Crohn's disease. Both trigger ongoing inflammation of the intestinal system, leading to pain, sometimes-debilitating diarrhoea and infections. For many, surgery to remove parts of the intestines brings relief. While most IBD begins in young adulthood, experts have noticed an upswing among people in their fifties and sixties. If you don't have IBD, the following strategies may lower your odds of getting it, which is very important if close family members do have it. If you have IBD, our advice may help you avoid relapses and complications.

Key prevention strategies

Stop smoking Smoking cigarettes tripled the risk of Crohn's disease in one Scandinavian study of 317 sets of twins. If you already have Crohn's, continuing to smoke raises your odds for relapses and needing bowel surgery or aggressive medical treatment. The reason? Experts suspect that smoking strangles blood flow to your intestines or somehow puts your immune system on high alert, making the intestinal walls extra sensitive. Oddly, smoking seems to slightly reduce the number of flare-ups for people with ulcerative colitis—but that's no reason to light up. Smoking is devastating for your health in every other way.

Eat more vegetables, fruit, olive oil, fish, grains and nuts
Eat less red meat and fatty foods (such as hot chips and nachos with cheese). Canadian researchers who studied 400 children found that those who had diets high in fruit and vegetables, whole grains, and good fats from fish, nuts and olive oil cut their IBD risk by two-thirds compared to those whose diets included more meat, saturated fats and sweets. Eating an unhealthy diet raised risk nearly five times higher than normal, according to researchers from the University of Montreal.

When the scientists looked more closely, they found that the most protective dietary components were fibre (think fruit, vegetables and whole grains) and omega-3 fatty acids. You'll find those in fish, walnuts, freshly ground linseeds, canola oil and, if you don't eat some source of good fats every day, in fish-oil capsules.

Kick the sugar habit Many people are addicted to sugar and don't even realise how much they're consuming. Instead of a biscuit or chocolate bar in the afternoon or cake for dessert, have fresh fruit instead. While eating more fruit cut the risk of IBD in several studies, eating more desserts and refined sugar tripled the odds of developing Crohn's disease and ulcerative colitis. In one study, people who developed Crohn's reported eating twice as much refined sugar in the months and years before their diagnoses as people without this painful condition.

Use pain relievers sparingly Aspirin and other nonsteroidal anti-inflammatory pain relievers such as ibuprofen (Nurofen) and naproxen (Naprosyn) can all raise the risk for a relapse of IBD, probably because they can damage the lining of the upper intestinal tract. In one study, 28 per cent of people with IBD taking these medications had a relapse within nine days. If you have IBD plus arthritis or another chronic pain condition (or just need relief for a headache), talk to your doctor about your options. There's some evidence that paracetamol and the prescription pain reliever celecoxib (Celebrex) don't trigger relapses.

Cut back on red meat and processed meats When researchers at the University of Newcastle in the UK followed 191 people with ulcerative colitis for one year, they found that those who ate red meat (roasts, hamburgers and steaks) and processed meats (sausages, bacon and salami) the most often were five times more likely to have painful relapses than those who ate very little of these foods.

Limit your alcohol intake In the same UK study, people who drank the most alcohol were four times more likely to have relapses of ulcerative colitis compared to those who drank little, if any, alcohol.

Skip cola drinks and chocolate When researchers from The Netherlands checked on the eating habits and relapse rates of 688 people with IBD and 616 people without it, they discovered that these two dietary splurges were big troublemakers. Drinking cola and nibbling on chocolate doubled the risk of both ulcerative colitis and Crohn's disease.

Got the gene?

Having a parent or sibling with Crohn's disease raises your own risk six times higher than normal; having a close family member with ulcerative colitis raises your risk two and a half times. Scientists have begun to identify the genes behind IBD, and they hope their discoveries will yield new treatments. In a study of nearly 2000 people, US researchers have uncovered a genetic variation that appears to play an important role in raising risk. Those with an 'unhealthy' version of a gene called IL23R were two to four times more likely to develop IBD than those with a 'healthy' variant. This gene helps regulate inflammation, the core problem in IBD.

Prevention boosters

Snack on yogurt Your intestines are home to millions of bacteria. Some of them are there to help digest the food you eat and keep your bowels healthy. But 'unhealthy' bacteria may contribute to or even cause IBD problems. Having enough beneficial bacteria in your body keeps the unhealthy types in check. You can make sure you have enough by eating yogurt that contains active cultures or by taking a probiotic ('healthy' bacteria) supplement.

When researchers at the University of Alberta in Canada gave a probiotic supplement to 34 people with mild to moderate ulcerative colitis, 53 per cent felt completely better after eight weeks, and 24 per cent felt somewhat better. The supplement, called VSL, contained eight species of lactobacillus bacteria, a type also found in yogurt with live active cultures. In another study, researchers found that when people with ulcerative colitis and Crohn's disease ate yogurt every day for a month, blood tests showed that inflammation levels in their intestinal tracts were reduced. Some studies suggest that probiotics are more helpful for preventing relapses of ulcerative colitis and less helpful for Crohn's.

Take a break Stress doesn't cause IBD, but it may make it worse. Some studies suggest that stress increases levels of inflammation in the intestines and that the inflammation persists even when your stress levels subside. It makes sense to find time to unwind on a regular basis, in whatever way works for you—time in the garden, yoga, a hot bath or breathing deeply as you let tension flow out of your body.

Drink lots of water If you already have IBD, you're at risk for dehydration due to frequent and severe diarrhoea, which flushes excess fluid from your body. Be sure to drink plenty of fluids every day; some experts recommend 30 ml for each kilo of body weight. If you weigh around 70 kg, that's about 2 litres—or eight 250-ml

Protect your bones

As many as 60 per cent of people with IBD may have low bone density, raising the risk of osteoporosis and bone fractures. The reason is that long-term use of glucocorticoid medications (such as prednisone and cortisone) that keep a lid on intestinal inflammation can also interfere with your body's ability to maintain healthy bones. And if you have severe IBD or have had surgery to remove part of your intestines, your body may not absorb enough calcium and vitamin D, nutrients essential for strong bones. It's a good idea to take 1000 mg of calcium a day (1200 mg a day after the age of 50). You'll get there with three serves of low-fat dairy foods a day or a mix of dairy plus calcium supplements (don't take more than 600 mg with a meal, since your body can't absorb more than that at once). And aim for 800 IU of vitamin D daily if your skin isn't regularly exposed to sunlight, to help your body absorb and use all that calcium. Weight-bearing exercise such as walking also helps. Talk with your doctor about whether you need a bone density test or are a candidate for bone-strengthening osteoporosis medications.

glasses of water or other clear fluids a day. And watch for signs of dehydration such as a dry mouth, extreme thirst or weakness.

Avoid dietary irritants If you have Crohn's disease that isn't improving, cutting back on sources of insoluble fibre—wholegrain bread, fruit and vegetable skins, nuts and seeds, and tough cuts of meat—could give your intestinal tract the break it needs. Instead, eat more soluble fibre (see below). However, consult a registered dietitian or a doctor before eliminating foods from your diet, as they may want you to slowly replace some of the foods once the inflammation subsides, and it's important to make sure that the diet you're getting is nutritionally balanced.

For ulcerative colitis, consider soluble fibre Soluble fibre forms a protective gel in your intestinal tract and releases compounds that soothe inflammation and promote healing of the intestinal wall. Ask your doctor or a registered dietitian if you should eat foods such as pasta salad, potato salad (with the skin off), barley, warm porridge and cooked legumes, or if you would be better off trying a fibre supplement with ingredients such as wheat dextrin (Benefiber) or psyllium (Metamucil).

Watch your reaction to dairy foods An estimated 35 per cent of people with Crohn's disease and 12 to 20 per cent of those with ulcerative colitis are lactose-intolerant (lactose is a sugar found in milk and milk products). If milk, ice-cream or cheese cause discomfort, try low-lactose milk (available from some supermarkets and health food shops). Yogurt and hard cheeses are usually low in lactose.

▶ WHAT CAUSES IT

Inflammation of the intestines. Experts don't know what triggers it, but suspect that genetics and an immune system response— perhaps to 'unhealthy' bacteria in the intestinal tract, or perhaps to nothing at all—are responsible.

▶ SYMPTOMS TO WATCH FOR

Diarrhoea, which can range from slightly loose stools to dozens of liquid bowel movements per day, abdominal pain and cramping, blood or mucus in the stool, lack of appetite, and weight loss. You may also have fatigue, night sweats and/or fever.

▶ LATEST THINKING

Doctors aren't screening enough people with IBD for colon cancer. If you have Crohn's disease or ulcerative colitis, your risk of developing colon cancer is up to five times higher than normal. Experts recommend early checks for this cancer, with a colonoscopy 8 to 10 years after you first have IBD symptoms.

Be sure to drink plenty of clear fluids every day.

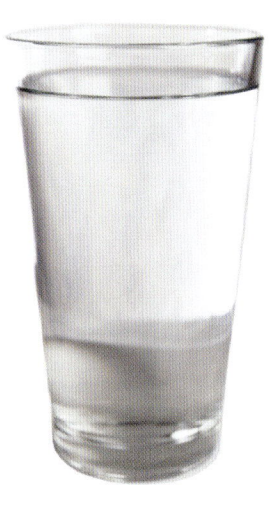

Insomnia

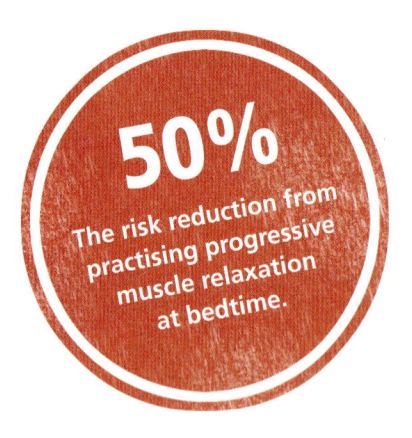

50% The risk reduction from practising progressive muscle relaxation at bedtime.

Having trouble falling asleep may seem minor, but insomnia raises the risk of depression, makes you more sensitive to pain, compromises concentration and memory, and significantly increases the risk of driving accidents. There's even evidence that it wreaks havoc with hormones that control appetite and metabolism, and may be partly responsible for obesity. To try to prevent or help with insomnia, follow our advice.

Key prevention strategies

Stick to a regular sleep schedule That means going to bed at the same time every night and waking up at the same time in the morning, even on weekends. Think of it as training your body to fall asleep when it should.

Create the perfect sleeping environment If you have bills stacked on your bedside table or piles of laundry collecting around the bed, your bedroom is hardly an oasis for sleep. Clear the clutter, then remove the TV and computer from the bedroom, because bedrooms are used only for sleeping and intimate time with your partner. Don't eat or work in there, either. Don't even talk on the phone in your bedroom. This way, as soon as you enter the room at night, your body knows it's time for sleep.

If your windows let in too much light, it may also help to invest in blockout curtains or blinds. And keep the room cool, which also helps to induce sleep.

Limit your time in bed The harder you try to fall asleep, the less likely you'll succeed. If you haven't fallen asleep after 15 minutes, get out of bed and move to another room. Do something quiet, such as reading or knitting, until you feel sleepy enough to nod off, then go back to bed. Continue this pattern until you finally fall asleep.

Take a walk outside Exercise can improve sleep, and doing it outside in bright sunlight can have an even greater effect by ensuring that your body clock is properly set. In one study, people who got 30 minutes a day of bright light therapy with full-spectrum lamps that mimic sunlight (available online and from lighting shops) increased their total sleep time by 44 minutes.

Go to the gym or take a jog One of the best ways to get a good night's sleep is to exercise. Studies find that in athletes, just one day without exercise leads to worse sleep, and increases the time they need to fall asleep. Most researchers think that exercise reduces insomnia, in part, by raising body temperature. If you exercise vigorously enough to raise your temperature in the late afternoon, it will fall around bedtime—and decreased body temperature naturally triggers sleep. Exercise also helps by lowering stress hormones. Most people with insomnia have high levels of these hormones, or they release them with very little provocation. Exercise initially increases the hormones, but a few hours later, seeking to return to balance, your body sends out signals to reduce them. That's why you shouldn't exercise in the evening; try to end your work-out at least 6 hours before bedtime.

Prevention boosters

Talk to a therapist A form of therapy called cognitive behavioural therapy (CBT) can help with insomnia by teaching you techniques to overcome it—and your anxiety about it. For instance, after a few sleepless nights, many people begin to stress about their ability to ever fall asleep, starting what becomes a self-perpetuating cycle. They may also underestimate how much sleep they actually get and over-estimate how much time they spend lying awake stressing about how to fall asleep. CBT helps put things into perspective by teaching you more about insomnia and how to address it.

Ten ways to fall asleep

1. **Sip on chamomile tea before bedtime**
2. **Cover your eyes** You can find eye masks in most pharmacies, or save one next time you're on a plane. They work wonders for banishing even the tiniest glow of a night-light.
3. **Cool down your bedroom** Open the windows, turn on a ceiling fan or run the airconditioner. Reducing your body temperature signals your brain to release the sleep hormone melatonin.
4. **Read a book of poetry** The cadences of the lines and the images the words invoke can be much more calming than a novel. Better yet, listen to poetry on CD or an MP3 player—it's almost like hearing a bedtime story.
5. **Make a list** Before you get into bed, make a list of everything that's on your mind. Then you don't have to lie awake worrying about it.
6. **Listen to white noise** Tune in to radio static or buy a white-noise machine.
7. **Spray lavender scent on your bedlinen** Lavender is known for its calming effects.
8. **Try progressive muscle relaxation** Starting with your feet and working up to your eyes, tense and relax one group of muscles at a time. This forces every muscle in your body to relax.
9. **Sleep in your underwear** It'll keep you cool.
10. **Wear earplugs** They block out snoring.

Limit alcoholic drinks While alcohol may help you fall asleep, you're likely to wake up again as the effects wear off and find yourself unable to fall back to sleep. If you want a drink, have it in the late afternoon or early evening.

Stay away from cigarettes Nicotine is a central nervous system stimulant, which means it keeps you awake. Even just being around cigarette smoke within a couple of hours of bedtime could interfere with your ability to fall asleep or stay asleep.

Check your medications Numerous medications, particularly some prescribed for attention deficit disorder (ADD), high blood pressure, asthma, underactive thyroid, depression and neurological problems such as Parkinson's disease, can keep you up at night. If you're having trouble drifting off or staying asleep, ask your doctor whether one of your medications may be to blame and what you can do about it.

Get treated for allergies Sneezing because of pollen and other seasonal allergens may keep you up at night. French researchers found that about 42 per cent of people with seasonal allergies said they had trouble falling asleep compared with around 18 per cent of those who didn't have allergies. The worse the allergies, the longer it took people to fall asleep, and the more sleeping pills they took.

Consider a sleeping pill To prevent occasional insomnia, over-the-counter or prescription sleeping pills can help and, if you use them only for the short term, probably won't hurt. Over-the-counter sleeping pills contain an antihistamine, either alone or together with a painkiller, but they can leave you with a sleep 'hangover' the next day. A better option is one of the newer prescription sleeping aids, such as zaleplon (Sonata) or zolpidem (Stilnox). These are sedatives. They work similarly and carry a risk of similar side effects, including performing activities such as eating or even driving while you're still asleep.

Turn on some music A study by Taiwanese researchers compared the effects of soft music on sleep in 63 people who had trouble sleeping. Half listened to 45 minutes of music when they went to bed; half listened to nothing. The result is that those who listened to music slept better and longer, took less time to fall asleep and functioned better the next day. Overall, sleep quality improved 45 per cent in the music group compared to the control group. Plus, the group's sleep quality improved more with each week of music.

Take an afternoon nap Long naps will only keep you up at night, but short naps could make a positive difference. A very small Japanese study found that a 30-minute nap after lunch, followed by some stretching and flexibility exercises in the early evening, significantly improved sleep quality and reduced the amount of time it took to fall asleep.

Join a tai chi class When researchers assigned 118 older adults to either a tai chi or another low-impact exercise class for three 1-hour sessions a week over 24 weeks, they found that people taking tai chi improved significantly more than the control group in quality of sleep, the time it took to fall asleep and the total time spent asleep. In fact, the tai chi participants fell asleep an average of 18 minutes faster than those in the other group and slept nearly an hour longer per night. The study authors theorise that tai chi helps in part by enhancing overall wellbeing through relaxation and diaphragmatic breathing.

▶ WHAT CAUSES IT

Anyone can have trouble falling asleep during a stressful time. Other causes include chronic pain, depression and anxiety disorders. You can also 'train' yourself to have insomnia by worrying so much about whether you'll fall asleep that you stress out when you hit the bed. Watch out for daytime sleepiness and snoring; the two together are often a sign of sleep apnoea, which contributes to numerous medical conditions.

▶ SYMPTOMS TO WATCH FOR

An inability to fall asleep or stay asleep, or waking up too early in the morning. Trouble falling asleep may be related to anxiety, whereas waking up too early could be related to depression.

▶ LATEST THINKING

Treating the insomnia that exists alongside medical or mental health conditions not only relieves the insomnia but can actually improve the coexisting condition. However, most doctors still treat only the coexisting condition, believing that once it improves, so will the insomnia.

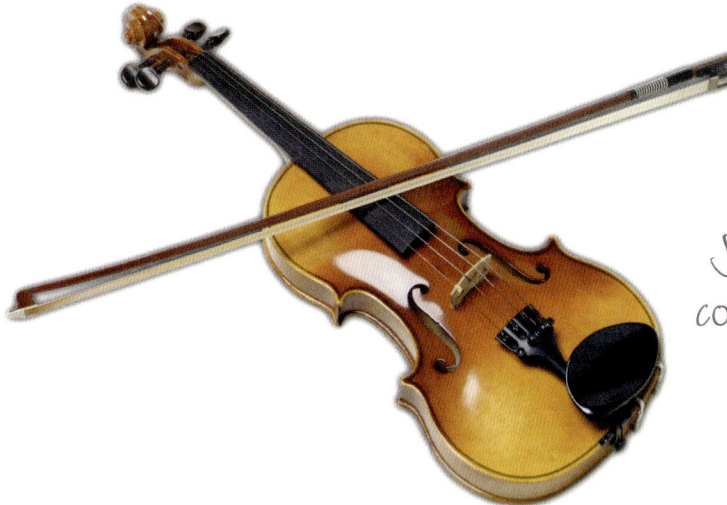

Soothing music really could succeed in sending you off to sleep.

Irritable bowel syndrome

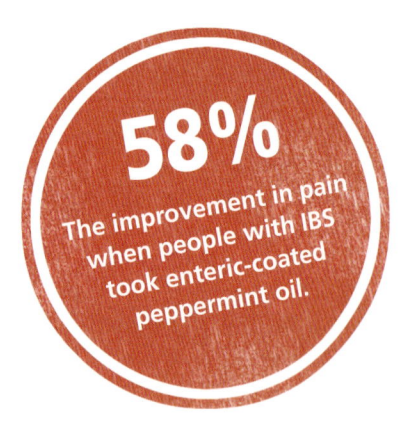

58%
The improvement in pain when people with IBS took enteric-coated peppermint oil.

Irritable bowel syndrome (IBS) is a frustrating mystery. Experts say that this digestive problem's pain, cramps, diarrhoea and constipation seem to be the result of bowels that move too quickly or too slowly and nerves that become exquisitely sensitive to the slightest pressure after you eat a meal. The following solutions will work, but be patient—you may have to try a few to find a plan that works for you.

Key prevention strategies

Pinpoint trouble foods Many people with IBS know from experience which foods trigger problems. Common foods include alcohol, chocolate, caffeinated beverages, dairy products and sugar-free sweeteners such as sorbitol and mannitol. People who have problems with wind and bloating may be bothered by beans, broccoli, cabbage and cauliflower, too. For others, high-fat foods can cause intestinal pain.

When researchers at St Georges Hospital Medical School in London tested the blood of 132 people with IBS and 42 healthy people who had been exposed to 16 common foods, people in the IBS group had higher levels of an antibody called IgG4 (associated with food intolerances) in response to beef, lamb, pork, soybeans and wheat—leading the scientists to say that if you have IBS, pay careful attention to how you feel in the hours after eating these foods. Here's how to pinpoint your trouble foods:

- **Step 1: Track your symptoms** Write down the date, the type of symptoms you're having, how long they last, what you ate (and how much) during the preceding day or two, any medications you took and what you were doing just before your discomfort began. After 14 days, look for patterns.
- **Step 2: Eliminate one suspected trigger food at a time** In another UK study, people who eliminated problem foods saw symptoms improve by 26 per cent. Cutting out one food at a time will give you a clearer picture of what helps and what doesn't.

Investigate antibiotics Digestive disease researchers are beginning to suspect that an overgrowth of bacteria in the upper intestines—a place where few bacteria should be living—may explain many of IBS's confusing and hard-to-treat symptoms. In one study, US researchers found evidence that 84 per cent of study volunteers with IBS had an overgrowth of bacteria in the small intestine. Those who took antibiotics to wipe out these unwanted bugs saw IBS symptoms improve by 75 per cent. (Other studies found a lower, 36 per cent improvement rate.)

Some doctors prefer to use a broad-spectrum antibiotic. Experts recommend that people with IBS may need to repeat the antibiotic treatment every two to three months to see an improvement.

Try a little fibre Until recently, digestive disease experts heartily recommended higher-fibre diets for people with IBS. Conventional wisdom said that soluble fibre—the type found in beans, pears, barley and some fibre supplements—could firm up the stools of people with diarrhoea, while soluble and insoluble fibre (the type found in wholemeal bread and many vegetables) would speed up bowels slowed by constipation. Sometimes it works; in one US study of 81 people with IBS, 26 per cent reported less abdominal pain and bloating when they switched to a diet with more than 25 g of fibre per day. But other studies show that fibre isn't a miracle fix. It makes pain worse for some people and has little effect for others.

If you'd like to give it a try, go slowly. Swap one low-fibre food for a higher-fibre one a day (replace white bread with wholemeal, for example) for a week and monitor how you feel. If you're feeling well, make another swap. And make sure you drink plenty of water so the fibre won't cause constipation.

DRUGS THAT PREVENT DISEASE

A wide variety of medications can help prevent and control the most difficult IBS symptoms, from constipation and diarrhoea to pain and cramps.

Antidepressants Even if you aren't depressed, antidepressants can block pain signals travelling between the intestines and brain, and can even help your bowel movements become more normal. In one study, people with IBS who took citalopram (Cipramil) reported that abdominal pain and bloating improved significantly in just a few days. Which one's best for you? Expect pain and cramp relief with any of them. Constipation seems to improve more with selective serotonin-reuptake inhibitors (SSRIs) such as citalopram, escitalopram (Lexapro), fluoxetine (Prozac), paroxetine (Aropax) and sertraline (Zoloft). Diarrhoea seems to ease more with tricyclic antidepressants such as amitriptyline (Endep), imipramine (Tofranil) and nortriptyline (Allegron).

Antispasmodic drugs These medications are useful in treating pain and cramping, and include hyoscyamine (Donnatab). They work by relaxing the walls of the intestines. You may have to try several to find one that's best for you.

Diarrhoea medications The over-the-counter diarrhoea medication loperamide (Imodium) works for many people. It shouldn't be used for acute infectious diarrhoea.

Mild laxatives Plain old milk of magnesia is often effective in treating constipation. If it doesn't help, see your doctor. If your constipation is severe, he or she may suggest medications that can help prevent future problems, such as Movicol.

Peppermint oil This old-fashioned remedy was effective in several clinical trials. Look for enteric-coated preparations.

Relax all over Progressive muscle relaxation eases stress, which in turn seems to reduce IBS pain sensitivity. In one small US study, people with IBS who practised this technique daily for a month were five times more likely to experience improvement in pain and cramping than those who didn't use the technique.

Sit or lie down in a comfortable place and shut your eyes, breathe deeply and imagine stress flowing out of your muscles. Beginning with your feet, tense each muscle group tightly, then let the tension go so the muscles feel more relaxed than when you started. Move on to your calves, upper legs and up to your neck, face and head.

Prevention boosters

Get moving Exercise eased gastrointestinal symptoms in one large US study. The researchers weren't looking specifically at IBS, but there's plenty of other proof that being active can help by relaxing your bowels. Intestinal activity often settles during exercise, allowing your body to shunt more blood to your legs and arms. It also relieves stress and boosts mood, making pain easier to cope with.

Take peppermint-oil capsules for spasms Peppermint oil relaxes muscles in your gastrointestinal tract. In one well-designed study of 57 people with IBS, 75 per cent of those who took peppermint-oil capsules saw symptoms improve by 50 per cent or more after four weeks, compared to 38 per cent who took a placebo. Study volunteers took two capsules twice a day. Use enteric-coated capsules so the oil is released in your intestines, not your stomach.

Try hypnotherapy In one UK study, people with IBS who tried five sessions of hypnotherapy had less pain and diarrhoea after three months than study volunteers who didn't have therapy. Benefits faded over time; after a year, the hypnosis group needed less medication to control IBS, but their symptoms were about the same as the non-hypnosis group. In another study, people who got 12 sessions over three months were still feeling better five years later. Ask your doctor for a referral to a practitioner trained in hypnotherapy who is familiar with 'gut-directed' hypnotherapy, a technique that teaches you how to ease your own symptoms.

Soothe with yoga In one study from India, men with IBS had equal reductions in diarrhoea after two months of daily yoga or two months of daily doses of the over-the-counter medication loperamide (Imodium). Yoga seemed to soothe overactive nerves that stimulate bowel activity, according to researchers from the All India Institute of Medical Sciences in New Delhi. Meanwhile, a Canadian study of teenagers with IBS found that doing yoga routines as instructed in a video daily for a month eased anxiety.

Talk with a cognitive behavioural therapist This practical type of counselling is aimed at helping you perceive and respond to everyday problems in new ways and to find solutions that really work. You may also work on relaxation skills. Some studies find a benefit for IBS, while others don't. Still others have found that it works for a little while, but then the effects wear off. It may be worth a try if you find that coping with IBS is overwhelming or if you just can't do all the things you want or need to do in your life. It seems to work best as an add-on therapy along with medications.

Try biofeedback If you're bothered by constipation, learning how to properly use your abdominal muscles during a bowel movement could improve results—and make you feel better. In one Australian study, 25 women with IBS used biofeedback to help them as a doctor and nurse gave them 'advanced training' in the proper way to push out stools without straining. (They practised with small water balloons, not the real thing!) This type of biofeedback uses a probe inserted into the rectum to measure pressure exerted on stools. The result: 75 per cent reported that things had improved. Other types of biofeedback can help people with IBS learn to control stress, too.

Send in the 'healthy' bacteria Probiotics—as supplements or in yogurt with active cultures—may help IBS symptoms by raising levels of healthy bacteria in your intestinal tract. In one study, 44 people with IBS took a supplement containing *Lactobacillus acidophilus* and *Bifidobacterium* (also found in yogurts containing live active cultures) for a week. Symptoms such as pain, spasms, constipation and diarrhoea improved by 50 per cent.

▶ WHAT CAUSES IT

The root cause of IBS remains a mystery. Experts suspect that an overgrowth of bacteria, a gastrointestinal infection or other factors make muscles in the intestinal wall move too quickly or too slowly; in addition, nerves in the intestines seem to become oversensitive.

▶ SYMPTOMS TO WATCH FOR

Abdominal pain and cramping, bloating, flatulence, diarrhoea or constipation (or alternating bouts of both), and mucus in the stools.

▶ LATEST THINKING

Slow down and rest when you have a stomach bug. There's new evidence that trying to 'tough out' a gastrointestinal infection raises your risk of developing IBS afterwards. When researchers at the University of Southampton in the UK contacted 620 people with past gastrointestinal infections, they found that those who had pushed themselves hard (for example, they kept working until they collapsed in bed) during their illnesses were more likely to develop IBS than those who took it easy.

Jaw pain

60% The amount you can reduce jaw pain by doing isometric jaw exercises and taking an anti-inflammatory for four weeks.

The joints responsible for your jaw 'popping out' when you open your mouth wide are the temporomandibular joints on each side of your head, and they keep your jaw attached to your skull. They're among the most complicated and commonly used joints in the body, able to move forwards and backwards and side to side. However, chewing too much, grinding your teeth or having a misalignment in your teeth and/or jaw can all stress the joints or the muscles and ligaments that control them, leading to temporomandibular joint (TMJ) disorder, more commonly known as jaw pain.

Key prevention strategies

Rest your jaw Minimise your chewing (stop crunching ice, for instance) and halve the size of your sandwiches so you don't have to open your mouth as wide. If you open your mouth wider than the width of three fingers, it's too wide. It also helps to avoid chewing gum and especially chewy foods such as toffees.

See the dentist Our teeth were not meant to grind, so if you grind your teeth (or, if you're not aware of it, your sleeping partner says you do), see your dentist, who can fit you with a mouth guard or splint to wear at night to prevent this major cause of TMJ. You're also more likely to develop TMJ if your teeth don't come together neatly. If you have this problem (called malocclusion), talk to an orthodontist about braces to realign your teeth, improve your bite and reduce your risk of TMJ.

Stop clenching Some people hold tension in their jaws without even realising it, especially when they're under stress. That tension can contribute to or even cause jaw pain to the extent that it becomes painful even to eat. The following tips can help you learn how to relax the muscles that control your jaw.

Put a cork in it Hold a wine bottle cork between your front teeth and relax the muscles around it. Do this whenever you feel yourself clenching or until relaxing those muscles becomes automatic.

Try biofeedback Electromyogram (EMG) biofeedback teaches you to relax your jaw and facial muscles. You start out with sensors attached to your forehead, jaw muscles and shoulder muscles that signal when they sense muscle tension. Then you're taught techniques to relax and reduce the tension. After practising for a few weeks, you're able to reduce the tension without the sensors. Ask your doctor or dentist for a referral.

See a cognitive behavioural therapist This type of therapy can help you realise and change factors, such as your response to stress and anxiety, that contribute to jaw pain. It may provide you with skills to reduce your response to pain and works well for many people when it comes to preventing jaw pain. You don't need many sessions; one study found that pain improved by 50 per cent in people who had just four sessions. Your doctor can help you find a specialist. Combining this type of therapy with biofeedback and a mouth splint works better than any of the three treatments alone.

Prevention boosters

Exercise your jaw Isometric jaw exercises can strengthen and stretch the muscles around the joints. Practise the exercises below several times a day. Try to hold each position for a full five seconds and repeat the exercise five times.
- **Opening** Hold the back of your hand underneath your jaw to create resistance. Open your mouth about 2.5 cm wide pushing against your hand.
- **Forward thrust** Hold the back of your hand against the bottom of your jaw to create resistance. Push your jaw forward against your hand.
- **Sideways thrust** Hold the palm of your hand against the side of your jaw that hurts. Push your jaw to that side.

▶ WHAT CAUSES IT
Stress, a misaligned jaw, clenching your jaw, grinding your teeth or degenerative joint disease.

▶ SYMPTOMS TO WATCH FOR
Jaw pain; neck, back and facial pain; pain in and around the ear; headaches; or ringing in the ear. You may hear a clicking sound when you chew.

▶ LATEST THINKING
Injections of botulinum toxin type A (Botox), the same substance used to erase frown lines, into the muscles used to move the jaw significantly reduce pain in people with TMJ.

Kidney disease

26% The amount by which you could reduce your risk of kidney disease by maintaining normal blood pressure.

Chronic kidney disease is on the rise in large part due to the prevalence of diabetes and hypertension, both of which are leading causes. One out of six adults has kidney disease, yet many people with weak or failing kidneys have no idea that anything's wrong. Chronic kidney disease (CKD) occurs when the kidneys gradually lose their ability to filter waste and toxins from the blood. It can eventually cause fatigue and shortness of breath, and it's the main reason people end up needing dialysis. Once you have CKD, you can't get rid of it, but you can halt or slow its progression.

Key prevention strategies

Prevent diabetes and hypertension Your risk of chronic kidney disease doubles if you have both of these conditions, which damage tiny blood vessels in the kidneys. If you already have high blood pressure, talk to your doctor about treating it with an ACE inhibitor. Studies find these medications work best at preventing kidney disease or at the very least preventing it from advancing to the point where dialysis or a transplant is required. If you already have diabetes, keep your blood sugar levels as normal as possible. (For more information on how to prevent these two conditions, see 'Diabetes', on page 164, and 'High blood pressure', on page 210.) If you have both conditions, talk to your doctor about a medication combining an ACE inhibitor and the diuretic indapamide. A study of 11,000 patients found it worked best to prevent kidney disease and its progression.

Get a simple kidney check-up If you're at risk for kidney disease—you have diabetes or high blood pressure, or a family history of kidney problems—your doctor should test your kidney function regularly. In the past, doctors used a blood test that measured a protein called creatinine. But because creatinine levels vary among individuals, the test can be somewhat unreliable. Now doctors screen kidney function with the glomerular filtration rate (GFR) test, a blood test that measures how well the kidneys filter waste from the blood.

Buy a home blood pressure monitor Pay special attention to your systolic blood pressure, the top number in your reading; it's a good indication of your vulnerability to kidney disease. A major study of 8093 men who were followed for 14 years found that a systolic pressure between 130 and 139 mmHg increased the risk of kidney disease by 26 per cent, and one of 140 mmHg or higher increased it by 69 per cent.

Prevention boosters

Prevent kidney stones Blockages caused by kidney stones can increase the risk of chronic kidney disease. (See 'Kidney stones' on the following page for some prevention tips.)

Spend the night in a sleep lab If you snore loudly, your partner says you make loud choking or gasping noises while you sleep, and/or you're exhausted during the day, you could have a condition called obstructive sleep apnoea, which may mean you're more likely to have chronic kidney disease, though experts aren't sure why. Being overweight and having high blood pressure increase the risk of both conditions, but researchers also note that people with sleep-related breathing disorders often have anaemia, or low levels of oxygen-carrying blood cells, which increases the risk of chronic kidney disease. It can't hurt—and will certainly help your overall health—to take care of your apnoea. The only way to diagnose obstructive sleep apnoea for certain is with polysomnography, a test that evaluates your breathing as you sleep.

Skip dessert Or find other ways to lose weight. While being overweight makes existing kidney disease worse, it can also increase the risk of developing the condition. A study in 11,000 healthy men that found those whose body mass indexes, or BMIs, increased 10 per cent or more over 14 years were 27 per cent more likely to develop chronic kidney disease than those whose BMIs either dropped or increased just 5 per cent. The risk remained even if the men had normal blood pressure and blood sugar, and exercised regularly.

▶ WHAT CAUSES IT

Damage to blood vessels in the kidneys. The damage is most often caused by high blood pressure or diabetes but may also be the result of lupus, infections, inherited diseases, long-term use of NSAIDs such as aspirin or ibuprofen, kidney stones, an enlarged prostate that obstructs urine flow from the kidneys, or cancer.

▶ SYMPTOMS TO WATCH FOR

The early stages have no symptoms. In later stages, you may experience fatigue, frequent hiccups, feeling 'fluey', itching, headache, foot and ankle swelling, nausea and vomiting, or weight loss. In the late stages, symptoms include blood in vomit or stools, decreased alertness, reduced feeling in your hands or feet, easy bruising, an increase or decrease in urine, muscle twitching or cramps, seizures, or white crystals in and on your skin.

▶ LATEST THINKING

A recent study found that people with gum disease were 60 per cent more likely to have chronic kidney disease. Researchers suspect that the chronic inflammation caused by gum disease may play a role.

Kidney stones

29–49% The risk reduction of having stones by drinking enough to urinate twice as much as most people do.

One out of every 10 adults will experience the excruciating pain of trying to pass a kidney stone at some point in their lives, and some say it's worse than the pain of childbirth. Kidney stones result from microscopic deposits in urine that eventually solidify, much like the salt left at the bottom of a glass of salt water after the liquid evaporates. There are several types of kidney stones. If you have passed a stone, your doctor can test its composition and measure chemicals in your blood and urine to decide on the best way to prevent stones from developing in the future.

Key prevention strategies

Drink lots of fluids Drinking more fluids is the best way to prevent all types of kidney stones. One study found that men who produced a prodigious 2.5 litres or more of urine a day (the average is 1.4 litres) were 29 per cent less likely to develop symptomatic stones than those who excreted 1.2 litres or less. In women, urinating 2.6 litres or more reduced their risk by 49 per cent compared with urinating less than 1.4 litres a day. You'll need to drink 3.5 to 3.8 litres of liquid a day to get there. This should make you urinate every 2 hours or so. Ask your doctor first about whether this strategy is safe for you to try out.

Eat yogurt Doctors used to warn all patients at risk for kidney stones to limit their calcium intake. But it turns out that people who have the least calcium in their diets can have the highest risk of kidney stones. (A few patients, those with absorptive hypercalciuria, are still asked to reduce their calcium intake.) Note that this relates to dietary calcium; there's no evidence that calcium supplements reduce your risk. In fact, in women, supplements could increase the risk of stones by about 20 per cent.

Researchers think that calcium protects against stones by binding to oxalic acid, a

DRUGS THAT PREVENT DISEASE

If you've had calcium stones before, talk to your doctor about taking a thiazide diuretic (which reduces the amount of calcium in the urine) with potassium citrate (to replace the potassium the diuretic depletes) to cut your risk of future stones. Studies show these medications are effective and can reduce new stone formation by 90 per cent or more. Uric acid stones can be treated with other medications.

salt found in certain foods that contributes to kidney stones, so preventing it from getting into urine. The best sources are low-fat milk, yogurt and cheese. Edamame (green soybeans) are also high in calcium. An unexpectedly good source is wholegrain cereal, which can contain up to 1000 mg in a single serve. Most people need 1200 mg of calcium a day to protect their bones, although there is no specific level recommended to reduce the risk of kidney stones.

Limit high-oxalate foods This is for people who have already had calcium stones. Researchers find that certain high-oxalate foods—spinach, rhubarb, beetroot, strawberries, figs, chocolate, wheat bran, peanuts and almonds—increase the risk of stones. If you can't bear to give up any of these foods, increase the amount of calcium you take in when you eat them. For instance, slice strawberries into a bowl of cereal with milk, sprinkle almonds over yogurt and top a spinach salad with low-fat grated cheese.

Prevention boosters

Drink a glass of orange juice every day Experts have long prescribed tart (very lightly sweetened) lemonade as a way to keep stones at bay. But recent studies suggest that orange juice may be an even better choice. Both are great sources of potassium citrate, which is often prescribed to prevent kidney stones. Just stay away from grapefruit juice: it seems that having as little as 250 ml a day can increase the risk of kidney stones, though researchers have no idea why. Apple juice may increase risk by 35 per cent.

Lose weight if need be When researchers analysed study results they found that men who were over 100 kg were 44 per cent more likely to develop kidney stones than those who weighed less than 68 kg. For women, the danger of being overweight was greater: those who weighed more than 100 kg were between 89 and 92 per cent more likely to develop kidney stones than those under 68 kg.

Avoid high-fructose corn syrup Numerous packaged foods and drinks contain corn syrup, but kicking the soft-drink habit, avoiding sweetened fruit drinks and eating fewer packaged snacks is a good start. Cutting back may significantly reduce your risk of stones. Researchers suspect the connection has to do with fructose's tendency to increase the amount of calcium in urine.

WHAT CAUSES IT

Genetic disposition, urinary tract infections, kidney disease, chronic dehydration and certain metabolic conditions that affect the make-up of urine. Certain medications, including diuretics and calcium-based antacids, can also contribute.

SYMPTOMS TO WATCH FOR

Initially, none. In fact, the majority of stones pass without any symptoms. Larger stones, however, can cause sudden, intense pain in your back, side and lower abdomen, as well as nausea and vomiting. You may also have some blood in your urine, feel that you have to urinate more often than usual and/or feel burning when you urinate.

LATEST THINKING

People with metabolic syndrome—a constellation of symptoms that include high blood pressure and triglycerides, abdominal fat, insulin resistance and low levels of 'good' HDL cholesterol—have a much higher risk of developing kidney stones.

Knee pain

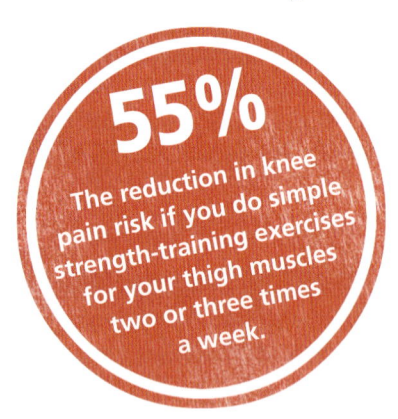

55% The reduction in knee pain risk if you do simple strength-training exercises for your thigh muscles two or three times a week.

The human knee is built to withstand forces four times greater than your body weight—and to support you as you bend, twist and jump. However, its rigging system of bones, ligaments and tendons works best when the muscles around it are also strong and flexible. If they go soft, then even carrying heavy bags around can lead to pain. And time isn't always kind to knees, either. Since ageing, genetics and injuries contribute to the wide variety of problems that can cause pain, it's no wonder that one in four people over the age of 55 complains of chronic knee pain. Here's how to avoid it.

Key prevention strategies

Drop extra kilos Each 500 g of excess weight you lose reduces the pressure on your knees by nearly 2 kg. On a 1-km walk, that translates to 1300 fewer kilos that your knees have to support.

Exercising while you diet not only makes permanent weight loss much easier but also translates into bigger benefits for knees. In a study that followed 316 women and men with painful knees, those who took a knee-friendly low-impact aerobics and strength-training class for an hour three times a week, and also lost weight, reported a 30 per cent drop in knee pain and a 24 per cent improvement in their ability to do everyday things such as climbing stairs.

Don't smoke Chemicals in tobacco smoke derail the process that heals torn ligaments, including those in the knees. US researchers found that smoking reduced the number of infection-fighting cells called macrophages that arrive at the site of ligament injuries. That's a problem because macrophages release chemical signals that summon other cells needed for making repairs. It matters because thousands of people endure knee pain each year due to torn ligaments. A symptom of a torn ligament is pain, tenderness or stiffness on the outside of the knee that you feel mostly when you're moving around.

Avoid high-impact exercise If running, step aerobics or even jumping jacks hurt, it's time to switch to a lower-impact fitness routine. Walking, swimming, cycling and water aerobics are great work-outs that burn kilojoules, boost cardiovascular fitness, and have even been shown to reduce knee pain in studies. Stop doing an activity if it hurts your knees and choose something different.

Strengthen all the muscles that support your knees Strong quadriceps (the big muscles that run down the front of your thighs) and hamstrings (at the back of your thighs) act as shock absorbers that take some of the pressure put on your knees when you walk, jump and bend. They also keep the bones in your knees better aligned, which reduces the risk of pain and excess wear and tear. In one study, women with stronger thigh muscles had 55 per cent less chance of developing knee pain. (See pages 110–113 for exercises to strengthen your quadriceps and hamstrings.)

But don't stop there. Strengthening your 'core' abdominal and back muscles, as well as those in your hips and buttocks, is equally important for decreasing knee pain. (See also pages 122–127 and 268–269 for helpful exercises.)

Prevention boosters

Wear joint-friendly footwear The best shoes for your knees are flat and flexible, according to researchers from Rush Medical College in the US. The scientists analysed pressure on the knees of 16 volunteers as they walked in clogs, thongs, walking shoes and 'stability' shoes (stiff shoes often worn by older people with balance problems). The surprise winners were thongs and walking shoes, which allowed the feet to bend and flex naturally with each step, taking pressure off the knees. We recommend the walking shoes. While thongs are comfortable on the beach, they don't protect your feet or stay in place very well as you walk.

If you have flat feet, slipping over-the-counter shoe inserts or custom-made orthotics into your shoes can help keep the bones in your knees better aligned, helping to prevent pain.

Measure your legs Or better yet, ask your doctor to do it. Legs of unequal length can contribute to osteoarthritis as well as knee and hip pain, say US researchers from the University of North Carolina at Chapel Hill School of Medicine. Apparently, having one leg just 8 mm shorter than the other can raise the risk of knee pain by 50 per cent. The answer is to ask your doctor about shoe inserts.

▶ WHAT CAUSES IT
Osteoarthritis, rheumatoid arthritis, overweight, falls and accidents, overuse, weak muscles, or not warming up before starting a challenging exercise routine.

▶ SYMPTOMS TO WATCH FOR
Knee pain due to osteoarthritis is usually deep and achy, is felt around the knee joint and is often worse at night. Sudden, severe pain can be the result of injured ligaments (which attach the bones in your upper and lower legs), irritation or inflammation of tendons (which attach muscle to bone), or a dislocated kneecap. Your knee may also lock in place, often due to a torn meniscus, the curved piece of cartilage inside your knee joint. If your knee swells (often called water on the knee), it may be a sign that fluid-filled sacs called bursae that act as joint cushions have become inflamed. You may also have pain just below the knee. See your doctor if your knee is hot, swollen or extremely painful, has locked in place or if you can't stand or walk.

▶ LATEST THINKING
Low vitamin D levels can make knee pain worse. If you have osteoarthritis of the knee, be sure you're getting 1000 to 2000 IU of vitamin D a day.

Lung cancer

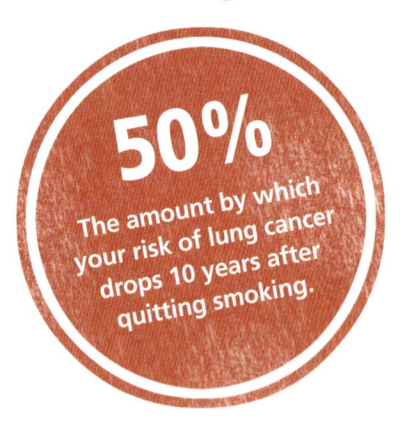

50% The amount by which your risk of lung cancer drops 10 years after quitting smoking.

Unless you've been on a desert island for the past 40 years, you know that smoking is the leading cause of lung cancer (although 2 to 10 per cent of lung cancers occur in people who have never smoked, particularly women). To help prevent lung cancer, don't smoke, and stay away from smokers—an hour spent inhaling someone else's cigarette smoke damages your lungs as much as smoking four cigarettes yourself!

Key prevention strategies

Quit smoking Your risk of developing lung cancer if you smoke a pack of cigarettes a day for 40 years is about 20 times that of someone who never smoked. We know it's not easy to quit; it typically takes several attempts before it sticks. Our advice is to make a doctor's appointment. Working with your doctor increases your odds of success by 75 per cent versus going solo. The doctor will probably prescribe a nicotine-replacement product. Whether you choose gum, a patch, lozenges or a nasal spray, studies find that the products can double the odds of quitting successfully (defined as being smoke free for a year). Your doctor may also prescribe bupropion (Zyban) or varenicline (Chantix), both of which help people quit. Only bupropion can be used in conjunction with nicotine-replacement products.

Should you try to quit slowly or all at once? Research shows that quitting cold turkey works better, but starting nicotine-replacement therapy a couple of weeks before you stop may help.

Test your house for radon Radon, a colourless, odourless gas that results from decaying radioactive elements in the earth, is found in most homes but in very low levels. If your home is poorly ventilated and

DRUGS THAT PREVENT DISEASE

Researchers evaluating the use of statins, medications widely prescribed to reduce cholesterol, in nearly half a million patients found that taking them for at least six months reduced the risk of lung cancer by 55 per cent. Researchers suspect that statins protect against lung cancer by taming inflammation in the body, which contributes to cancer development. The next step is clinical trials to confirm the findings.

Another drug that may help prevent lung cancer is the pain reliever celecoxib (Celebrex). In one study, researchers found that heavy smokers who took a high dose were less likely than those who didn't get the medication to develop the kind of precancerous cellular changes seen in smokers. Like statins, celecoxib reduces inflammation. Both have potential side effects, so talk to your doctor.

is built on a cement slab, radon levels may be a bit higher, but in Australia and New Zealand house levels are lower than in most other countries. It is the second leading cause of lung cancer (albeit way behind smoking). The way to find out if you have radon in your house is to test for it by calling in a professional.

Prevention boosters

Eat lots of vegetables Start with broccoli, cabbage and brussels sprouts. These cruciferous vegetables are high in compounds called isothiocyanates, which prevent lung cancer in animals. In humans, researchers find that eating these vegetables at least once a week could cut your risk of lung cancer by 33 per cent.

Avoid hamburgers, steak and ice-cream Sticking to poultry, fish and low-fat or fat-free dairy foods, and using olive oil instead of butter could reduce your lung cancer risk threefold, and nearly fivefold if you're a smoker. Researchers don't know why saturated fat has such a strong impact on lung cancer risk; it could be related to high levels of inflammation seen in people who eat too many of these fats.

Brush and floss regularly Losing your teeth, which is usually due to bacterial infection in the mouth, increases your risk of lung cancer by 54 per cent even if you don't smoke. The reason? It could be related to the inflammation that leads to gum disease and tooth loss, or to the fact that people who lose their teeth more often don't have as healthy a diet as people with a full set.

Broccoli is high in compounds called isothiocyanates, which prevent lung cancer in animals.

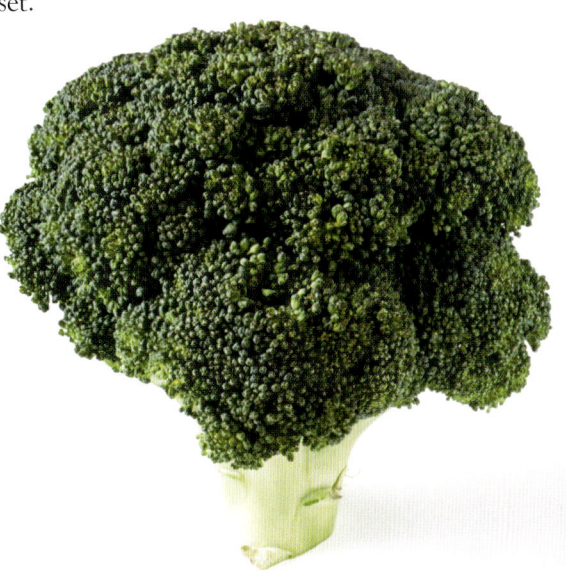

▶ WHAT CAUSES IT
Smoking causes 90 per cent of lung cancers. Other causes are radon and exposure to asbestos, other chemicals, and breathing in secondhand smoke.

▶ SYMPTOMS TO WATCH FOR
Chronic cough, hoarseness, coughing up blood, weight loss, loss of appetite, shortness of breath, fever for no reason, wheezing, bouts of bronchitis or pneumonia, or chest pain.

▶ LATEST THINKING
Vitamin E supplements don't protect against lung cancer and may even increase your risk. A large study involving more than 77,000 people found that taking a 400-mg daily dose increased risk by 28 per cent over 10 years. Don't worry about dietary vitamin E, though; there's no evidence that it—or levels of any other vitamin or mineral in food—increases the risk of lung cancer.

Macular degeneration

35% The drop in your risk of progressive vision loss if you keep your plate loaded with colourful fruit and vegetables.

There's no cure for age-related macular degeneration (AMD), so called because it usually strikes after age 60. It destroys the macula—the centre of the retina, a whisper-thin layer of light-sensitive tissue deep in the eye. People who have it find that vision erodes so gradually that it's easy not to notice anything at first, and, in fact, most people with AMD have this slow-moving 'dry' form. However, 1:10 develop 'wet' AMD, in which blood vessels in the macula leak, and vision deteriorates rapidly. The best advice is to have regular eye exams and try the following tips, to reduce your risk.

Key prevention strategies

Don't smoke The more you smoke, the higher your risk. In fact, when US scientists at the University of Wisconsin tracked the health of nearly 5000 women and men for 15 years, they found that smoking raised risk by 47 per cent. Smoking robs your eyes of anti-oxidants that protect against cell damage, reduces blood flow to the eyes and may even affect the pigments in your irises, which not only determine your eye colour but also act as a natural sunscreen.

Eat the right vegetables Spinach, buk choy and silverbeet are rich in the eye-protecting nutrients lutein and zeaxanthin. These compounds concentrate in the macula of the eyes, filtering out the sun's destructive blue light before it can harm delicate light-sensitive cells deeper in the retina. They also neutralise damaging free radicals produced when light hits the eye. Other good food sources include brightly coloured fruit and vegetables such as corn, orange capsicum and mandarines.

At this point, experts say there's no evidence that anti-oxidant supplements help prevent AMD, though they may slow its progression if you already have it.

Supplements for vision loss

If you already have macular degeneration, taking an anti-oxidant supplement could cut your risk of deteriorating vision by 33 per cent, according to a recent UK review of eight well-designed studies. (They didn't help prevent AMD in people whose eyes were healthy.) You may want to consider taking a supplement if you have been diagnosed with intermediate or advanced AMD. The formula recommended by experts contains 500 mg of vitamin C, 400 IU of vitamin E, 15 mg of beta-carotene, 80 mg of zinc (as zinc oxide) and 2 mg of copper (as cupric oxide). The latter is added to prevent copper deficiency, which can occur if zinc intake is high.

Eat smarter carbs 'White' foods such as white bread, white rice and pasta, and potatoes, baked goods or sweetened fruit drinks may be harming your eyes because of blood sugar spikes. When US researchers checked the diets of 526 people with AMD, they found that those who ate the most foods that make blood sugar spike were 2.7 times more likely to develop AMD than those who ate the fewest.

The answer is to eat fresh fruit, vegetables and dried beans; choose wholegrain bread and cereal; drink water or unsweetened tea; and avoid chips, crackers and biscuits. Experts think that lower blood sugar helps to maintain a healthy flow of blood and oxygen to the eyes, keeping them healthy.

Eat fatty fish, not fatty meats In one Harvard Medical School study, eating two or more fish meals a week cut the risk of AMD by an impressive 60 per cent. The researchers think that the omega-3 fatty acids in fatty fish promote good blood flow to the eyes and cool inflammation, an emerging risk factor for AMD. The catch is that fish helped only those people who also limited their intake of omega-6 fatty acids. These are found in corn, safflower and sunflower oils as well as fried foods and margarines made with these oils.

Other foods to avoid include cheese, ice-cream, hamburgers and anything else rich in saturated fat, and also alcohol. People who ate these foods had twice the risk that early macular degeneration would progress compared to people who ate a healthier diet.

Prevention boosters

Snack on nuts The same Harvard study found that people with AMD who ate more than one serve of nuts each week cut their risk for the progression of AMD by 40 per cent. (A serving is a small handful of any type of nut.) What is it about nuts that helps? Scientists speculate that it could be resveratrol, an anti-oxidant found in nuts and other foods that can protect against cell damage, soothe inflammation and promote healthy blood flow.

Watch your weight Overweight people with AMD worsen up to twice as fast as people of normal weight. Research shows that exercising as part of your weight-control strategy pays dividends for your eyes. In one study, people with early AMD who got at least half an hour of vigorous exercise three times a week cut their risk of developing advanced AMD by 25 per cent.

▶ WHAT CAUSES IT
Experts don't know what triggers the damage, but smoking and being over age 60, Caucasian or female raises the risk.

▶ SYMPTOMS TO WATCH FOR
Distorted vision in one or both eyes; or straight lines that look wavy. Over time, central vision grows worse, and it becomes difficult to see objects far away, to read or do close work, or even to distinguish faces and colours.

▶ LATEST THINKING
Avoid second-hand smoke. Nonsmokers who lived with smokers raised their risk of AMD by 87 per cent in one recent UK study. Don't wait for your someone to quit in order to clear the air and guard your eyesight: ask them to smoke outside to protect your health.

Menstrual problems

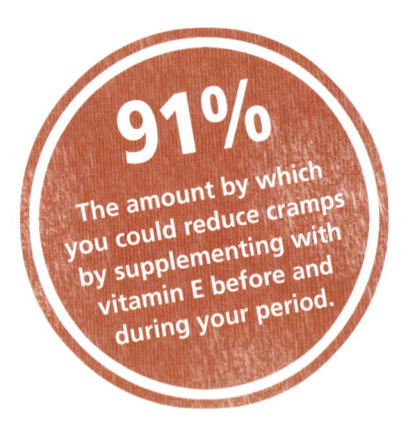

91% The amount by which you could reduce cramps by supplementing with vitamin E before and during your period.

Compared to their ancestral grandmothers, who spent most of their reproductive years pregnant or breastfeeding, women today have about three times as many menstrual periods. The reality is that we don't *need* to menstruate. In fact, the manufacturers of birth control pills originally included one week of placebo pills mainly because they thought that women would find it 'reassuring' to have a regular period. Today women can choose a range of treatments for painful or heavy periods. And there are always new approaches and treatment options being trialled to help women with heavy menstrual bleeding. One such technique currently being researched is using sound waves from high-intensity ultrasound to destroy fibroids, which are a common cause of heavy bleeding.

Key prevention strategies

Use the birth control pill to treat painful periods If you're not trying to get pregnant, starting on oral contraceptives is the most effective way to prevent menstrual cramps. Standard birth control pills contain progestin, a synthetic hormone that thins the lining of the uterus over time. A thinner lining produces less arachidonic acid, which contributes to the production of prostaglandins, hormone-like chemicals that cause cramps.

However, if you want to avoid having a regular period (and the resulting cramps) altogether, talk to your doctor about continuous oral contraception, in which you use the Pill for up to a year without a break, or extended oral contraception, in which you use the Pill for three months at a time, then have a period. Other contraceptive options that can reduce or prevent menstrual cramping include the vaginal ring (NuvaRing), contraceptive implant (Implanon), injectable contraception (Depo-Provera) and the hormone-impregnated IUD (Mirena).

Take painkillers early Start taking an over-the-counter anti-inflammatory such as ibuprofen or naproxen, following the label directions, one to two days before your period is due. A review of

51 studies involving 1649 women found that 72 per cent experienced significant pain relief with this approach compared to women taking a placebo. Continue for the first two or three days of your period. These pain relievers prevent your body from making prostaglandins, which cause cramping.

Ask your doctor about prescription medication Tranexamic acid (Cyklokapron) is the most effective medical treatment available for preventing heavy bleeding. It is an antifibrinolytic, which means it prevents blood clots from disintegrating. It also stimulates clot formation. And more clotting means less bleeding. Studies find this medication can reduce heavy menstrual bleeding by as much as 50 per cent.

Try an NSAID Over-the-counter painkillers such as ibuprofen (Nurofen) and naproxen (Aleve) and the prescription medication diclofenac (Voltaren)—all known as nonsteroidal anti-inflammatory drugs, or NSAIDs—can help prevent heavy menstrual bleeding by reducing levels of prostaglandins, hormone-like chemicals that interfere with blood clotting. Mefenamic acid (Ponstan), a non-prescription NSAID, may be less likely to irritate the stomach and reduces bleeding by 22 to 46 per cent. Avoid aspirin, which may increase bleeding.

Consider an oral contraceptive or an IUD for heavy bleeding
Because oral contraceptives thin the lining of the uterus, there is less lining to shed and therefore less bleeding. Studies find that the oral contraceptive pill can reduce menstrual bleeding by up to 60 per cent. Taking continuous contraceptive pills, which skip the week of placebo pills that trigger a period, often prevent menstruation altogether and can significantly reduce heavy bleeding even if your periods continue each month. An alternative is a 24-day pill.

A hormone-impregnated implant or IUD is another option. The IUD Mirena releases a progestin hormone called levonorgestrel, while the Implanon implant releases the progestin etonogestrel. Progestins help prevent heavy bleeding by reducing the growth of the uterine lining. Numerous studies find that Mirena works as well as surgery for controlling heavy menstrual bleeding. It may even stop your periods altogether. The DMPA injection (Depo-Provera) is yet another option—many women stop having their period while on this therapy, and for months afterwards.

'Menstrual bleeding can be reduced by up to 50% by taking prescription medication.'

Prevention boosters

Try a low-fat vegetarian diet Researchers asked 33 women with bad cramps to follow such a diet (no animal products, fried foods, avocados, olives or nuts, but plenty of grains, vegetables, legumes and fruit) for two menstrual cycles, then eat their regular diet for two cycles and take a placebo pill. During the vegetarian diet phase, the duration and intensity of the women's menstrual pain dropped by about a third. And there was a bonus: they lost weight. The diet probably triggers beneficial changes in the metabolism of oestrogen and/or cuts down on the production of prostaglandins.

Feast on fish or take fish oil Fish rich in omega-3 fatty acids, such as salmon, trout, sardines and mackerel, may help ease menstrual cramps and have the added benefit of improving your levels of blood fats, including cholesterol. A study of 181 Dutch women found that those with the lowest levels of omega-3 fatty acids in their diets had the greatest amount of menstrual pain.

Even if you don't like fish, you can still get your omega-3s by taking fish-oil capsules. A study of 70 women, half of whom received fish oil, found that pain levels in those taking the oil dropped by 33 per cent compared to a 20 per cent improvement in the women who took placebos. The women took 2 g of fish oil every day for a month. The next month, they took 2 g a day for eight days before their period and two days after their period. Check with your doctor before taking fish oil.

Supplement carefully with vitamin E Regular long-term use of vitamin E supplements, which may slightly increase the risk of early death, are not recommended. But some research suggests that taking vitamin E just before and after your period begins can bring significant relief from cramps. One study involving 278 adolescent girls found that taking 400 IU of vitamin E a day, beginning two days before their period began and for the first three days of their period, relieved cramps better than a placebo. After four months, girls who took the vitamin E had average pain scores nearly six times lower than those who took placebos, and their pain lasted an average of 1.6 hours compared to 17 hours in the placebo group. Vitamin E may work to relieve cramping by affecting prostaglandins.

Run (or walk) off cramps Chances are strong that women who are physically active regularly simply don't have debilitating menstrual cramps. Studies find that women who exercise regularly—regardless of what kind of activity they do—are less likely to have pain during their period, so make an effort to be active throughout the month, and try to keep it up during your period.

Try chasteberry to stem heavy bleeding *Vitex agnus castus*, better known as chasteberry, is a herb often used by naturopaths to treat reproductive issues in women. Studies find that as little as 15 drops of a tincture of extract can significantly reduce the number of days of heavy bleeding, though it may take several months before you see a benefit.

Get tested for a bleeding disorder Blood clotting disorders such as von Willebrand's disease often underlie heavy menstrual bleeding, yet many doctors don't always think to check for them. Women who have had heavy periods since they were young girls are most likely to have bleeding problems. If you have a clotting disorder, regular injections or infusions of missing clotting factors could make your heavy periods a thing of the past.

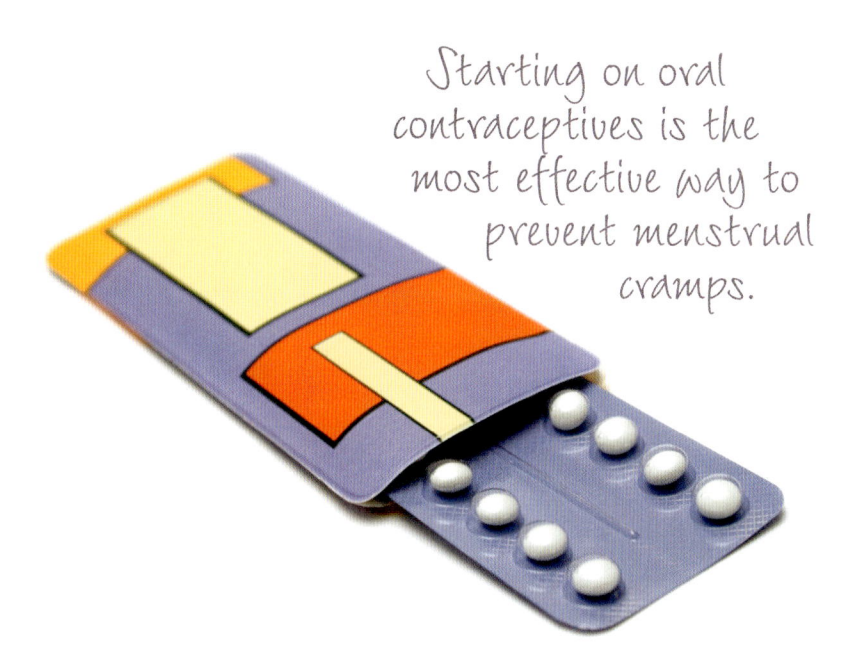

Starting on oral contraceptives is the most effective way to prevent menstrual cramps.

▶ WHAT CAUSES IT

Hormonal changes during your menstrual cycle trigger the production of hormone-like chemicals called prostaglandins that make the uterus contract, causing cramps. Endometriosis, a condition in which the tissue that lines the uterus grows outside the organ, also causes cramping. Heavy periods are caused by an imbalance between oestrogen and progesterone, most often during puberty and the years just before menopause; fibroids; and, rarely, endometrial cancer.

▶ SYMPTOMS TO WATCH FOR

Lower-abdominal pain during your period is a sign of cramps. With heavy bleeding, if you are changing your tampon and/or pad every hour during the first couple of days of your period, you have an abnormally heavy flow. Also watch out for any unusual fatigue or dizziness—a heavy menstrual flow could lead to anaemia from iron loss. But don't take supplemental iron on your own; always talk to your doctor first.

▶ LATEST THINKING

Menstrual blood may someday provide a rich source of stem cells, which can be used to create a variety of tissue including insulin-producing cells for people with Type 1 diabetes.

Migraines

40% The drop in the number of migraines among people who switched to a low-fat diet for eight weeks.

Migraines are a problem for 1 in 6 women and 1 in 16 men. But half of all sufferers don't realise what's behind the head pain, and, as a result, they're missing out on strategies that might stop the downward spiral before it starts. If your symptoms match some or all of those listed on the opposite page, then try the following prevention measures.

Key prevention strategies

Avoid your personal migraine triggers Certain foods, some medications, stress, changes in sleeping patterns, cigarette smoke and a variety of other things can result in a migraine. Triggers vary, so keeping a headache diary may help you to determine yours (and note that some triggers are unidentifiable). Record when you get a migraine and what you were taking, eating, drinking, feeling and doing for the 24 hours before the pain began.

Common medication culprits include some antidepressants, bronchodilators, contraceptives containing oestrogen, and diet pills. Food triggers include caffeine, most alcoholic drinks, aged cheese, processed meats, MSG, nuts, dairy foods, tropical fruits and most dried fruits, onions, fresh yeast breads and aspartame.

Step off the painkiller merry-go-round Taking any painkillers more than twice a week can be problematic. These medications constrict swollen blood vessels, which makes your head feel better. But when they wear off, blood vessels swell again, and you could end up with a migraine as a result. End the cycle by stopping your pain medications. It will probably hurt at first, but experts say you'll start feeling better after a week to 10 days. Then you can focus on prevention strategies such as the ones outlined here. However, when you do need to take a painkiller, take it promptly, because the longer you leave it, the less effective it will be.

DRUGS THAT PREVENT DISEASE

If you get two or more migraines a month, ask your doctor if you might benefit from taking migraine medication such as propranolol (Inderal). The right treatment could cut your risk of future migraines in half, but it can take four weeks to begin seeing improvements and up to six months to know whether a medication is really working for you.

You may even find relief by taking a low-dose aspirin every day or every other day, studies show, provided your doctor gives you the OK.

Cut back on dietary fat Drastically reducing the amount of fat you eat could cut the number of migraines you have by 40 per cent. That was the finding from a US study that followed 54 migraine sufferers who stuck with extremely low fat diets (they got just 10 to 15 per cent of their kilojoules from fat each day) for eight weeks. When study volunteers did get headaches, they were 66 per cent less intense and about 70 per cent shorter than before. The participants also used 72 per cent less headache medication.

The researchers suspect that eating less fat improves the flexibility of blood vessels so they expand and contract more easily. They also discovered that study volunteers replaced fat with carbohydrate-rich foods like bread and pasta, which raise levels of the brain chemical serotonin, linked to lower migraine risk.

Not ready to go so low fat? Work on cutting back on saturated fat—the kind found in fatty meats, full-fat milk and cheese, and tropical oils (like palm and coconut oil)—and getting most of your fat from fatty fish, canola or olive oil, walnuts and linseeds. In some studies, these good fats reduced the frequency of migraines, perhaps by keeping blood vessels flexible.

Prevention boosters

Give ginger a try Research shows that this warming spice contains potent compounds that are similar to the ones in NSAIDs. It may work against migraines by blocking inflammatory substances called prostaglandins. Although ginger hasn't been rigorously tested for its ability to subdue a migraine, it may well relieve the nausea that often comes with severe headache. Try taking ginger as a tea made by steeping fresh ginger root in boiling water, or in cooking.

Ask your doctor about supplementing with riboflavin In one Belgian study, 60 per cent of people who took 400 mg of riboflavin (vitamin B_2) every day for three months had half as many migraines as they had before the study started.

Relax your mind and body You can do this with yoga, meditation, deep breathing or any other therapy that helps relieve tension. In one promising study from India, 72 migraine sufferers who practised yoga for an hour five days a week reduced the frequency and intensity of their migraine attacks.

▸ WHAT CAUSES IT

No one's sure. Experts suspect that the trigeminal nerve system, which sends and receives pain signals involving the face and head, is involved, as is the brain chemical serotonin. Levels of serotonin fall during a migraine and may prompt the trigeminal nerve to send out chemicals that dilate blood vessels, causing pain.

▸ SYMPTOMS TO WATCH FOR

Moderate to severe pain on one or both sides of the head. It may throb or pulse, feel worse with physical activity and come with nausea, vomiting and sensitivity to light and sound. Some people experience auras just before the pain begins. These can include flashing lights, blind spots, tingling in arms or legs, or feeling extremely weak. (Migraines with auras also raise risk for cardiovascular problems, studies show, so follow our advice for preventing heart disease and stroke.)

▸ LATEST THINKING

Think twice before using feverfew. It probably won't do any harm, but this popular anti-migraine herb did little to prevent migraines or lessen pain in a UK review of five well-designed studies.

Mouth ulcers

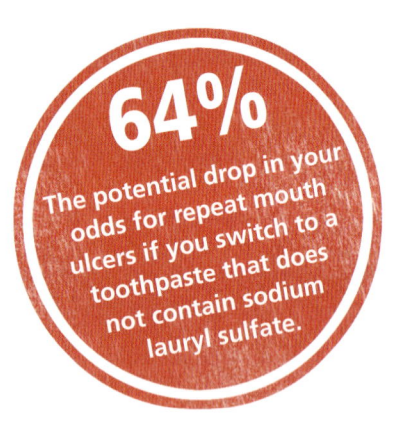

64%
The potential drop in your odds for repeat mouth ulcers if you switch to a toothpaste that does not contain sodium lauryl sulfate.

Mouth ulcers are tiny white sores inside your mouth or along the gums, and they can be painful, not to mention making it difficult to eat or even to talk. Mouth ulcers are triggered by everything from food to toothpaste ingredients and sharp-edged potato chips to stress. Researchers aren't sure what causes them, but the following tips may help you avoid them.

Key prevention strategies

Avoid toothpaste containing sodium lauryl sulfate (SLS)
This ingredient can irritate the delicate lining of the mouth and trigger mouth ulcers in some people. In a Norwegian study of 10 people who got recurring mouth ulcers, switching to an SLS-free toothpaste cut their rate of new sores by nearly two-thirds. But don't skimp on dental hygiene. Brushing and flossing twice a day can keep your mouth free of tiny food bits and bacteria that can irritate the lining of your mouth and kick-start a new mouth ulcer. Scrub gently to avoid activating a new sore.

Swish with an antibacterial mouthwash Rinses containing triclosan, chlorhexidine and other antibacterial ingredients have significantly reduced the number of mouth ulcers in people who get them repeatedly, several studies show. They may work by washing away debris from hard-to-reach spots, preventing the flare-up of tiny infections that could trigger a mouth ulcer, or by helping to prevent infection if you do get a sore.

Avoid these food culprits Some mouth ulcers are caused by a food or food additives. Citrus fruits, tomatoes, eggplant, tea and cola drinks all triggered mouth ulcers in one study from Turkey, presumably because these foods irritated the lining of the mouth. Benzoic acid (a food preservative), cinnamon, milk, coffee, chocolate, potatoes, cheese, walnuts and figs are said to be other culprits. Avoid spicy foods, which

The gluten connection

An estimated 1 in 20 people who get regular mouth ulcers have coeliac disease, an intolerance to the gluten protein found in wheat and some other grains. But don't give up wheat yet. If you think you may have coeliac disease, talk to your doctor about testing and treatment. Other symptoms of gluten intolerance include diarrhoea, abdominal pain, weight loss, fatigue and wind.

can also irritate sensitive mouth tissue. And skip sharp-edged foods such as corn chips, potato chips and crackers.

Before eliminating these foods from your diet, look for connections between foods you've eaten recently and the onset of a new sore. Experts recommend removing a food for a few weeks, taking note of whether you get fewer sores, and then introducing the food again to see if it triggers a sore.

Ask about levamisole This prescription-only medication stimulates the immune system in ways that can help prevent mouth ulcers. In four studies of people who got frequent sores, the number of repeat attacks was cut in half for 43 per cent of volunteers who took it. Some experts consider this the safest and most effective medication for preventing mouth ulcers.

Prevention boosters

Be calm Stress seems to be a classic instigator of mouth ulcers. In one study of people with mouth ulcers, 16 per cent said that extreme stress triggered outbreaks. Experts think stress may be a factor in up to 60 per cent of first-time mouth ulcer episodes. Irish researchers have found higher levels of the stress hormone cortisol in the saliva of people who get the sores, too. Try a relaxation technique like yoga.

Take a supplement When Israeli researchers gave 15 people with recurring mouth ulcers either an injection of vitamin B_{12} or a daily vitamin B_{12} tablet, mouth ulcers dropped from an average of 10 per month to about one every three months. Several studies have found low levels of vitamin B_{12} in people who get mouth ulcers regularly. People in the study took 1000 mcg of vitamin B_{12} daily, but talk to your doctor before taking that much. (Some experts recommend a more conservative 100 mcg per day.) Top sources include fortified cereals, lamb or veal kidney, mussels, chicken liver and salmon.

Clear up other nutritional deficiencies About one in five people with recurring mouth ulcers has a nutritional deficiency. Some need more B vitamins or have iron-deficiency anaemia. Correcting low iron could cut your odds for more mouth ulcers by 71 per cent, studies show. We don't recommend that you take extra iron on your own; for some people, it can be harmful. Ask your doctor whether you need a blood test to check for deficiencies.

▶ WHAT CAUSES IT

No one knows. Experts suspect that mouth ulcers are caused by several factors, including tiny immune system attacks on healthy mouth tissue, allergic reactions, low levels of B vitamins and iron, injury and irritation of the lining of the mouth, additives in foods and toothpaste, menstrual cycle hormone changes in women, and stress.

▶ SYMPTOMS TO WATCH FOR

Small round sores under your tongue, inside your cheeks or lips, or at the base of your gums. Most are less than 1 cm in diameter, but some mouth ulcers can be large and can take up to a month to heal.

▶ LATEST THINKING

Some children get recurring mouth ulcers along with a fever and sore throat on a regular basis between the ages of three and ten. This newly recognised condition, called periodic fever, aphthous-stomatitis, pharyngitis and adenitis (PFAPA) syndrome, returns like clockwork every few weeks or months. No one's sure what causes it, and there's no recognised treatment, though new research from Children's Hospital Boston in the US suggests that removing the tonsils of a child with PFAPA can stop future attacks.

Neck pain

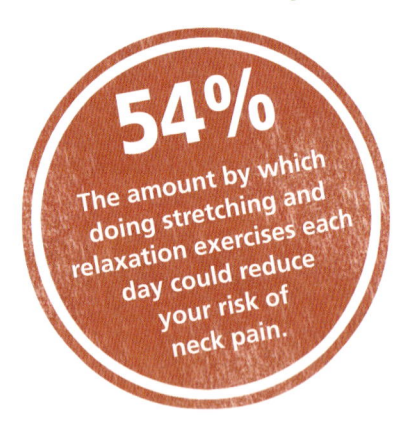

54% The amount by which doing stretching and relaxation exercises each day could reduce your risk of neck pain.

The average human head weighs about as much as a bowling ball, yet it rests atop seven of the smallest, lightest vertebrae in your spine. Nature designed your neck to curve slightly backwards to keep your head from flopping over, but years of bad posture, computer work, driving and sleeping on saggy mattresses or big pillows can erase that curve, leading to pain. Injuries, such as whiplash, and stress also contribute. Here's how to reduce your risk for neck pain.

Key prevention strategies

Pull up on your string Think of yourself as a puppet with a string coming out of the top of your head. Now imagine that someone's pulling on that string, causing you to sit (or stand) straight and hold your head high, with your chin tucked in slightly. That's the position you want to be in most of the time. Instead, many of us sit, drive and even walk on the treadmill with our heads thrust forward, which puts added strain on the neck. To help you sit up straight at the computer, use armrests and adjust your monitor so that your eyes are looking near the top of the screen. While driving, adjust your seat and headrest so you don't have to crane your neck forward to see the road.

Keep your head held high by balancing an object Most music CDs come in hard plastic cases that are quite light, so place one on top of your head and see how long you can balance it there. Eventually, sitting straighter should become second nature.

Help for a stiff neck

Wet a towel, wring it out and warm it in the microwave for 30 seconds on *High*. Then wrap it around your neck and keep it on until it loses its heat. Do this before performing neck exercises to loosen up the muscles. (Never put a dry towel in a microwave oven.)

Downsize your pillows Sleeping on a big pile of pillows or just one high pillow inevitably means your neck will be out of line with the rest of your spine while you sleep. It's better to use a small pillow and sleep on your back or side, not on your stomach. If you're prone to neck pain, a neck pillow is the best way to go (you'll need to sleep on your back to use it).

Move every 20 to 30 minutes If you're sitting at the computer surfing the Net, knitting a jumper or painting at an easel, it's easy to get lost in the flow and sit in an unnatural position for too long, straining your back, shoulder and neck muscles. Set an alarm or kitchen timer to ring every 20 to 30 minutes. Each time it goes off, stand up, walk around for a few minutes and practise the neck exercises on the following pages. An Italian study found that when office workers were trained to practise relaxation and stretching exercises several times a day to stop 'clenching' their neck and shoulder muscles, they had 54 per cent less neck and shoulder pain compared with a control group, whose pain dropped by 4 per cent.

Prevention boosters

Lighten the load Carrying an overstuffed bag slung over one shoulder is a leading cause of neck pain for many women because it pulls the body out of balance. One doctor, tired of hearing his patients complain about neck pain, started weighing their bags and found that many tipped the scales at 3 to 4.5 kg. If you carry a lot of stuff, use a backpack to distribute the weight evenly.

Watch your phone posture If you're talking on the regular home phone often, avoid scrunching the phone between your ear and shoulder. And when using a mobile phone, use an earpiece.

▶ WHAT CAUSES IT

Trauma, such as whiplash from a car accident; excessive strain on the neck or shoulder muscles; emotional stress that causes you to tighten your shoulder or neck muscles; and degenerative changes in the vertebrae and disks in your neck, which are common with age.

▶ SYMPTOMS TO WATCH FOR

Pain and difficulty turning your head to the right or left or moving it up or down; frequent headaches.

▶ LATEST THINKING

Stainless steel discs can replace worn-out cervical discs in your neck, relieving pain while retaining mobility. The first one was approved in the US in late 2007. Surgery is a last resort when nothing else helps.

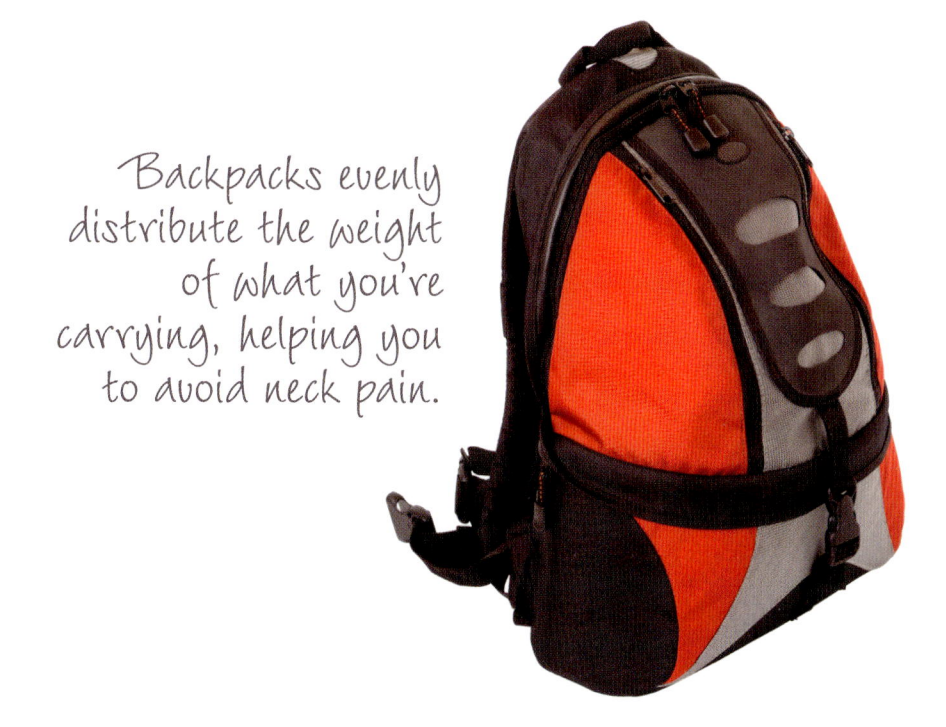

Backpacks evenly distribute the weight of what you're carrying, helping you to avoid neck pain.

Stretch and strengthen your neck

Often, pain in the neck area is related to unconsciously tensing your neck, particularly when you're spending hours at the computer or in the car. Next time you're online playing Scrabble, or sitting and knitting for hours at a time, remind yourself to do these easy stretching exercises to relieve the tension and to help keep your neck limber. You can strengthen your neck simply by resisting all these motions with your hand.

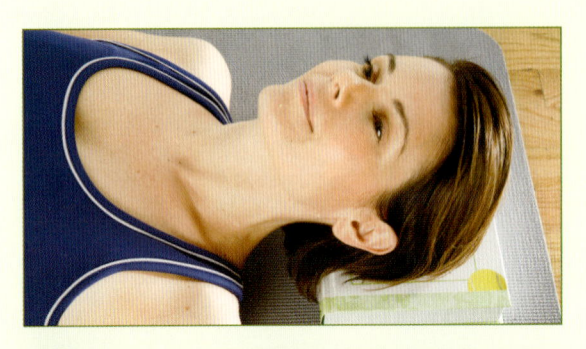

Neck rotation

1 Lie on the floor with a thick book under your head (a phone book is perfect).

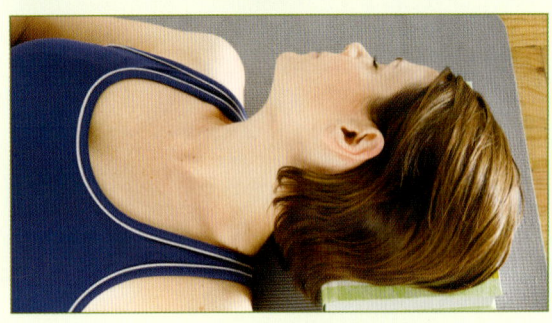

2 Slowly turn your head to one side and hold in that position for 10 to 20 seconds. Repeat on each side three to five times.

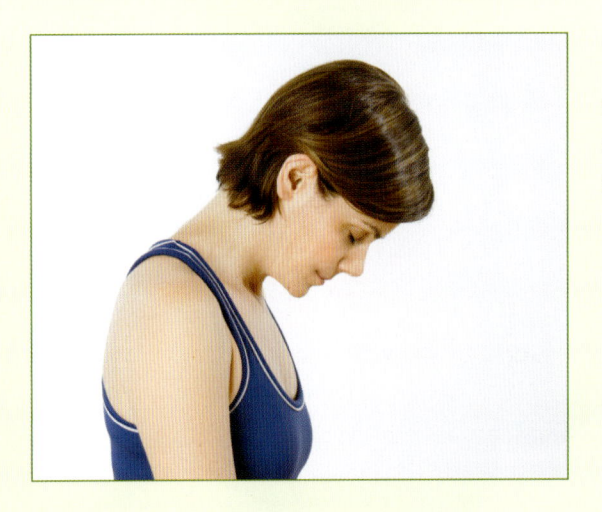

Head tip

Sit straight and gently tilt your head forward as far as it will go. Hold for 10 seconds, then return to the starting position. Repeat five times.

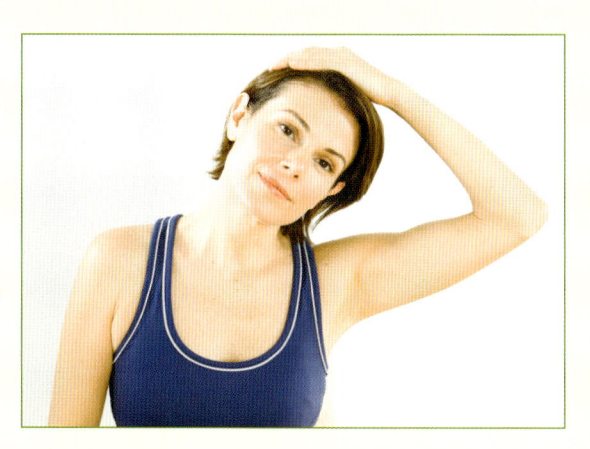

Head tilt

Stand or sit straight and hold the right side of the top of your head with your left hand. Let your right arm hang loosely at your side. Slowly pull your head to the left until you feel a gentle stretch in your neck. Hold for 10 seconds, then repeat on the other side.

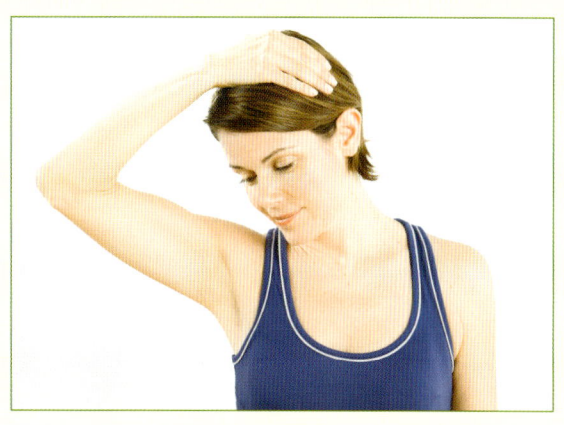

Armpit stretch

Stand or sit straight and hold the left side of the top of your head with your right hand. Let your left arm hang loosely at your side. Slowly pull your head to the right and down, stopping when you feel a gentle stretch. Hold for 10 seconds, then repeat on the other side.

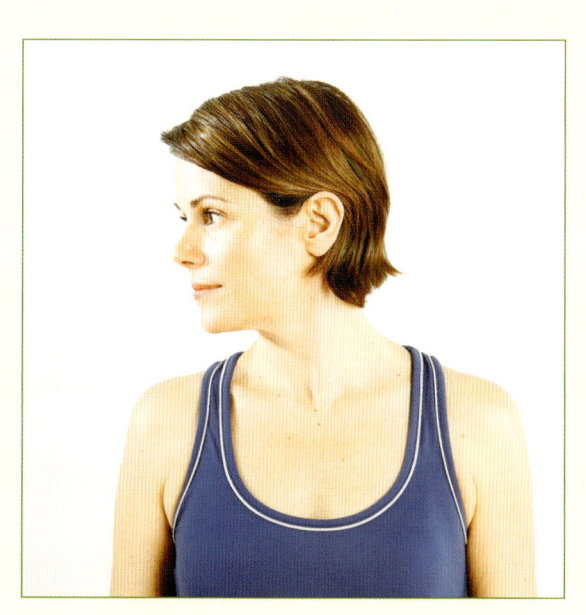

Side tip

Sit straight and turn your head to the right as far as it will go. Gently tilt your head forward until you feel the stretch. Hold for 10 seconds, then return to the starting position. Repeat five times on each side.

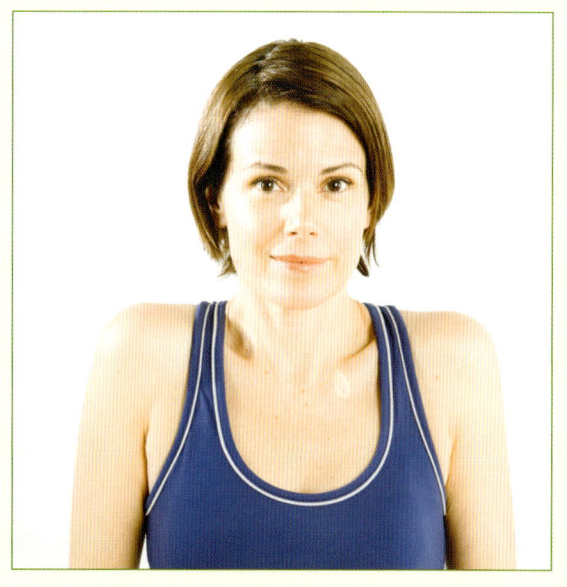

Shoulder shrug

Stand or sit straight and raise your shoulders up towards your ears until you feel slight tension in your neck and shoulders. Hold for 5 seconds, then relax. Repeat five times.

Obesity

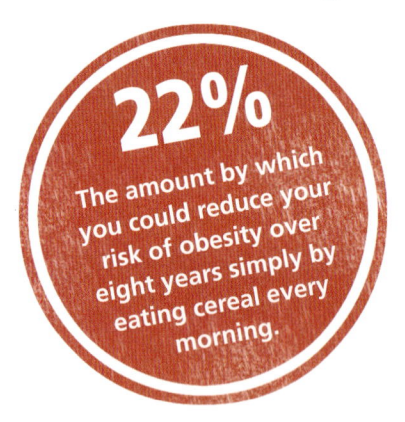

22%
The amount by which you could reduce your risk of obesity over eight years simply by eating cereal every morning.

Obesity is one of the most devastating conditions when it comes to your health. It's linked not only to an increased risk of the problems you'd expect—heart disease and diabetes, as well as joint pain—but also to numerous others you may not think of, such as cancer, hearing loss, Alzheimer's disease and gastrointestinal problems. For some people, keeping extra weight off seems almost impossible—but it's not. Just don't make the mistake of relying on short-term dieting, which is surprisingly ineffective. The trick is to combine balanced nutrition and smart portion control with exercise—something you simply can't leave out of the equation.

Key prevention strategies

Exercise 30 minutes a day Exercise, even more than cutting kilojoules, is key to losing weight and keeping it off. Any amount helps, but a good, easily reached goal is 30 minutes on most days. Surprisingly, a 30-minute work-out is almost as effective as a 60-minute work-out, according to a study published in the Journal of the American Medical Association. When 184 women walked either outside or on a treadmill at various intensities for 30 or 60 minutes a day, five days a week for a year, researchers found that it didn't matter how hard or how long the work-out was—the women still lost nearly the same amount of weight. Those who exercised for an hour a day lost about 10 per cent more than those who did it for half an hour a day. Given that the average weight loss was 8.5 kg, that's a difference of only about a kilogram. But why? The researchers speculate that the more you exercise, the more you think you can eat—and by eating more, you offset some of the weight loss you would have achieved. The moral of the story is to go ahead and get as much exercise as you can (some people will need more than 30 minutes a day to get rid of stubborn fat or keep weight off); just don't raid the fridge as a reward.

Don't skip breakfast We've known for a long time that people who eat breakfast every day (a wholegrain cereal with at least 4 g of fibre per serve) are more likely to maintain a healthy weight or, if they're trying to lose weight, drop more kilos than those who don't have breakfast. The reason has to do with how your body reacts to any shortage of food, even a brief one. If you skip breakfast in the morning, not only do you feel like you're starving by lunchtime, your body actually thinks it's starving and reacts by slowing down metabolism to conserve energy. Most experts agree that eating breakfast every day is simply one of the best things you can do for your weight.

Some researchers now even think that your breakfast should be a big one—your biggest meal of the day, in fact. They point to research that suggests a big breakfast does a better job of controlling appetite and cravings for sweets and starches later in the day, helping you keep weight off.

Practise portion control In the developed world, we're eating as much as 25 per cent more food per person than we did 40 years ago. One reason is 'portion distortion'—we've become used to the vastly oversized servings at fast-food and sit-down restaurants, making it difficult for us to recognise a 'normal' portion at home. Here's a new mindset to adopt: when you eat, think about quality over quantity, and consider yourself done eating when you're only 80 per cent full. The point is to give your body the nutrition it needs, not to overstuff yourself as if food may never again be available. Try these tips:

- **Use smaller plates** Studies find that if you use large plates, you not only put more food on the plate but eat more of what's in front of you.
- **Eat in the dining room** Serve in the kitchen, then go to another room to eat. You'll be less likely to go for seconds if you have to get up and return to the kitchen to get them.
- **Slow down** Most of us eat too fast. This doesn't give the brain time to receive the hormonal signals from the stomach that

'Fast food' in the freezer

Eating out—particularly fast food—is a major cause of weight gain. One study found that people who ate fast food more than twice a week gained 4.5 kg more over a 15-year period than those who ate fast food less than once a week. To reduce the incentive to eat out, keep the freezer stocked with these 'convenience' foods.

- **Frozen prawns**
- **Frozen fish (no sauce)**
- **Frozen vegetables (no sauce)**
- **Frozen edamame (green soybeans)**
- **Boneless skinless chicken breasts**
- **Homemade soup**
- **Turkey mince meatballs**
- **Frozen ravioli**
- **Pork loin (thinly sliced for quick cooking)**

Combine them with pantry items such as wholegrain pasta, brown rice, olive oil, homemade pesto, canned tomatoes, miso, beans and lentils, along with washed salad greens from the fridge, and you have the makings of countless emergency meals.

it's full. Along those lines, wait at least 20 minutes after eating before helping yourself to seconds or dessert. Chances are, you won't want to have either.

Fill half of your plate with nonstarchy vegetables Most vegetables, not including corn and potatoes, fill you up on very few kilojoules—far fewer than whatever other food your plate contains. Fill another quarter of your plate with a carbohydrate such as wholemeal pasta, brown rice or corn and the rest with lean meat, chicken, fish or another protein food. It's the easiest, simplest way we know to keep a lid on excess kilojoules.

Join a weight-loss support group If you've managed to lose weight and want to keep it off, it helps to have support, preferably in person (think Weight Watchers). When researchers compared people who attended support groups with those who received online help or just a newsletter about maintaining weight loss, they found that the live-meeting group regained an average of 2.5 kg; the other two groups regained an average of under 5 kg. The online support did have some benefit, however: just 54.6 per cent of those participants regained weight compared with 72.4 per cent in the newsletter group.

Prevention boosters

Support healthy-weight habits One major study that followed a group of people for more than 30 years found that a person's risk of obesity increased by 57 per cent if a close friend became obese and by 37 per cent if their spouse became obese. So if you or your spouse or close friend is gaining weight, join the work-out/weight-loss group together (there are lots of groups out there); studies find that buddying up like this can lead to both of you shedding more kilos than either of you would if you tried alone.

Weigh yourself often It's much easier to lose 1 kg than 10, and unless your clothes are tight-fitting you may not notice that

---

DRUGS THAT PREVENT DISEASE

Researchers are still searching for a 'miracle' diet pill that works, but some medications—coupled with lifestyle changes—can help you lose more weight than lifestyle changes alone.

One of those drugs is sibutramine (Reductil). It works like many antidepressants by increasing the amount of serotonin and norepinephrine in your brain. These chemicals are involved in regulating not only mood but also appetite. Increasing them helps you feel full sooner, thereby reducing the amount you eat.

If you take sibutramine, it's important to eat well and exercise. In one study, people who took it and changed their lifestyle lost an average of more than 12 kg compared with the 5 kg lost by those who only took the medication and nearly 7 kg lost by those who only made lifestyle changes. The researchers found similar results in people using the medication to maintain weight loss.

you've added a few. A study of more than 3000 people found that the more often people weighed themselves, the more weight they lost or the less weight they gained.

Watch it when you're pregnant It's important to be careful about exactly how much weight you gain during pregnancy. It turns out that pregnancy itself may leave a 'legacy' of extra kilos. For instance, in one study, a year after women delivered, they still weighed between 2 and 3 kg more than women of the same age who had not been pregnant. To maintain a healthy weight during pregnancy, keep being physically active, weigh yourself regularly and don't pretend that you need to eat more 'for the baby'.

Eat less and exercise more when you quit smoking Nicotine suppresses weight gain, so if you're quitting smoking, plan to get more exercise and stock up low-kilojoule foods that you can use to help you through the times when you really want to light up. Also, weigh yourself regularly to catch the kilos before they accumulate. The prescription medication bupropion (Zyban) may help you quit without gaining weight. (See page 62 for more information.)

Seek professional advice A registered dietitian will evaluate how you eat and live, help you set weight and health goals, and design a customised eating plan and exercise program to help you reach your goals and stay on track. A US study from the University of Minnesota found that adults who met with a dietitian once a week for nearly three months lost 67 per cent more weight than those who attended semi-weekly weigh-in meetings that didn't involve a dietitian. Your health insurance may help cover the cost, but even if you have to pay out of pocket (figure about A$110 for a one-hour appointment), it's still less than the costs associated with obesity.

▶ WHAT CAUSES IT

While genetics plays a role in weight, the greatest contributor is eating more kilojoules than your body burns as energy. The excess is stored as fat.

▶ SYMPTOMS TO WATCH FOR

A body mass index (BMI) of 30 or more, which indicates obesity. Find out what your BMI is at www.bmi-calculator.net/metric-bmi-calculator.php.

▶ LATEST THINKING

A virus known as human adenovirus-36 may be partly responsible for obesity in some people. A study involving 502 unrelated thin and obese people found that 30 per cent of those who were obese had at one point been infected with adenovirus-36 compared with 11 per cent of those who were not obese. The researchers also looked at 28 pairs of twins and found that people with antibodies to the virus (meaning that they had been infected at some point) tended to weigh more than their identical siblings who didn't have the antibodies.

Osteoporosis

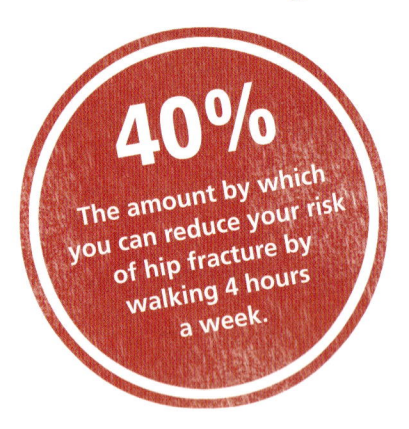

40% The amount by which you can reduce your risk of hip fracture by walking 4 hours a week.

After about the age of 30, the body breaks down old bone faster than it can build new bone. And since the hormone oestrogen works to keep bones strong, women have even more rapid bone loss after about 50, or when they reach menopause, but men get osteoporosis, too. Medications are available to slow the process in people at high risk of fractures, but generally speaking, once bone is lost, it's gone for good. (And some bone-building medications come with serious side effects, including an *increased* risk of certain fractures.) That's why prevention is so important. While about 60 per cent of your bone density is determined by genetics, that still leaves 40 per cent you can affect.

Key prevention strategies

Get enough calcium and vitamin D If you're not getting enough calcium in your diet, your body takes what it needs from your bones, putting you at risk for osteoporosis. To protect your bones, add more low-fat dairy foods, such as low-fat or skim milk and low-fat yogurt, to your diet. Aim for about 1200 mg a day (200 g of low-fat yogurt or a 250-ml glass of skim milk has 300 mg). Spread your intake out through the day in amounts of 500 mg or less for the best use of calcium (See 'Getting your calcium from food' on page 266 for other good dietary sources.)

It's also critical to get enough vitamin D, which helps your body use calcium. Sunlight is the best source, but because we're wearing more sunblock these days, some of us run low. Experts sometimes recommend getting 10 or 15 minutes of sunlight—without sunblock—a day. Unfortunately, as you age, your body's ability to synthesise vitamin D from sunlight decreases, so you may want to think about taking a daily supplement of 400 IU

DRUGS THAT PREVENT DISEASE

If you're a postmenopausal woman with a high risk of osteoporosis—because it runs in your family, you're underweight, you smoke or used to smoke, and/or you don't get much weight-bearing exercise (being Caucasian is also a risk factor, as is long-term use of corticosteroids for diseases such as asthma or arthritis)—talk to your doctor about taking either raloxifene (Evista) or one of the bisphosphonate medications, including risedronate (Actonel) and alendronate (Fosamax). Raloxifene works by mimicking oestrogen in your body, which slows bone-destroying cells. Bisphosphonates work by suppressing the bone-destroying cells directly. These medications have side effects, so ask your doctor for an assessment of their risks and benefits.

of vitamin D, especially if you don't want to expose yourself to sunlight because of fears about skin cancer.

Although getting calcium from food is best, as insurance you might also consider calcium supplements. In the massive US Women's Health Initiative study, women who took 1000 mg of calcium and 400 IU of vitamin D every day for seven years had a hip bone density 1.06 per cent higher than that of those who took a placebo, plus a 29 per cent lower risk of hip fracture. You can take up to 1200 mg of calcium a day in two doses (up to 600 mg each, which is all the body can absorb at one time). Calcium citrate, though it costs more than other forms of calcium, is absorbed better by your body, especially if you're taking a proton-pump inhibitor such as omeprazole (Losec) or esomeprazole (Nexium) or an H2 blocker such as famotidine (Pepcid) or ranitidine (Zantac), which reduce stomach acid that breaks down nutrients.

Strengthen your bones through exercise When astronauts go into space, they lose up to 1.5 per cent of their total bone mass for each month in orbit. Why? Because at zero gravity, there's no weight pressing on their bones, and bone-building cells do their work only when they feel some 'strain'. That, in a nutshell, sums up the reason why exercise is so important to bone strength. An analysis of 25 major studies on the effect of exercise on bone found it could prevent or reverse almost 1 per cent of bone loss a year in the lower spine and hip for pre- and postmenopausal women. That may not sound like a lot, but it's enough to make a huge difference in your risk of fracture, given that with age, between 0.5 and 1 per cent of bone density is lost per year.

The best kinds of exercises are those that tax muscle (and therefore bone), such as heavy gardening, lifting weights or jogging. You can even just hop up and down. When UK researchers had premenopausal women hop on one leg for a few minutes (50 hops) for six months, they found increased hipbone density on the side of that leg compared to no change in the other hip. Plain old walking also helps. A study of more than 61,000 postmenopausal women found those who walked for 4 hours or more a week had a 40 per cent lower risk of hip fracture than those who walked an hour or less a week.

Get treated for depression If you have even mild depression—feeling less interested in things you usually enjoy, changes in your sleep and eating patterns, fatigue and so on—your bones may suffer.

'The best kinds of exercises are those that tax muscle.'

It turns out that premenopausal women with even mild depression have less bone mass than women of the same age who aren't depressed. It doesn't seem to be related to antidepressants but to changes in the immune system that increase inflammation. In fact, some experts suggest that depression should be viewed as an early symptom of osteoporosis, which typically has no symptoms. It appears to be just as serious a risk factor as low calcium intake, smoking and lack of exercise.

Prevention boosters

Stop smoking Studies find that smoking increases the risk of a spinal fracture by 13 per cent in women and 32 per cent in men and ups the risk of a hip fracture by 31 per cent in women and 40 per cent in men. Once you quit, that risk begins to drop quickly.

Getting your calcium from food

Getting calcium from food sources is generally better for your bones than getting it from supplements. Here are some easy ways to get more calcium every day, and to reach your daily target of 1200 mg.

- **Start with cereal** Just 1 cup (40 g) of fortified breakfast cereal contains up to 200 mg. Add a cup of fat-free milk and you'll get 500 mg.

- **Snack on low-fat dairy** A 200 g low-fat yogurt, 250 ml low-fat milk or 200 ml fortified soymilk provide about 300 mg of calcium.

- **Eat your greens** One cup of cooked spinach contains 120 mg of calcium, although only 5 per cent of this may be absorbed because spinach contains calcium oxalate—a salt that makes calcium less available to your body. Pair it with a vitamin C source, such as red capsicum, to absorb more of the calcium. One cup of cooked soybeans contains about 260 mg and a cup of cooked broccoli has about 45 mg.

- **Lunch on canned fish** About 100 g of sardines, with bones, provides 370 mg of calcium, and 100 g canned salmon, with bones and liquid, has about 310 mg.

- **Look for fortified foods** About ½ cup (100 ml) of fortified orange juice has up to 80 mg calcium. And some breads are calcium-fortified, with around 30 g providing 200 mg.

- **Opt for low-fat cheese** About 50 g of low-fat cheese (less than 10 per cent fat) on wholegrain crackers or toast makes a calcium-rich healthy snack or breakfast, and contains about 400 mg of calcium, whereas 50 g of full-fat cheddar cheese has less than that—only 355 mg.

- **Snack on nuts** Eating almonds is an easy way to get more calcium in your diet; a small handful (about 15 nuts) provides about 40 mg. Brazil nuts and tahini are other good sources.

- **Whip up a smoothie** Blend a banana, 1 cup low-fat milk or calcium-fortified soy milk, ½ cup strawberries and 1 tablespoon honey on *High* for 30 seconds for a delicious drink that is full of bone-strengthening calcium.

Stock up on spinach Spinach is packed with vitamin K, an often-forgotten vitamin important for preventing fractures. One study found that taking 45 mg of vitamin K a day reduced the rate of spinal fractures by 65 per cent in women with osteoporosis compared to women who didn't supplement. Aim for 90 to 120 mcg of vitamin K daily, about the amount in 2 tablespoons of chopped parsley and a quarter of the amount in 1/2 cup of spinach.

Reduce your risk of falls Taking a few simple precautions can dramatically decrease your risk of falls, thereby reducing your risk of fractures to areas such as the wrist and hip. Try these tips:

- **Get your vision checked** If you have vision problems, you're two and a half times more likely to fall. This means that getting glasses, increasing the strength of prescription glasses or having your cataracts removed could prevent a fractured hip.
- **Review your meds** Certain medications, including some anti-depressants, anti-arrhythmia medication, diuretics and sleeping pills significantly increase the risk of having a fall. Regardless of what you're taking, if you take three or more medications regularly, you're also more likely to fall than someone who takes fewer. Discuss your regular medications with your doctor to see whether they may be contributing to an increased risk of falling, but never stop taking any medication without first talking to your doctor.
- **Declutter the house** Throw rugs, pot plants and badly positioned end tables can all trip you up as you move around your home. Talk to your doctor about having an occupational therapist do a home visit in order to assess these things.
- **Install bright bulbs** No matter how good your eyesight is, if it's too dark to clearly see obstacles in your way you're more than likely headed for a fall. Make sure all reading lamps have at least the equivalent of 60-watt bulbs, and preferably 75 watts. Put the equivalent of 100-watt bulbs in all overhead fixtures and turn on the lights when you enter a room. Make sure the path to the bathroom is well lit if you usually have to get up during the night to go to the toilet.

▶ WHAT CAUSES IT

Bone is constantly being built up by cells called osteoblasts and broken down by cells called osteoclasts. Until about your thirties, the osteoblasts are in the lead, but sometime during that decade you reach 'peak bone mass', and for the next decade or so, the two run neck and neck. From about the age of 50 onwards, as levels of oestrogen (in women) and testosterone (in men) drop, the osteoclasts pull ahead.

▶ SYMPTOMS TO WATCH FOR

None. Osteoporosis is typically identified with a bone density scan or when you fracture a bone. If you have a fracture, particularly if it occurred as a result of something relatively simple, such as tripping over a step, ask your doctor for a scan to measure your bone density. Consider having a bone scan at least once at the age of 65, or earlier if your GP recommends it.

▶ LATEST THINKING

Men should also be screened for osteoporosis. If risk factors exist, men should consider having a scan to measure bone density and start on medication if it's low. About 6 out of 100 men will have osteoporosis by sixty-five.

Balance exercises

One of the best ways to prevent falls—and therefore hip fractures—is by improving your balance and strengthening the muscles in your legs and around your hips. The following exercises are designed to do just that, and are not difficult. Start out by holding onto a sturdy chair or table. As you get stronger and your balance improves, hold on more loosely and then with just one finger; finally, don't hold on at all.

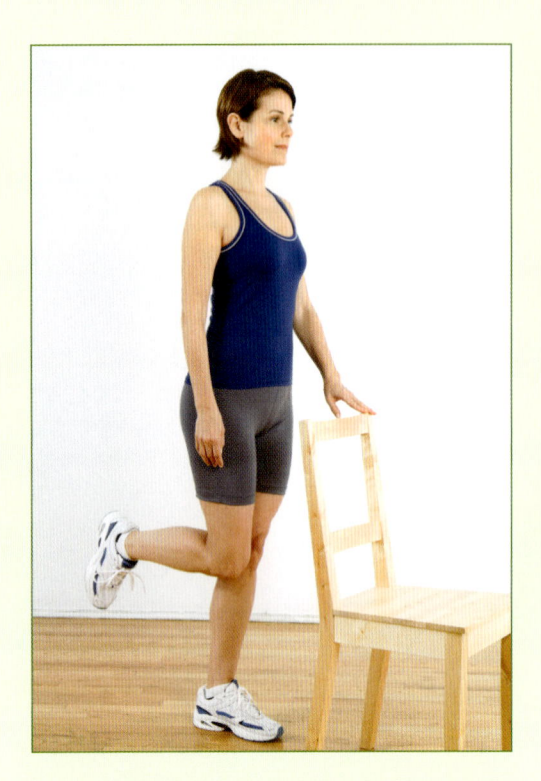

Knee bend

1 Stand straight with one hand on a table or chair back for balance.

2 Bend your right leg at the knee, bringing your foot as far up behind you as possible. Hold for 5 seconds, then lower your foot and repeat with your left leg. Repeat 10 times on each side.

Heel raise

1 Stand straight with one hand on a table or chair back for balance.

2 Rise on the balls of your feet as high as possible. Hold for 5 seconds, then lower your heels to the floor. Repeat 15 times. Rest for a minute, then repeat another 15 times.

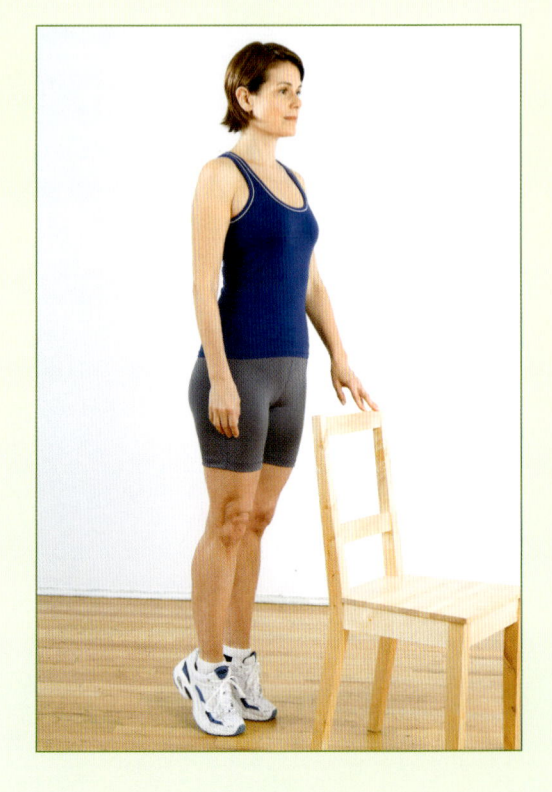

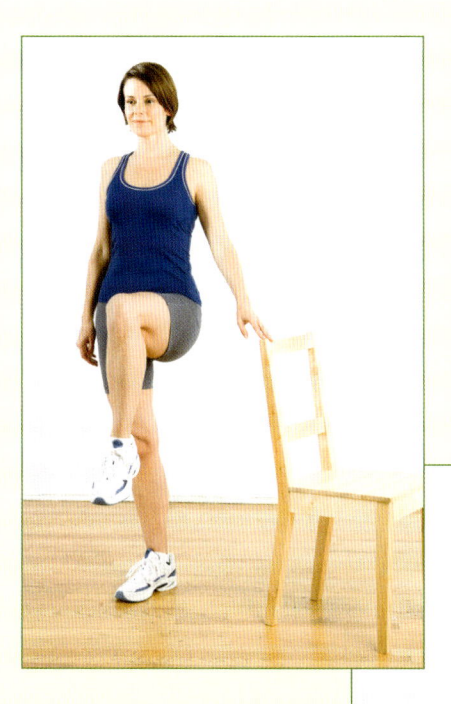

Hip stretch

1 Stand straight with one hand on a table or chair back for balance.

2 Slowly raise one knee towards your chest while keeping your waist and hips straight. Hold for 5 seconds, then slowly lower your leg and repeat with the other leg. Repeat 10 times on each side.

Hip strengthener

1 Stand 30 to 45 cm away from a table or behind a chair. Lean forward and hold onto the table or chair with both hands.

2 Slowly lift one leg back and up without bending the knee. Hold for 5 seconds, then slowly lower your leg and repeat with the other leg. Repeat 10 times on both sides.

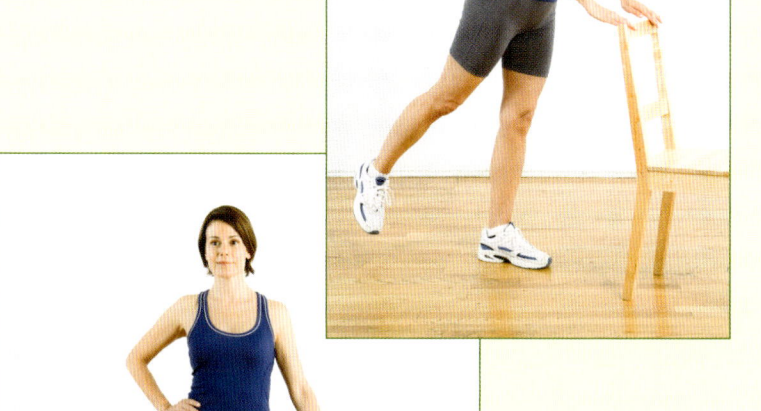

Side leg raise

1 Stand straight and hold onto a table or chair back for support.

2 Keeping your back straight, slowly raise one leg to the side as far as you can. Hold for 5 seconds, then slowly lower your leg and repeat with the other leg. Repeat 10 times on each side.

Ovarian cancer

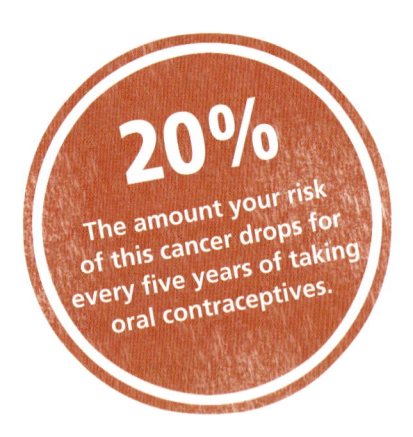

20%
The amount your risk of this cancer drops for every five years of taking oral contraceptives.

Don't shrug off persistent back or abdominal pain, especially if you've also been feeling bloated and tired. It could be a signal of ovarian cancer. While breast cancer is far more common in women, ovarian cancer is far more deadly. That's because most of the time, it isn't discovered until the late stages, when it's much more difficult to treat. However, this cancer isn't inevitable for women; researchers have found numerous steps you can take to reduce your risk.

Key prevention strategies

Take oral contraceptives The link between oral contraceptives and a reduced risk of ovarian cancer is so strong that a recent editorial in a leading medical journal suggested that all women who can take the Pill should. Just how strong is the link? An analysis of 45 studies from 21 countries found that women who had ever used oral contraceptives had a 27 per cent lower risk of developing ovarian cancer than women who had never used them. Every five years of use reduced the risk by about 20 per cent; after 15 years of use, the risk was halved. And the protective effect of oral contraceptives lasts 30 years after a woman stops taking them. The downside is that they include a higher risk of blood clots.

Breastfeed if you can Because breastfeeding suppresses ovulation, it can also reduce your risk of ovarian cancer. One study of nearly 150,000 nurses found that women who had ever breastfed a baby—no matter for how long—reduced their risk by 14 per cent. Those who breastfed for 18 months or longer cut their risk by one-third. Overall, each month of breastfeeding reduced the risk of ovarian cancer by 2 per cent.

Prevention boosters

Get your tubes tied Many studies find that having a tubal ligation—an operation in which the fallopian tubes are cut and sealed shut—reduces the risk of ovarian cancer by at least one-third overall and by up to 60 per cent in women who carry the

Got the gene?

If your mother, sister or mother's sister had ovarian cancer or breast cancer before menopause, talk to your doctor about the possibility that you might carry a mutation of the BRCA1 or BRCA2 gene. These mutations significantly increase your risk of getting ovarian cancer as well as breast cancer. If genetic screening shows you do carry the gene, you may want to consider having your ovaries removed, which studies find can reduce your risk of ovarian cancer by 96 per cent and of breast cancer by 50 per cent.

BRCA1 genetic mutation. One reason may be that when the tubes are closed off, cancer-causing chemicals and other toxins can't travel from the vagina and cervix through the tubes to the ovaries.

Avoid talcum powder Made from magnesium silicate, talcum powder has been controversially linked with an increased risk of ovarian cancer in some studies and has even been found embedded in some ovarian cancers. One study found that women who used talcum powder in the genital area or on sanitary pads had a 50 to 70 per cent increased risk of developing ovarian cancer. The link may be related to the inflammation that results if particles of talc travel through the reproductive tract to the ovaries or to the fact that, decades ago, the powder was contaminated with asbestos, a known carcinogen. While today's manufacturers are careful to keep any asbestos fibres out of the powder, it's still worth finding another alternative for staying dry.

Shed a few kilos If you have a body mass index (BMI) of 30 or more, you also have about a 30 per cent increased risk of developing ovarian cancer. And if you do get the cancer, your risk of dying from it is 50 per cent higher than that of women with a healthier BMI. The reason is probably related to the fact that fat cells release chemicals that are eventually converted to oestrogen, a hormone that fuels the growth of reproductive cancers like ovarian cancer.

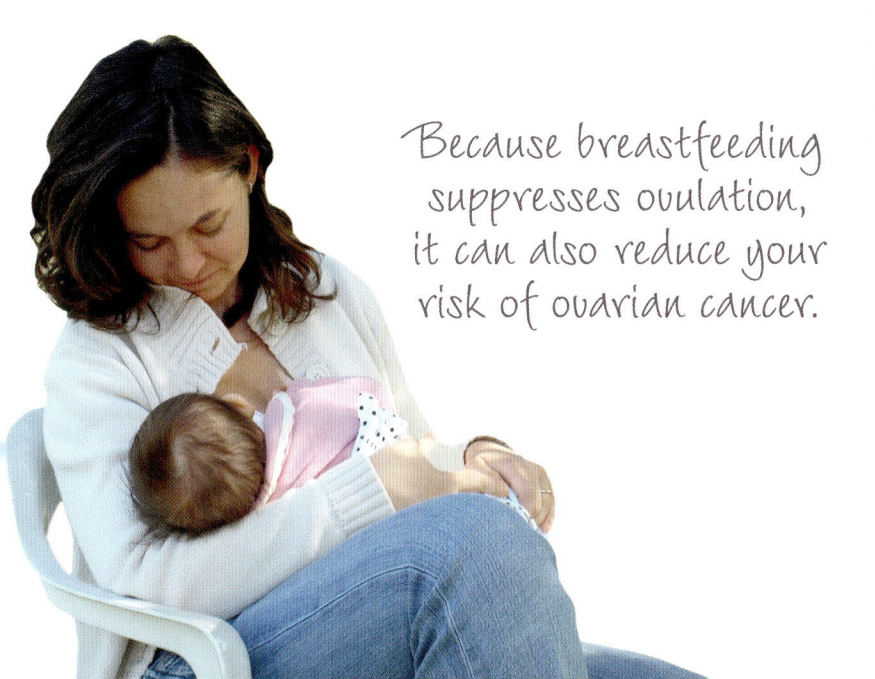

Because breastfeeding suppresses ovulation, it can also reduce your risk of ovarian cancer.

▶ WHAT CAUSES IT

The precise cause is still under investigation, but there are two main theories. One is that ovulation leads to trauma and repair of ovarian cells; the more you ovulate, the more repair is required, providing more opportunities for genetic errors to occur when cells divide. The other theory suggests that long-term exposure to reproductive hormones like oestrogen, which contribute to cell division, triggers those cellular errors.

▶ SYMPTOMS TO WATCH FOR

Bloating; persistent pain in the pelvis, abdomen or lower back; feeling full quickly; urinary symptoms, such as the urgent or frequent need to urinate; and persistent fatigue. If these symptoms occur suddenly and are present nearly every day for several weeks, see your doctor.

▶ LATEST THINKING

A simple screening test for early ovarian cancer is every doctor's dream, but so far no test or combination of tests (e.g. regular pelvic ultrasound or blood tests for a cancer marker called CA125) has proven reliable.

Peripheral vascular disease

33% The reduction in your risk of peripheral vascular disease if you get 29 g of fibre per day.

Think of peripheral vascular disease (PVD) as heart disease in your legs. The same factors that clog your coronary arteries with plaque, from eating saturated fat to being inactive, also pad the walls of your leg arteries with plaque. This can eventually shut off the blood supply to leg muscles and trigger intense pain when you walk. PVD is a problem for two reasons: it causes circulation problems that keep you off your feet and raise your risk of getting hard-to-heal sores on your feet, and it's a warning sign that arteries throughout your body are being narrowed by plaque. People diagnosed with PVD have a one-in-five chance of having a heart attack or stroke within a year. The following advice will help to keep the blood vessels in your legs clear.

Key prevention strategies

Stop smoking Nothing's worse than tobacco smoke for the arteries in your legs. The thousands of toxic chemicals in cigarettes narrow your arteries so much that smokers have a tenfold higher risk for PVD than nonsmokers do. Nicotine and other chemicals in tobacco also stiffen the normally flexible inner lining of artery walls, raising blood pressure and helping to trigger changes in your cholesterol that prompt the buildup of plaque in artery walls. If you already have signs of PVD, such as leg pain, stopping smoking can double or triple the distance you could walk pain free.

Control your blood sugar Having diabetes raises your risk of PVD two and a half times higher than normal (see 'Diabetes', starting on page 164). But if your blood sugar remains high (7 mmol/L or higher on a fasting blood sugar test), it's time for blood sugar-lowering medication. In a UK study of people with diabetes, those who kept their blood sugar under tight control cut their risk of serious PVD problems, such as leg pain or the need for blood vessel surgery or even amputation, by 22 per cent.

Lower LDL, raise HDL Unhealthy cholesterol levels clog the walls of arteries in your legs (or arms) just as they do in your heart.

Having high total cholesterol (over 5.5 mmol/L) increases your odds for PVD by an incredible 90 per cent. The best fix is to use the same strategies that protect the arteries in your heart and brain: reducing your 'bad' LDL cholesterol and boosting your 'good' HDL cholesterol (see 'High cholesterol' on page 214 for more information) and eating more healthily—choose heart-healthy salmon instead of steak, switch from refined grains to whole grains, eat plenty of fresh fruit and vegetables, drink lots of water, and get at least 30 minutes of exercise on most days of the week.

Follow advice if you've had a stroke or have heart disease A history of heart attack or stroke more than triples your risk of PVD. If you've survived one of these life-threatening events, it's time to pamper your entire cardiovascular system so that you can live well. That means getting regular physical activity, eating well, trying not to get stressed and taking any medications your doctor prescribes.

Get rid of that spare tyre If you have a beer belly or any other form of extra fat around your middle, it's time to get rid of it. When Spanish researchers weighed and measured 708 men with and without PVD, they found that those carrying more fat around their waistlines had a 32 per cent higher risk than those with trim waistlines. Experts recommend waist measurements less than 102 cm for men and 88 cm for women. (For people of Asian descent, risk rises with measurements over 95 cm for men and 80 cm for women.)

Prevention boosters

Go high fibre Men who consumed 29 g of fibre a day had a 33 per cent lower risk of developing PVD compared to men who had just 13 g a day (closer to the amount the average person eats), according to US researchers from the Harvard School of Public Health who tracked the health of more than 44,000 men for 12 years. The men who ate high-fibre foods got lots of whole grains, fruit and vegetables; compared to men who ate low-fibre foods, they also tended to exercise more and eat less fat, all strategies that also help to keep blood vessels healthy.

▶ WHAT CAUSES IT

Deposits of plaque in the walls of the arteries that supply blood to your legs and/or arms. They narrow arteries and restrict the flow of blood to your muscles. They can also trigger the formation of artery-blocking clots.

▶ SYMPTOMS TO WATCH FOR

Numbness or weakness in your legs; cold feet or legs; sores that won't heal on your toes, feet or legs; hair loss or changes in the colour of the skin on your legs and feet; pain or cramping that starts when you're active and disappears at rest. Half of the people with PVD have very mild symptoms or no symptoms at all.

▶ LATEST THINKING

Exposure to lead and cadmium could raise PVD risk. In one US study, researchers found that those with the highest lead exposures—from sources such as lead paint, lead-glazed pottery and contaminated drinking water—had a 65 per cent higher risk than people with the lowest exposures. High exposure to cadmium, found in the emissions from coal-fired power plants and garbage incinerators and in cigarette smoke, raised risk 86 per cent compared to people with the lowest exposures. Steering clear of cigarette smoke and following safety advice for removing lead paint are some ways to limit exposure.

Premenstrual syndrome

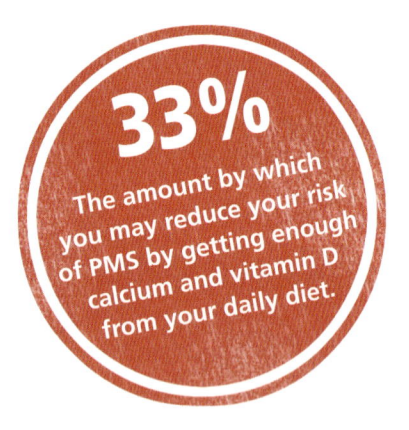

33% The amount by which you may reduce your risk of PMS by getting enough calcium and vitamin D from your daily diet.

About one in three women experiences the bloating, breast tenderness, insomnia, headaches and other symptoms of premenstrual syndrome (PMS) in the five to seven days before their period. Another 3 to 8 per cent experience a more severe version, premenstrual dysphoric disorder, or PMDD. Given that women will have, on average, 451 menstrual cycles in their lifetimes, feeling lousy for four or five days before each cycle adds up to more than six years of misery. Find out how to beat the averages with the following tips.

Key prevention strategies

Follow a bone-strengthening diet That means one rich in calcium and vitamin D, which helps the body absorb calcium. No one is certain exactly why this combination works—it's possible that PMS actually stems from a lack of calcium—but it does help some women. A large study of about 3000 women found that those who got about 1200 mg of calcium and 400 IU of vitamin D from food were about a third less likely to have PMS than those who got considerably less. Low-fat dairy foods such as milk and yogurt are great sources, as is fortified orange juice. You can read more about good food sources of each on pages 264 and 266.

While getting calcium from food provides the greatest benefit (both for preventing PMS and helping to keep bones healthy), there is also evidence that supplementing can help. One study of 248 women found that supplementing with 1200 mg of calcium carbonate for three months cut PMS severity nearly in half compared to taking a placebo.

Turn to chasteberry Several studies find that an extract from the fruit of chasteberry trees works fairly well at preventing PMS symptoms. In one study of 170 German women, 86 received the dried herbal extract and 84 got a placebo. Researchers tracked six PMS symptoms—irritability, mood swings, anger, headache, breast fullness and bloating—and found that symptoms improved by more than 50 per cent in the majority of the women taking the extract compared to no improvement in those taking the placebo.

Got the gene?

In late 2007, researchers identified the first genetic link to PMS and its more severe cousin, premenstrual dysphoric disorder (PMDD). The gene in question affects how women respond to changes in oestrogen levels; in women with PMS, mutations in the gene make them respond abnormally. The mutations also lead to reduced levels of dopamine, a brain chemical involved in mood. The findings may provide some peace of mind to women who now know that the mood swings and other symptoms of PMS are not in their heads but at least partly in their genes.

Prevention boosters

Eat less fat and more vegetables A study of 33 healthy women found that reducing the amount of fat in their diets—from the typical 40 per cent to 20 per cent—by following a vegetarian diet, reduced duration and intensity of pain, improved concentration and reduced mood swings and bloating prior to menstruation. Overall, bloating incidence dropped from nearly three days to just over a day, mood swings from nearly two days to one day, and concentration problems from nearly two days to less than a day.

Why does this type of diet help? It could be that it flattens the hormone rollercoaster by lowering levels of oestrogen in the blood.

Consider these supplements Various studies suggest that taking either 100 mg of vitamin B_6 a day or 200 to 360 mg a day of magnesium (in divided doses taken three times a day beginning 15 days after your period starts) can also relieve PMS symptoms. Check with your doctor before taking any of these supplements long term in case it is contraindicated.

DRUGS THAT PREVENT DISEASE

Some medications are approved for preventing the more severe form of PMS known as premenstrual dysphoric disorder (PMDD). However, some doctors will prescribe them if you have PMS. One is a low dose of the antidepressant fluoxetine (Prozac). In numerous studies, it relieved 60 to 75 per cent of PMS/PMDD symptoms. You take it only during the 14 days prior to your period. Another medication, YAZ, is an oral contraceptive that combines oestrogen with a new form of progestin. It may help with premenstrual symptoms, and some studies find that it significantly decreases PMDD symptoms. Both medications carry a risk of side effects.

Even regular oral contraceptives, if taken for 24 days with 4 days off rather than the typical 21 days on and 7 days off, can reduce PMS symptoms. Discuss this option with your doctor.

▶ WHAT CAUSES IT

There is probably a link between hormonal changes during the menstrual cycle and mood-related chemicals in the brain called neurotransmitters, particularly serotonin and endorphins. There's some evidence that the autonomic nervous system, which manages involuntary processes such as breathing and heart rate, also plays a role.

▶ SYMPTOMS TO WATCH FOR

Bloating, fatigue, breast tenderness, headaches, mood swings, irritability, depression, increased appetite, forgetfulness, trouble concentrating.

▶ LATEST THINKING

Severe PMS may be a sign of a permanently depressed nervous system. Japanese researchers proposed this theory in late 2007 after measuring heart rates and hormone levels in 62 women and evaluating their physical, emotional and behavioural symptoms before and during their period. Women with PMS showed significant drops in heart-rate variability, a sign of how well the autonomic nervous system functions.

Prostate cancer

73% The amount by which drinking three cups of green tea a day could reduce your risk of prostate cancer.

If you're a man and you live long enough, you'll develop prostate cancer. That's just one of the downsides of the hormone testosterone, which fuels the growth of prostate cells. The key is to keep this typically slow-growing cancer at bay long enough so that if you do get it, it remains so minuscule that it doesn't need treatment.

Key prevention strategies

Follow a prostate-protective diet Eating the right kinds of food can be protective. Here's what a typical day might look like:

BREAKFAST

- **Half a grapefruit** It turns out that the pectin in citrus fruits—the substance used to make jam 'set'—destroys prostate cancer cells. It's also an important form of soluble fibre, one that binds to hormones like testosterone to reduce the amount circulating in your body—and the amount your prostate cells are exposed to. Studies find lower levels of prostate-specific antigen (PSA), a protein released by prostate cells and often used to detect prostate cancer, in men whose diets are rich in soluble fibre (also found in legumes and oats). Researchers suspect that high-fibre diets are one reason why vegetarians are so much less likely to develop prostate cancer than meat-eaters.

- **A cup of green tea** Green tea contains hefty amounts of a powerful antioxidant called EGCG, which protects prostate cells from the type of biological damage that can lead to cancer. One study found that men who drank three cups of tea a day were 73 per cent less likely to develop prostate cancer than those who didn't drink tea at all; men who drank this much tea for more than 40 years were 88 per cent less likely to develop the cancer. Overall, the more tea the men drank and the longer they drank it, the lower their risk of prostate cancer. This area is so

DRUGS THAT PREVENT DISEASE You may have heard of finasteride (Proscar), the medication used to treat prostate enlargement. It may help prevent prostate cancer, too. A major prostate cancer prevention trial involving nearly 20,000 men who didn't have prostate enlargement found that men who took finasteride for seven years had about a 25 per cent reduced risk of prostate cancer compared to men who took a placebo.

promising that the US National Institutes of Health is studying a green tea extract as a way to prevent prostate cancer.

LUNCH

- **Soup or salad with edamame** People in Asian countries tend to eat a lot of soy, and men there don't develop prostate cancer as often as Western men do. Soy products such as edamame (immature soybeans still in their pods), tofu and soy milk contain plant-based hormones called isoflavones that help reduce levels of sex hormones like testosterone. The less testosterone, of course, the less fuel is available to drive prostate cancer cell growth. Buy edamame frozen, thaw, then add to soups and salads, or steam lightly and enjoy them as a tasty snack.

SNACK

- **A handful of nuts** Next to tahini, hazelnuts and almonds are great food sources of vitamin E, providing 6 mg and 4 mg, respectively, in just a small handful—and vitamin E may reduce your risk of prostate cancer. A major study of 29,000 Finnish males found that men who took 50 IU of vitamin E (about 33 mg) in supplement form were 32 per cent less likely than men not taking the supplement to develop prostate cancer and 41 per cent less likely to die from it during a five- to eight-year period. Vitamin E supplements have, however, been linked to premature death, so stick to natural food sources.

DINNER

- **Roasted salmon** Salmon is an excellent source of heart-healthy omega-3 fatty acids, which are also strongly linked to a lower risk of prostate cancer. A 30-year study of 6000 Swedish men found that those who ate little or no fatty fish had two to three times the risk of developing prostate cancer compared to those who ate moderate or high amounts of fatty fish. Trout, sardines and mackerel are other good sources of omega-3s.
- **Broccoli sautéed in olive oil** Broccoli, along with cauliflower, cabbage and brussels sprouts, contains the anticancer compound sulforaphane. One study found that men who ate three or more serves a week of these vegetables were 41 per cent less likely to develop prostate cancer than those who ate less than one serve a week. Use olive oil to sauté because it's made primarily of healthy monounsaturated fat, versus the polyunsaturated fat in corn,

'The more tea the men drank and the longer they drank it, the lower their risk of prostate cancer.'

safflower and sunflower oil. Several studies found that men whose diets were high in polyunsaturated fats were more likely to develop prostate cancer.

Get enough selenium The trace mineral selenium, found in brazil nuts, many white fish, salmon, oysters, wheat flour and pearled barley, is linked to lower rates of prostate cancer. But since levels of selenium in the soil vary widely throughout the world, they vary widely in much of the food we eat. For example, a study conducted with people living in the south-eastern US, where soil levels of selenium are very low, found nearly half the rate of prostate cancer in people who supplemented with 200 mcg of selenium compared to those who didn't supplement. This and other studies find the benefits of selenium are even greater in ex-smokers.

Taking individual selenium supplements can be risky, though, since they can raise the risk of diabetes, according to new research (and side effects of excess selenium can include hair loss and brittle nails). We recommend sticking with the amount in a multivitamin, if you take one, and adding more fish to your diet, if you haven't already. Your doctor can check your selenium levels through a blood test if you suspect they are low.

Get 10 minutes of sunshine (without sunscreen) a day You'll get valuable vitamin D, which the body manufactures when the sun's UVB rays strike the skin. Men in the UK—a place where vitamin D deficiency is fairly common—who took regular holidays in sunny climates, sunbathed regularly and had more overall exposure to ultraviolet rays had far less risk of prostate cancer than men who didn't do these things. Men with low levels of sun exposure also developed cancer younger (age 67.7) than those with more exposure (age 72.1). Of course, sun exposure raises your risk of skin cancer, so don't take this news as an excuse to sunbathe; 10 minutes is all you need. If you spend most of your time indoors or dress modestly for cultural reasons, you may want to consider supplementing with 1000 IU of vitamin D a day; it's also good for your bones.

Prevention boosters

Ask your doctor about a PSA test If your doctor suspects you have prostate cancer (or even if not), he or she may order a PSA test. This blood test measures levels of a protein called prostate-

---

Got the gene?

Many researchers are studying genes that may be linked to prostate cancer. A company in Iceland recently discovered a genetic mutation that may provide an early warning of risk—and help explain why black men are more likely than white men to develop the disease. The mutation is carried by about 13 per cent of men of European ancestry and 26 per cent of men of African ancestry. It increases the risk of prostate cancer by 60 per cent in either group, accounting for about 8 out of every 100 cases of prostate cancer overall. The mutation also appears to be associated with more aggressive forms of the disease. A test for the gene is in the works. If doctors find that men have the gene, they might take action, perhaps with medication, to prevent prostate cancer; if they discover that a man with prostate cancer has the genetic mutation, they might decide to treat his cancer more aggressively.

specific antigen, which is produced by prostate cells. The higher your levels, the more likely it is that you have prostate cancer. But the test isn't definitive; it sounds a lot of false alarms that can result in unnecessary needle biopsies. And since prostate cancer often grows so slowly that treating it isn't necessary, finding it early doesn't necessarily affect your risk of dying from it. That's why there's no consensus on whether doctors should use the test to screen men for the disease. Should you get screened? That's a decision you and your doctor should make based on your family history and your overall risk.

Another test that's used to detect prostate cancer is the digital rectal exam, often used in conjunction with the PSA test.

Order the chicken If you are black skinned, eating 650 g or more of red meat a week—no matter what type—means you are more than twice as likely to develop prostate cancer than if you eat less than 255 g. (The study showed a difference only in African-American men.) Bacon, sausage and salami pose the greatest risk. So load up on chicken and turkey instead.

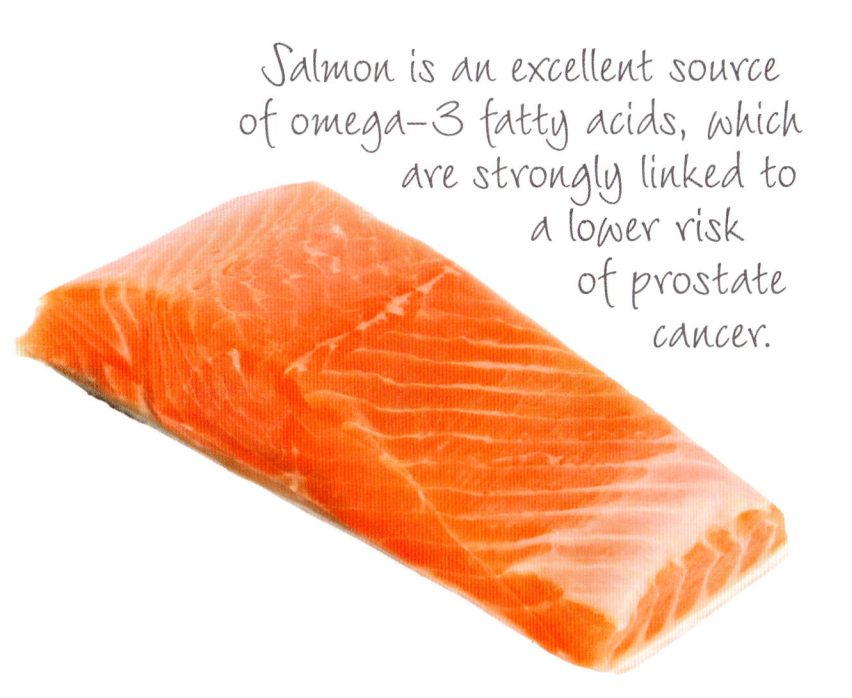

Salmon is an excellent source of omega-3 fatty acids, which are strongly linked to a lower risk of prostate cancer.

▶ WHAT CAUSES IT

Ageing. Over time, the cellular mechanisms that prevent abnormalities in dividing cells and destroy aberrant cells weaken. This increases the risk of cells whose 'off buttons' don't work. When that happens, the cells divide relentlessly, fuelled in part by male hormones such as testosterone. Two out of every three prostate cancers are found in men over the age of sixty-five.

▶ SYMPTOMS TO WATCH FOR

Frequent urination, particularly at night; problems urinating (starting or stopping the flow); painful urination; or blood in the urine or semen.

▶ LATEST THINKING

Prostate cancer in many men does not require treatment. Older men with less aggressive forms of cancer can be simply monitored through check-ups and blood tests. In a major study of 9000 men, average age 77, with early-stage prostate cancer who did not undergo treatment, researchers found that 72 per cent either died of other causes or didn't have enough cancer growth to warrant treatment. For the rest, about 10 years passed before the cancer grew enough to require treatment. Men with more aggressive forms of the cancer, however, do require treatment.

Psoriasis

57%
The likelihood that using the drug etanercept will help prevent new psoriasis flare-ups.

In psoriasis, skin cells mature almost 10 times faster than normal. They pile up, creating silvery scales and patches of thick, red, scaly skin on the elbows, knees, legs, scalp, and elsewhere. These steps can help you avoid the condition and, if you have it already, lower your odds of a flare-up.

Key prevention strategies

Quit smoking Tobacco use triples your risk of plaque psoriasis, the most common form of this condition, according to Swedish research. And if you already have psoriasis, smoking destroys your chances of having clear, calm skin. When researchers asked 104 people if their psoriasis had ever gone into remission, 77 per cent of nonsmokers said yes, compared to just 9 per cent of smokers.

Think before you drink Alcohol boosts psoriasis risk. And Finnish scientists have found that, for people who already had psoriasis, the amount of skin affected increased as their alcohol intake rose. If you're in the midst of a flare-up, abstaining makes sense. If your psoriasis is under control, and you find that an occasional drink doesn't aggravate your skin, enjoy in moderation.

Maintain a healthy weight Gaining extra kilos raised risk by 40 per cent in one Harvard Medical School study of more than 78,000 women. Doctors aren't certain how excess body fat contributes to psoriasis, but they do know that it can make existing skin problems worse and render psoriasis treatments less effective.

Try one of the newer treatments If you have psoriasis, your goal is to prevent flare-ups. Older medications were often too messy or risky for many people. For people with just a few spots of psoriasis, newer sprays or foam products may be preferable. For more severe forms of psoriasis or for psoriatic

Dead Sea magic?

A month of sunbathing and swimming at one of the psoriasis spas along Israel's scenic Dead Sea is virtually guaranteed to improve or completely clear up your skin, studies show. A more affordable option is to fill a bath with warm water, sprinkle in Dead Sea salts (available from some health food shops), and soak. In one German study, almost everyone who did this three or four times a week for a month saw their psoriasis improve significantly.

arthritis, newer injectable medications are available. One of them, etanercept (Enbrel), improves psoriasis symptoms by 75 per cent in 57 per cent of the people who use it. Two others, adalimumab (Humira) and infliximab (Remicade), are even more effective.

Moisturise well Lubricating your skin every day can also help cut your odds for flare-ups prompted by dry skin.

Stress less Stress can trigger new flare-ups, so try to break the cycle by building relaxation into your day, even if it's just 10 minutes of quiet, calm breathing. Or try mindfulness-based stress reduction (MBSR). In one US study, people with psoriasis who listened to a MBSR tape while undergoing light therapy saw their skin clear up twice as fast as those who didn't hear the tape, researchers report.

Sunbathe, but safely Exposing your skin to sunlight for a few minutes each day can reduce inflammation and scaling. Eighty per cent of people with psoriasis who try daily sunbaths see an improvement. Don't overdo it, though; for about 1 in 10 people, exposure to sunlight makes skin problems worse, and getting sunburnt raises the risk of skin cancer. Use a broad-spectrum sunscreen on skin that's not affected by psoriasis. Commercial tanning beds may help, but talk to your doctor first, as their usefulness is controversial.

Steer clear of these medications Some prescription medications can trigger a flare-up. If your doctor recommends anti-malaria medication, beta-blockers, indomethacin (Indocin) or lithium, ask whether a substitute is possible.

Prevention boosters

Baby your skin For about half of all people with psoriasis, it worsens 10 to 14 days after any sort of cut, bruise, insect bite or scrape. Even shaving or removing an adhesive bandage could trigger a flare-up, so take care with your skin.

Check your reaction to gluten In studies, people with coeliac disease who avoided gluten—a protein found in wheat, barley and rye—saw their psoriasis improve. Symptoms of gluten intolerance include diarrhoea, abdominal pain and wind.

▶ WHAT CAUSES IT

Genes raise your risk of psoriasis, but experts aren't certain what triggers the immune system malfunction that leads to the condition. It begins when infection-fighting T cells in the skin become too active, stimulating the overgrowth of skin cells.

▶ SYMPTOMS TO WATCH FOR

Patches of thick red skin with silvery scales on the back of the elbows, front of the knees, other parts of the legs, scalp, lower back, face, palms and soles of the feet. Less often, they appear on the fingernails, toenails and genitals, and inside the mouth.

▶ LATEST THINKING

In a recent survey, over half of people with moderate to severe psoriasis weren't getting the treatments that prevent future flare-ups. If your psoriasis isn't improving with lotions and topical medications, ask about light therapy and oral or injectable medications that help normalise the overactive immune responses that trigger psoriasis.

Rosacea

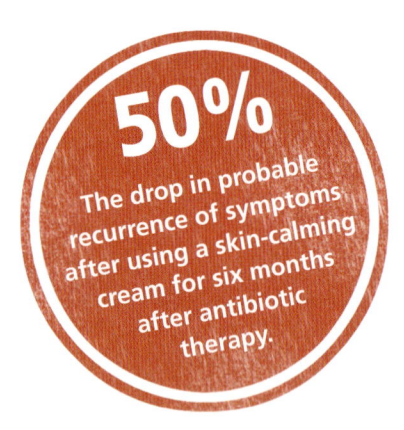

50% The drop in probable recurrence of symptoms after using a skin-calming cream for six months after antibiotic therapy.

Avoiding and treating flare-ups of this adults-only skin condition can help keep it from getting worse. Yet three out of four people don't recognise the early signs and symptoms. Flushing, blushing and persistently red skin on your cheeks and nose are major clues, but other hints are burning, stinging or itching facial skin as well as raised red patches and even swollen spots. In one survey, one in four people had signs of rosacea on the neck, chest, scalp or ears, too. You may be more prone to rosacea if other family members have it or if you're of Irish or English descent.

Key prevention strategies

Avoid rosacea triggers The most important step in avoiding outbreaks is learning what triggers them. Heading up most people's lists are sun exposure, emotional stress and hot weather, but there are plenty more. In a survey of people with rosacea, about half said that wind, heavy exercise, drinking alcohol, taking a hot bath, cold weather and spicy foods (including chillies and Indian food, as well as vinegar, white pepper and garlic) set off a reaction.

To pinpoint your triggers, keep a rosacea diary (use a small notebook or even a desk calendar). Write down common triggers you're exposed to and record days when symptoms flare up. After two to four weeks, you should see a pattern; triggers usually encourage redness within a few minutes to a day.

Avoid the sun The sun's ultraviolet rays aggravate rosacea simply by reddening the skin, but that's not all. US dermatologists from Boston University have found that sunlight also seems to trigger the production of compounds that spur the growth of blood vessels close to the surface of the skin. So stay in the shade during the brightest hours of the day and wear a broad-brimmed hat and apply sunscreen to your face when you leave the house.

Don't let your sunscreen aggravate your skin, though. Choose a formula that contains dimethicone and cyclomethicone. In one study, these additives protected against the irritation caused by the sun-blocking ingredient Padimate O. Or try a sunscreen formulated for babies, which may be milder. Also look for the ingredients zinc oxide and micronised titanium oxide, which deflect some of the sun's heat and therefore help prevent rosacea flare-ups.

Maintain healthy skin with a prescription cream or gel Many doctors begin treatment by prescribing antibiotics such as tetracycline for 12 weeks or so to help reduce bumps and redness. But that's not a cure. In one study, two-thirds of the people who took a course of tetracycline for rosacea saw skin problems return within six months. That's why doctors also prescribe a skin-calming cream or gel containing metronidazole (Rozex) or azelaic acid for long-term use. In one study, people who used metronidazole for six months after antibiotic treatment were about half as likely to have redness or bumps return as those who didn't use it.

Consider laser therapy This may be the best way to treat broken blood vessels, persistent redness and a rosacea-induced large nose.

Prevention boosters

Pamper your skin Skin-care products such as cleansers, moisturisers, sunscreens and make-up can easily irritate and redden your skin if you have rosacea. To avoid irritation, choose mild, hypoallergenic cleansers and moisturisers, wash with lukewarm (not hot) water, and avoid contact with rough materials such as scratchy face washers, loofahs and abrasive skin-care products such as grainy skin scrubs and exfoliators. If your skin tends to sting when you apply sunscreen, make-up or medicated creams and gels, wait half an hour after washing so that your skin is completely dry.

▶ WHAT CAUSES IT
Swelling of tiny blood vessels near the surface of the skin. Experts say that genetic factors and sun damage both play a role. There's also some evidence that microscopic mites that live in human hair follicles may clog oil glands and inflame skin.

▶ SYMPTOMS TO WATCH FOR
Reddened skin, especially on your cheeks and nose. As rosacea progresses, you may notice small, spidery blood vessels appearing in these areas as well as bumps on your nose, cheeks, forehead and chin. You may also notice a gritty or burning feeling in your eyes. For a few people, rosacea triggers the buildup of tissue on and around the nose, too.

▶ LATEST THINKING
Ask your doctor about a retinoid product. These vitamin A-based skin creams and gels speed cell turnover and are usually used to control acne and reduce wrinkles. Recent studies suggest they may reduce two visible signs of rosacea: redness and tiny blood vessels near the surface of the skin. Proceed with caution, though; retinoids can irritate the skin at first, so start with a low-dose product.

Sexually transmissible infections

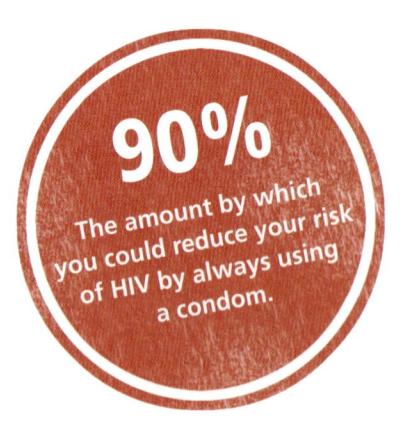

90% The amount by which you could reduce your risk of HIV by always using a condom.

Sexually transmissible infections (STIs)—including genital warts, herpes, chlamydia, gonorrhoea and syphilis—are common in young people, but increasingly common among people over forty-five. Since most STIs have no symptoms in the early or even late stages, simply asking or looking at your partner won't help you avoid them, but these tips might.

Key prevention strategies

Don't have sex It's that simple. If you abstain from anal, oral or vaginal sex until you are in a long-term monogamous relationship with someone who has tested negative for any sexually transmissible infections, it's highly unlikely you'll get an STI.

Use condoms These simple sheaths have been around for more than 300 years, and they're still the best thing we have to protect against many STIs, including HIV, gonorrhoea, chlamydia and trichomoniasis (caused by a parasite). They're not completely foolproof, but in the case of AIDS, for instance, properly used latex condoms could prevent 80 to 90 per cent of HIV infections. However, it's important that a condom fits properly. If it doesn't, it's much more likely to slip off or break during intercourse. If you try a regular size first, you'll get a good idea of whether you need a bigger or smaller size.

Limit your partners The fewer people you have sex with, the fewer of their sexual partners you're exposed to. And the less exposure, the less likely you are to catch an STI. Stick with one partner at a time.

The kindest cut?

A growing body of evidence suggests that circumcision may reduce the risk of STIs, particularly HIV, in men. For instance, a large Kenyan study showed that circumcision reduced men's risk of HIV infection from men or women by 53 per cent, while a Ugandan study showed a reduced risk of 51 per cent. Researchers think that circumcision protects against HIV because the foreskin of the penis contains a rich source of cells the virus likes to target; remove the foreskin, and you remove vulnerable cells. Other studies find that circumcised men have a lower risk of infection with syphilis and chancroid (a bacterial infection). There is still no good evidence that circumcised men are less likely to infect women with HIV than uncircumcised men are.

Get vaccinated for HPV While progress on an HIV vaccine has been dismal, we do have a vaccine that prevents four of the most common types of human papillomavirus (HPV), including the ones that cause the majority of cervical cancers, not to mention genital warts. Called Gardasil, the three-dose vaccine is recommended for girls from the age of 11, before they become sexually active, and is approved for women up to 26 years.

Prevention boosters

Get tested If you're sexually active and not in a monogamous relationship, you should be screened at least once a year for STIs, particularly gonorrhoea, chlamydia and trichomoniasis. A large multinational study found that women infected with trichomoniasis are 50 per cent more likely to acquire HIV. Researchers don't know why, but they suspect that the infection may lead to minuscule areas in the vagina that provide more entry points for the HIV virus.

Stop smoking We already know that smoking increases the risk of cervical cancer, but there's also intriguing evidence that smokers have a greater risk of HIV infection than nonsmokers, with the increase ranging from 60 per cent to more than threefold. Researchers suggest that the effects of tobacco smoke on the immune system may reduce the ability of immune cells to fight off the virus.

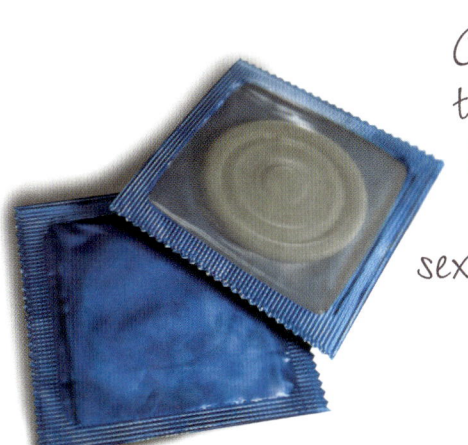

Condoms are still the best thing we have to protect against many sexually transmissible infections.

▶ WHAT CAUSES IT
Viruses, bacteria or protozoa (in the case of trichomoniasis) that are spread through sexual intercourse, oral sex or even skin-to-skin contact. Some, like HIV, are also spread through blood.

▶ SYMPTOMS TO WATCH FOR
Many STIs don't cause any symptoms in the early or even late stages; infections like chlamydia can spread and permanently damage parts of your reproductive system without you being aware of it. See your doctor if you have genital itching or discharge; painful sex or urination; pelvic pain; a sore throat (if you have oral sex) or a sore anus (if you have anal sex); sores, blisters or scabs on your genital area, anus, tongue and/or throat; a scaly rash on the palms of your hands and soles of your feet; dark urine, light-coloured loose stools and yellow eyes and skin; swollen glands, fever and body aches; or unusual infections, unexplained fatigue, night sweats and weight loss.

▶ LATEST THINKING
One reason that men are at greater risk for AIDS than women are may be an enzyme produced by the prostate and found in semen; it appears to increase the risk of HIV infection. The finding, from German researchers, could open up a new avenue for prevention.

Shingles

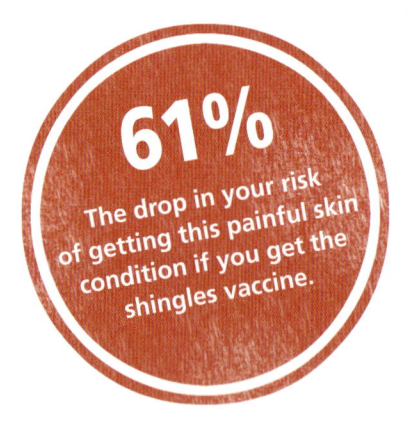

61% The drop in your risk of getting this painful skin condition if you get the shingles vaccine.

If you had chickenpox as a child or adult, the virus responsible remains in your body. Called the varicella zoster virus, it can lie dormant for decades in a bundle of nerves at the base of your spine, only to raise a new red rash and blisters in middle age or later—and possibly cause excruciating skin pain. An estimated one in five older adults will develop this infection, called shingles. However, there's a new vaccine and a host of immunity-bolstering strategies to lean on.

Key prevention strategies

Get the shingles vaccine Australian, New Zealand and South African infants now receive a chicken-pox vaccine (adults who have never had chickenpox need two doses rather than one), and so should be protected against shingles later in life. For everyone else, there's a shingles vaccine (Zostavax), a higher potency form of the chickenpox vaccine, and it cuts your risk of developing shingles by 61 per cent. In studies of more than 38,000 women and men, the vaccine also reduced the severity of shingles outbreaks for people who developed it. And it cuts the risk of the agonising chronic nerve pain that sometimes occurs after an outbreak by two-thirds.

You'll need a prescription for the vaccine from your doctor, and it isn't subsidised in Australia by the Pharmaceutical Benefits Scheme (PBS), so check with your pharmacist about cost and ask if your health fund will contribute to at least partially cover the cost if you're privately insured. The shingles vaccine isn't recommended for people with weakened immune systems and is only recommended for people over 50 years of age.

Act fast if you notice shingles symptoms Shingles blisters heal in three to five weeks, but pain can linger for months or even years. Called post-herpetic neuralgia (PHN), this sharp, throbbing or stabbing pain affects up to 40 per cent of people who get shingles. PHN can make your skin so sensitive that wearing even the softest, lightest silk or cotton is agony. A kiss or a cool breeze can be excruciating. Living with this chronic pain can lead to depression, anxiety, sleeplessness and even weight loss.

Your best option for avoiding PHN is getting the shingles vaccine if you can afford it. Your second-best strategy is recognising the early symptoms of a shingles outbreak and getting to your doctor for treatment within 72 hours. Studies show that the antiviral drugs aciclovir (Zovirax), famciclovir (Famvir) or valaciclovir (Valtrex) can lessen PHN pain and shorten its duration if taken early. These medications seem to work by reducing the nerve damage caused by the virus. They also speed healing of the original shingles outbreak.

It sounds odd, but adding a tricyclic antidepressant, such as amitriptyline (Endep), can help, too. In one study, people who took 25 mg of amitriptyline daily were 50 per cent less likely to have lingering PHN pain after six months than those who got a placebo. Study volunteers began taking the antidepressant, which stabilises nerve cells, two days after the rash came and continued for 90 days.

Prevention boosters

Feed your immune system more fruit and vegetables In a UK study of 726 people, those who ate more than three serves of fruit a day cut their risk of shingles in half compared to people who ate fruit less than once a day, report researchers from the London School of Hygiene and Tropical Medicine. Study volunteers who ate five daily serves of vegetables reduced their odds by 70 per cent compared to people who had just one or two daily serves.

Learn the ancient art of tai chi In one US study of 112 healthy adults aged 59 to 82, this gentle, flowing exercise form boosted immunity against shingles dramatically. Compared to participants who took health-education classes, volunteers who practised tai chi three times a week for four months developed antibodies to the shingles virus on a par with those found in 30- and 40-year-olds who had had the shingles vaccine.

No one's saying this type of exercise is a replacement for the vaccine, however; it works best in combination with immunisation. When the researchers gave the shingles vaccine to everyone in the study and rechecked their immunity a few weeks later, they found that the tai chi group's immunity was 40 per cent higher than that of the vaccine-only group.

WHAT CAUSES IT
The varicella zoster virus, the same virus responsible for chickenpox. Once you've had chickenpox, the virus lies dormant in a bundle of nerve cells called the sensory ganglia, located near the spinal cord. It can re-emerge as shingles decades later, often triggered by lowered immunity, physical or emotional stress, an injury, or even dental work.

SYMPTOMS TO WATCH FOR
Burning, tingling or numb skin plus chills, fever, upset stomach and/or headache; after a few days, a red rash develops on your body (especially the torso), neck or face. The rash morphs into fluid-filled blisters, which dry up in a few days. Shingles clears up completely in three to five weeks, but for 25 to 50 per cent of people who get it, severe nerve pain can linger for months or years afterwards.

LATEST THINKING
If you have a family history of shingles, don't put off getting the vaccine. Having just one close family member with shingles increases your risk of developing it fourfold, according to US dermatologists from the University of Texas Medical School in Houston. They quizzed 500 people with shingles about their relatives and discovered that, for 39 per cent, it ran in the family. The more relatives who've had it, the higher your risk.

Sinusitis and sinus infections

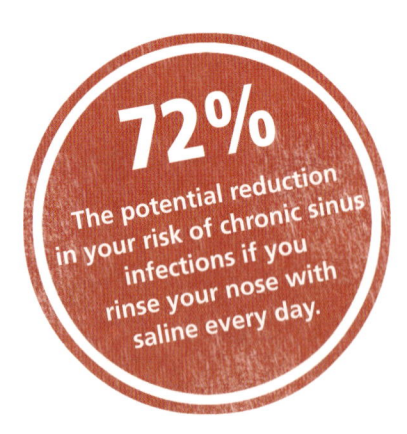

72% The potential reduction in your risk of chronic sinus infections if you rinse your nose with saline every day.

The purpose of sinuses—hollow cavities under facial skin and bones—remains a mystery, but their serious design flaw is well known. When tiny sinus drainage holes swell shut, trapped mucus causes pressure and pain—and provides a home where viruses and bacteria can breed. Stop your next sinus infection before it starts by avoiding colds and flu, and treating or preventing respiratory allergy attacks. Follow these tips to ease congestion and promote drainage.

Key prevention strategies

Rinse with saline For thousands of years, people have used saltwater or seawater rinses to prevent sinus problems. Now there's hard science to recommend this practice. When researchers from the UK's Royal National Throat, Nose and Ear Hospital reviewed eight well-designed studies, they concluded that a daily saline rinse cuts the risk of chronic sinus infections by up to 72 per cent. A rinse can also help prevent a cold from turning into a sinus infection. (Experts say you should use a decongestant first to reduce swelling so the fluid can drain out easily.)

You can buy a sinus-rinsing tool called a neti pot—it looks like a tiny watering can—at a health food shop, or use a bulb syringe to deliver the saline solution to your nose. Mix $1/4$ teaspoon of table salt and $1/4$ teaspoon of bicarbonate of soda in 250 ml of lukewarm water. Lean over the sink. Tilt your head sideways and pour some of the solution into your upper nostril. Relax and keep breathing through your mouth as the liquid makes its way into the other nostril and back out. Spit out any that solution that drains into your mouth. Repeat until you've used all the solution.

Don't be a blowhard

Blowing hard into a tissue is counterproductive because it triggers 'reflex nasal congestion', experts say. This natural reaction, which happens when you sneeze, increases blood flow and makes nasal tissues swell. It serves a purpose by preventing anything going back up your nose or from travelling further up your nose. But it also happens if you blow too vigorously. The result is that your nose becomes even more stuffy. Blowing gently is a better way to keep nasal passages open.

Thin nasal mucus Mucus trapped in your sinuses during a cold, flu or allergy attack is a breeding ground for viruses and bacteria. To keep it thin so it can drain, drink six glasses a day of water, hot tea or other clear liquids, unless your doctor has you on fluid restrictions. Also consider an over-the-counter remedy that contains the mucus-thinner guaifenesin, such as Robitussin. If you prefer a natural approach, inhale some steam for 10 minutes. Simply lean over a bowl of hot water with a towel over your head to trap the steam, stand in a steamy shower or sit in the steam room at the gym.

If your home or office is very dry, increasing the humidity can help. Use a humidifier or vaporiser, and clean it regularly.

Warm your sinuses Placing a hot face washer on your cheeks feels good if sinus pressure is building. It may also nudge microscopic hairs in your sinuses into action. Called cilia, they normally sweep back and forth at a brisk 700 beats per minute to whisk mucus along. When you have a cold or flu, the hairs move at a sluggish 300 beats per minute. Warmth seems to help them pick up the pace.

Use over-the-counter decongestants sparingly These tablets and sprays make blood vessels in your nose constrict, opening swollen nasal passages. Early in a cold or flu, using a decongestant could help promote drainage but it can backfire quickly, causing 'rebound congestion' as each dose wears off. Few experts believe decongestants should be used to help prevent sinus infections at all. The best advice is to never use an over-the-counter decongestant spray for more than three days, and use decongestants in tablet form sparingly; they can thicken mucus.

See your doctor for severe acute or chronic infections If you develop severe pain in your face or jaw and/or a fever higher than 38.5°C when you have sinus congestion, talk with your doctor. You may need an antibiotic, although this requires careful consideration.

Ask about preventive meds If you have multiple episodes of sinus congestion or sinusitis in a year, or your colds or allergy attacks tend to turn into sinus infections, you may benefit from long-term courses of appropriate antibiotics or from prescription steroid nasal sprays. The sprays soothe inflammation, shrinking swollen nasal and sinus passages so they can drain, without the side effects of over-the-counter decongestant sprays.

WHAT CAUSES IT

When swollen nasal and sinus passages cause congestion, trapped mucus can become a breeding ground for viruses and bacteria.

SYMPTOMS TO WATCH FOR

Pressure and pain in your cheeks or behind your eyes (often on just one side) or in the upper teeth or jaw; green, yellow or brownish nasal discharge; fever higher than 38.5°C; extreme fatigue; reduced sense of taste and/or smell; cough from post-nasal drip; and new or unusual bad breath.

LATEST THINKING

Antibiotics inhaled as a mist via a device called a nebuliser could help if sinus surgery and other medical treatments don't cure chronic sinus trouble. In one US study of 42 people with repeated sinus infections, 76 per cent saw significant improvement with three weeks of nebulised antibiotics, and they remained infection free for an average of 17 weeks. Before treatment, infections recurred every six weeks or so.

Skin cancer

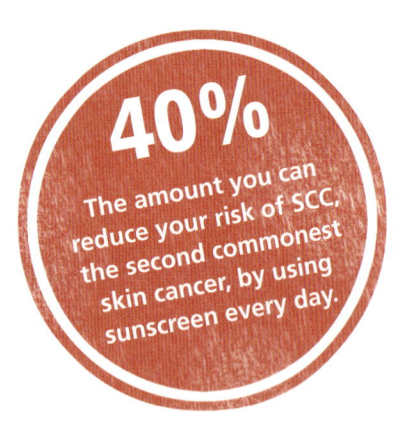

40% The amount you can reduce your risk of SCC, the second commonest skin cancer, by using sunscreen every day.

Sunlight improves our mood and provides us with all-important vitamin D. But everyone knows the downside of getting too much: skin cancer. Just consider the difference in skin cancer rates in different parts of the world. Australia has a rate of about 1035 cases per 100,000 men and 472 per 100,000 women, while Finland's rate is about 6 out of 100,000 in men and 4 out of 100,000 in women. UVB rays cause the majority of skin cancers, along with UVA rays, which make the damage worse (and may even cause cancer in their own right). Follow these strategies to keep your skin healthy.

Key prevention strategies

Slather on the sunscreen If you're going to be out in the sun for more than 10 or 15 minutes, make sure you're wearing sunscreen. Slather it on generously; most people don't use enough. It takes about a shot glass-full to cover you completely (for a day at the beach or pool) and about 2 tablespoons to cover your face and neck (don't forget the ears). And pay special attention to the danger areas; 55 per cent of skin cancers occur on the head or neck (balding men take note), followed by the hands, forearms and legs. Also use lip protection with an SPF rating of 15 or higher, and reapply sunscreen to all parts of your body every 2 hours (more often if you're in and out of the water).

Stay covered up Wearing protective clothing and a hat when you're in the sun is also important. These days, you can even find clothing with built-in sun protection; it's not cheap, but it's an excellent long-term investment in your health. Regular cotton or linen clothing

Shopping for sunscreen

Stymied by the plethora of sunscreens on the supermarket shelf? Look for the following.

- **An SPF of at least 15** These block 93 per cent of all incoming UVB rays, assuming you reapply often. SPF 30 blocks an extra 4 per cent, and SPF 50 an extra 6 per cent. SPF doesn't measure protection from UVA rays, only UVB.

- **UVA-filtering ingredients** Most sunscreens today offer 'broad-spectrum' protection, meaning they protect against both UVA and UVB rays. But some may not provide adequate UVA protection. For extra insurance, look for avobenzone or ecamsule, both of which absorb UVA light. (Unfortunately, they also add—sometimes significantly—to a product's price tag.) Also look for titanium dioxide or zinc oxide, which both scatter rather than absorb UVA light. If you have sensitive skin, look for a PABA-free sunscreen.

may not provide the physical protection from the sun that is necessary during prolonged periods of exposure, for instance while playing or watching sport.

In Australia, the Cancer Council has retail shops in various locations, as well as an online shop, where you can purchase sun-smart clothes that provide good protection. And since the most common form of cancer for Australians aged between 15 and 40 is melanoma, it makes good sense to protect your children's skin from an early age by covering up. Don't forget the sunglasses, too.

Use self-tanners, not tanning beds Tanning beds, which use UVA rays to darken your skin, can increase your risk of melanoma by up to 75 per cent, boost your risk of basal cell cancer (BCC) by 50 per cent, and more than double your risk of squamous cell cancer (SCC). Stick to topically applied self-tanning products, which safely provide a bronze glow.

Prevention boosters

Quit smoking As with nearly every other cancer, your risk of skin cancer is higher if you smoke, with one study finding that the risk doubled in smokers.

Cook with turmeric This yellow spice, prominent in curry powder, contains the chemical curcumin, considered a strong cancer-fighting agent. Lab studies suggest it may help protect against melanoma in particular.

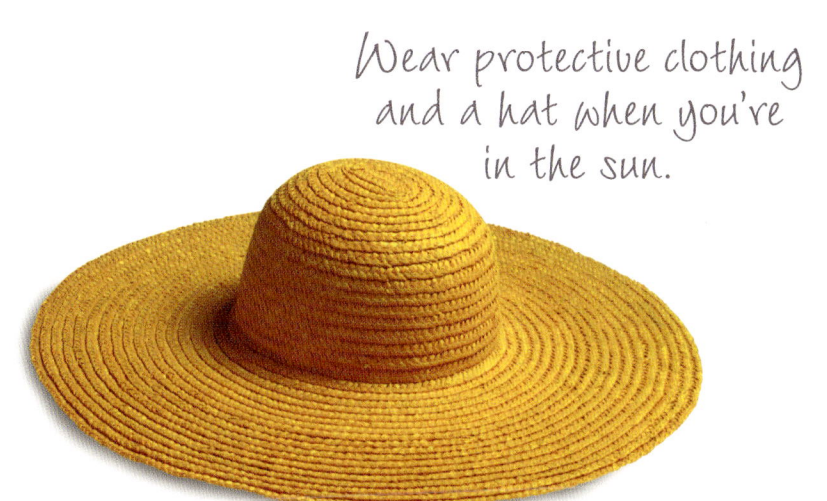

Wear protective clothing and a hat when you're in the sun.

▶ WHAT CAUSES IT

UV rays from the sun or radiation. Your risk of basal cell skin cancer, the most common type, and squamous cell skin cancer, the second most common type, depends on cumulative sun exposure throughout your life. Your risk of melanoma, the deadliest form of skin cancer, seems to depend more on the intensity of the sun exposure. Even a single bad sunburn could lead to melanoma.

▶ SYMPTOMS TO WATCH FOR

Pearly or waxy bumps; a flat, flesh-coloured, or brown scar-like lesion on your chest or back; a red nodule on your face, lips, ears, neck, hands or arms; a flat lesion with a scaly, crusted surface on your face, ears, neck, hands or arms; an ulcer that won't heal; a large brownish spot with darker speckles; a mole that has one of the ABCDEs—asymmetrical shape, irregular border, a variety of colours, a diameter greater than 6 mm or evolution (changes over time); dark lesions on your palms, the soles of your feet, fingertips and toes, or on mucous membranes lining your mouth, nose, vagina or anus.

▶ LATEST THINKING

A prescription skin cream in the works could protect against certain types of skin cancer by making the outer layers of skin less vulnerable to damage from UV rays. The active ingredient, myristyl nicotinate, is derived from the vitamin niacin.

Snoring

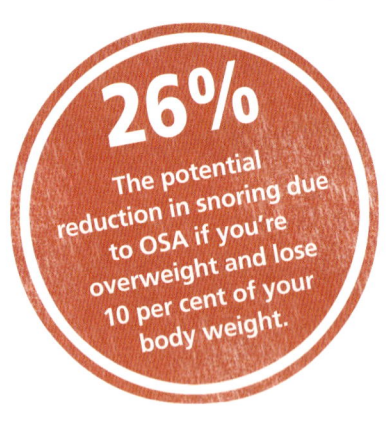

26% The potential reduction in snoring due to OSA if you're overweight and lose 10 per cent of your body weight.

If you've ever been banished to another room for snoring too loudly, it's time to take action. Loud night-time snorts and snuffling are a sign that tissue in the airway is vibrating with each breath at decibel levels that can keep a sleeping partner awake for hours. An estimated 50 to 60 per cent of loud snorers also have obstructive sleep apnoea (OSA), in which flabby tissue blocks the airway over and over throughout the night, leading to dozens or even hundreds of unrecognised partial awakenings and an increased risk of diabetes, high blood pressure, heart disease, depression, weight problems and dangerous daytime fatigue. OSA requires medical evaluation and therapy, though some of these measures may also help.

Key prevention strategies

Prop yourself up Instead of lying flat on your back, sleep with your head, shoulders and upper back elevated on extra pillows or a foam wedge. Or elevate the entire head of your bed by about 10 cm by putting two wide, flat lengths of board (such as short pieces of a two-by-eight from a hardware shop or timber yard) under the legs at the top end of your bed. Elevating your head may keep flabby tissue in your throat from collapsing into your breathing passages and vibrating all night, alleviating regular snoring and even mild obstructive sleep apnoea.

Try the tennis ball cure Snoring tends to be worse when you sleep on your back because your tongue and soft palate crowd the back of your throat, blocking your airway. Sleeping on your side can help. To keep you there, wear an old T-shirt (back to front) to bed, and put a tennis ball in the pocket (now at back), or put a ball in a bumbag and wear it to bed.

Solving sleep apnoea

In a recent Hungarian study of 12,643 people, those with obstructive sleep apnoea had increased odds of high blood pressure (40 per cent higher), of heart attack (34 per cent higher) and of stroke (67 per cent higher). The condition can also increase your odds for diabetes. A night of monitored sleep either with special devices brought to your home or in a sleep clinic, with monitoring of your breathing pattern, heart rate and blood oxygen levels, can help doctors determine whether you have apnoea. If you do, talk to your doctor about the advice outlined here that may improve mild cases. If you're overweight, losing weight will help, but it may take months or years, and treatment with medical solutions such as the ones here shouldn't wait.

Lose weight When US researchers tracked 690 Wisconsin residents for four years, they found that, for people who started out without OSA, a gain of at least 10 per cent in body weight increased the odds of developing it by sixfold. In people who already had it, whenever weight increased by 10 per cent, OSA worsened by 32 per cent. A 10 per cent weight loss lessened apnoea by 26 per cent.

Almost any amount of weight loss helps OSA and regular snoring. Extremely overweight people who underwent surgical weight-loss procedures to drop 25 to 50 per cent of their body weight had a 70 to 98 per cent drop in OSA in one study. And among people who lost just 7 to 9 per cent of their body weight (5.5 to 7 kg for someone weighing 80 kg), OSA fell by about 50 per cent.

Avoid alcohol, sleeping pills and antihistamines at night
All act as sedatives, which trigger snoring and apnoea by relaxing muscles in your mouth and throat. Sedatives such as these also make OSA worse, possibly by altering your ability to rouse yourself when your airway is blocked and making it more difficult to fall into deep, restorative stages of sleep.

Relieve congestion before going to bed Inhale steam—in a hot shower, from a dish of hot water or from the type of steam vaporiser that you can use as a facial sauna—to loosen mucus, then gently blow your nose. If you have seasonal allergies, keep the windows shut in your bedroom and use an airconditioner to filter the air. Keep pets out, too, and remove throw rugs—they can harbour allergens. Also, the next time you get new floor covering, choose something other than carpet.

Stop smoking Tobacco smoke from cigarettes, cigars and pipes irritates mucous membranes in your throat. The result is that tissue swells, narrowing your airway and making snoring more likely. Smoking also increases your risk of heart disease, breathing problems and the irritation of seasonal allergies.

Sleep with an oral appliance These devices, which look like a cross between a sports mouthguard and braces, reposition your jaw to prevent tissue in your mouth from flapping as you breathe. Custom-made versions, available from dentists, have a success rate of 70 to 80 per cent for regular snoring (and may also be effective for mild to moderate OSA). In South Africa, TheraSnore is one such

'Elevating your head may keep flabby tissue in your throat from collapsing into your breathing passages and vibrating all night.'

device available through dental and medical practices (visit the website at www.snore.co.za for more information). Off-the-shelf versions, sold online and in pharmacies, are less effective, according to dental experts from the US Academy of Dental Sleep Medicine.

Ask about surgery If you have a deviated septum, two surgical procedures—a submucous resection (SMR) and a septoplasty—can fix the ultra-loud snoring this nasal defect can trigger. Both involve removing cartilage from the bony divider between your left and right nasal cavity. In one small study from Thailand, septum surgery significantly reduced snoring for 28 out of 30 study participants.

Try continuous positive airway pressure (CPAP) The 'gold standard' treatment, CPAP uses a small, quiet air compressor to gently push air through a mask over the sleeper's nose and keep the airway open during sleep. Studies show that CPAP can ease daytime sleepiness by about 50 per cent, boost blood oxygen levels, reduce high blood pressure, improve heart function, reduce memory problems related to apnoea, lower blood sugar levels in people with diabetes and apnoea, and cut the number of sleep disruptions.

Consider other surgical options If CPAP and oral appliances don't work, surgical removal of excess tissue from your nose or throat might. The most widely used technique, uvulopalatopharyngoplasty (UPPP) trims tissue from the rear of your mouth and top of your throat; tonsils and adenoids are usually whisked out at the same time. UPPP improves apnoea for just 40 to 60 per cent of those who try it, say Israeli researchers who reviewed many apnoea studies—and it's impossible to predict who it will work for.

Prevention boosters

Try a nasal strip These adhesive strips improve airflow through your nose by lifting the top of each nostril. Some research has found no benefit for snorers, but in one Swiss study, the strips reduced snoring after about two weeks of use. This inexpensive solution could work for you, especially if your snoring is caused by nasal congestion or mouth breathing. It may be worth a try.

Sing loud, long and low When 20 chronic snorers practised singing techniques that shaped up their throat muscles, their snoring reduced, report researchers from the UK's University of Exeter. The snorers agreed to keep voice-activated tape recorders by their beds for a week before and after their three months of daily 30-minute singing sessions.

Belting out your favorites from *The Sound of Music* won't do the trick. Exercises that work—such as energetically singing 'ung-gah' to familiar tunes—build strength in muscles that support your soft palate, the tissue at the back of your mouth that vibrates if you snore. You can order the program at www.singingforsnorers.com.

Play a wind instrument When 25 snorers at a Swiss sleep clinic started playing the didgeridoo, daytime sleepiness improved by 12 per cent and snoring was reduced by about 22 per cent. If you don't have access to a didgeridoo, get that old clarinet, flute or tuba out of storage and start playing!

Rest your head on an anti-snore pillow These pillows have many different designs; some elevate the head, while others have a hump in the middle and slanting sides so that you simply cannot sleep on your back. Do they work? Experts say there's no guarantee, but some types may work for some people.

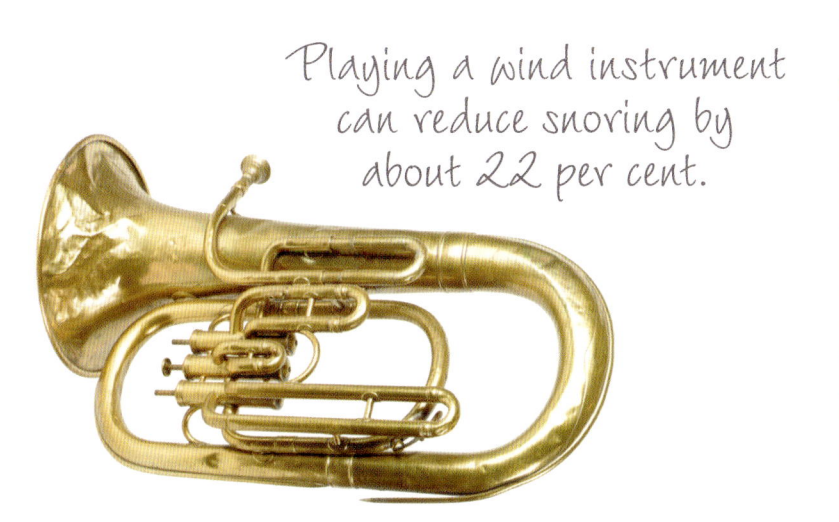

Playing a wind instrument can reduce snoring by about 22 per cent.

WHAT CAUSES IT
The relaxation of your tongue as well as muscles in the roof of your mouth and throat during sleep, which causes throat tissues to vibrate as you inhale and exhale. They may even collapse against your airway, restricting or blocking the flow of air. Being overweight or having enlarged tonsils, thick tissue on the roof of your mouth or an extra-long uvula increases the chances that you'll snore.

SYMPTOMS TO WATCH FOR
Light snoring may not disrupt your sleep or your partner's. But if you snore loudly and feel tired or have a headache when you wake up in the morning, or you gasp and choke or stop breathing for short periods of time during sleep, you may have obstructive sleep apnoea and should ask your doctor about testing and treatment.

LATEST THINKING
Obstructive sleep apnoea's immediate health risk is traffic accidents. People with OSA are twice as likely to be involved in crashes as those without the disorder, according to Canadian researchers who tracked the car insurance records of 1600 people. And they're not just fender-benders: OSA increased the odds of severe car crashes that caused physical injury and death three to five times higher than normal.

Stomach bugs

96% The percentage of stomach-bug virus particles removed when you wash with soap and water for 20 seconds.

All of us have, at some time, been hit by stomach bugs that cause cramping, fever, vomiting and diarrhoea. The germ most responsible for this misery is norovirus—a super-contagious virus that causes 90 per cent of 'stomach flu' outbreaks. Other viruses and bacteria can cause distress, too, so take precautions to help sidestep the next outbreak. And don't rely on the 'sniff' test to tell if a food is OK; you can smell rotten food, but you can't smell bacteria.

Key prevention strategies

Wash your hands You can easily get a stomach bug by touching a contaminated doorknob or shaking hands with someone who's sick. Soap, water and 20 seconds of vigorous scrubbing and rinsing can almost eliminate this risk. In one study, hand washing removed 96 per cent of viral particles compared to just 46 per cent removed with an alcohol-based hand sanitiser, although they're a good alternative.

If you're sick, stay out of the kitchen Many stomach-bug outbreaks have been traced to food prepared by people who had active or waning stomach infections. To avoid this, wipe down benchtops and other kitchen surfaces with disinfecting wipes or a solution of 1 teaspoon bleach in 1 litre warm water. And if a friend or relative who has been sick brings homemade food along to a function, don't eat it.

Clean up fast after someone is sick After a bout of vomiting and/or diarrhoea, fast clean-up can help prevent the spread of germs. Wipe down exposed surfaces with a mixture of bleach and water. Wear rubber gloves and use paper towels—and dispose of them outside the house. Wash

Infection know-how

Why are stomach bugs so contagious? For starters, norovirus, a family of hardy germs responsible for most cases of stomach flu, which isn't really the flu because it's not caused by the influenza virus, is highly contagious before anyone has warning signs. Here are some good reasons to protect yourself all the time:

- **Number of viral particles it takes to become infected** Less than 10
- **Percentage of infected people who are contagious but never have symptoms** 30
- **Length of time someone is contagious after vomiting ends** 2 to 3 weeks
- **Lifespan of the virus on floors, benchtops and other hard surfaces** 3 days
- **Lifespan on 'soft' surfaces like rugs** Up to 12 days

the gloves before taking them off. The person who's sick should also wash themselves and their clothes as soon as possible. Use a hot wash with bleach, if possible.

Wash fruit and vegetables and handle food safely Viruses and bacteria that trigger vomiting and diarrhoea can live on virtually any food. Prevent trouble by washing, storing and cooking foods safely. Don't let other foods touch raw poultry or other raw meats; don't put cooked meats, fish or poultry back on the plate that held the raw product; wash cutting boards and knives in hot, soapy water after using them for raw meats (wash the sink, too); wash your hands frequently during and after handling raw meat; don't eat or serve food that's been out of the refrigerator, off the stove or out of the oven for more than 2 hours; and if food looks or smells bad, throw it out. Use a meat thermometer to be sure meats are heated to the proper internal temperature to kill bacteria. Examples include beef steaks, 65°C; hamburger patties and rissoles, 70°C; and chicken breasts, 80°C.

Eat more 'good bacteria' Antibiotics can reduce the volume of beneficial bacteria in your intestinal tract, and getting more of these bacteria by eating yogurt with live active cultures or taking a probiotic supplement can help. When UK researchers studied 135 people taking antibiotics, those who also had a yogurt drink daily cut their risk of diarrhoea by 21 per cent compared to those who had a placebo drink. The yogurt drink contained the bacteria strains *Lactobacillus casei*, *L. bulgaricus* and *Streptococcus thermophilus*, commonly found in commercial yogurts and in probiotic supplements available from health food shops and some pharmacies.

Prevention boosters

Separate meat, chicken and seafood from other groceries Put meat in plastic bags, to contain any juices, and use separate bags at the check-out, too. At home, use containers or sealable plastic bags to store raw meats, poultry and seafood in the refrigerator.

Refrigerate meats properly Store meats on the bottom shelf so juices can't drip onto other foods. Freeze poultry and mince that won't be used within one or two days; freeze other meats within four or five days.

'About 97% of cases of foodborne illness could be avoided if home cooks followed safe handling rules.'

Don't defrost on the benchtop Germs grow quickly on fish, chicken, turkey and other meats left at room temperature even while they're defrosting. Use these techniques instead:

- **Plan ahead and defrost in the fridge** Put the frozen item in a zip-lock bag or wrap well to contain juices, then store on a plate or in a bowl in the refrigerator until defrosted.
- **Use the microwave** Set your microwave to *Defrost* or *Low* so the thinner edges of the meat won't cook while the middle thaws, then cook straight afterwards.
- **Dunk in cold water** Seal food in a zip-lock bag and place in a large bowl of cold water until just thawed. Cook immediately.

Marinate safely Keep marinating foods in the refrigerator. Don't use the marinade from raw seafood, poultry or meat during cooking or on cooked food unless you've brought it to a full boil first to kill any bacteria. Toss the rest away after use.

Wash before cooking and again as needed Scrub your hands vigorously with soap and water for 10 to 15 seconds immediately before handling food, then dry thoroughly. Wash your hands after handling raw foods and again before eating. Surveys show that 25 per cent of cooks do not wash their hands after handling raw meat and fish, and 66 per cent don't wash up after handling raw eggs.

Guard against cross-contamination Keep raw meat, poultry, seafood—and their juices—away from ready-to-eat foods. Do not reuse knives, cutting boards or other kitchen equipment that has been exposed to raw meats before washing them thoroughly. Always serve food on a clean dish or platter—not one that held raw food.

Clean up carefully When US researchers watched 100 home cooks prepare meals, they found that just 29 per cent cleaned benchtops and refrigerator doors adequately after being in contact with raw meat. An antibacterial cleanser or a solution of 1 teaspoon bleach to 1 litre hot water will do the trick; dry with a clean paper towel.

Leftovers 101

Refrigerate or freeze foods promptly Discard perishable food left at room temperature for longer than 2 hours, or 1 hour in temperatures above 30°C.

Divide and conquer Split large amounts of leftovers into small shallow containers for quick cooling in the refrigerator. Remove the stuffing from poultry and other meats immediately and refrigerate it in a separate resealable container, if possible.

If in doubt throw it out If you suspect food may have been sitting out for too long, toss it.

Cook it through Research reveals that colour isn't a good indicator that meat or poultry is fully cooked; beef mince may look fully browned when the internal temperature is just 60°C—far from the 70°C needed to kill disease-causing bacteria. To add to the confusion, some lean beef mince and some poultry may look pink even after it's reached a safe temperature, so use a food thermometer.

With seafood, look for signs that it's done Fish flesh should be completely opaque and flake easily with a fork. Cook lobsters or crabs until the shells turn red; their flesh—and also that of prawns—should be pearly and opaque. Cook mussels or oysters until the shells open; don't eat any that stay shut.

Keep hot foods hot and cold foods cold If food won't be served and eaten immediately—such as at a picnic or buffet—keep hot food at or above 60°C in warming trays and/or slow cookers. To keep cold foods at or below 4°C, put food in containers on ice.

Keep your refrigerator cold Many fridges aren't cold enough to keep foods safe. Set your fridge at 5°C or lower and the freezer at –18°C. To make sure your fridge is cold enough, check the refrigerator thermometer. And don't overpack the fridge—air needs to circulate in order to chill food quickly.

Keep fresh produce safe Despite news stories about food-poisoning outbreaks, most fresh fruit and vegetables are relatively safe. However, using these strategies will ensure that they are kept bacteria-free:
- Buy freshly cut produce, such as half a watermelon, only if it's refrigerated or surrounded by ice.
- Always store fruit and vegetables that are perishable, precut or peeled in the fridge.
- Wash fruit and vegetables under running water before eating, cutting or cooking, even if you're going to peel them. Dry with a clean paper towel when possible, as this may remove even more germs. Don't use washing-up liquid or soap to clean fresh produce.
- Remove the outer leaves of head vegetables such as lettuce.
- Make sure fresh sprouts are really fresh; it's easy for bacteria to flourish in the warm moist conditions they're grown in.

▶ WHAT CAUSES IT
Viruses and bacteria. Most 'stomach flu' is the result of infection with norovirus.

▶ SYMPTOMS TO WATCH FOR
Nausea, vomiting, stomach cramps and diarrhoea that last for 12 hours to 3 days. Usually a bout of gastroenteritis is uncomfortable but not serious, but young children, older people and anyone with a weakened immune system should be watched for signs of dehydration or lingering infection. Drink plenty of clear fluids and call the doctor if you have these signs: extreme thirst, dry mouth, dark or scanty urine, few tears, weakness, lethargy, or dizziness.

▶ LATEST THINKING
The largest stomach-bug outbreak in the history of New Zealand sickened 350 people who ate raw oysters during a party at a rugby match. While any food can carry viruses and bacteria that cause stomach troubles, bivalve shellfish can pose a special threat if they're uncooked. Substances in the oyster's gastrointestinal tract allow the norovirus to bind and accumulate, a recent US study showed, meaning you could get a big dose of the virus if you eat a contaminated one. So eat your oysters steamed, boiled, baked or fried, because thorough cooking destroys the virus.

Stomach cancer

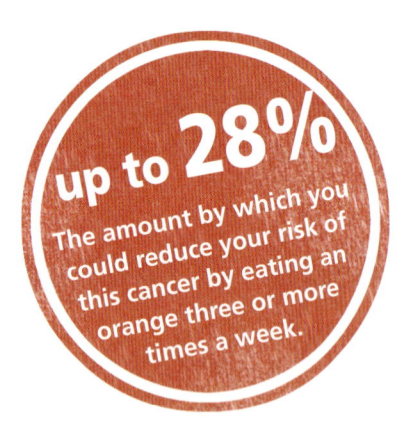

up to 28% The amount by which you could reduce your risk of this cancer by eating an orange three or more times a week.

Here's the good news about stomach cancer: ever since we discovered that most ulcers and the most common form of stomach cancer (non-cardia cancer) are caused by the bacterium *Helicobacter pylori* and began treating people who are infected with it with antibiotics, rates of stomach cancer have plummeted in most countries. The not so good news is that, at the same time, rates of the other form of stomach cancer (cardia cancer) are rising.

Key prevention strategies

Avoid foods high in nitrites Most studies evaluating what people eat and their risk of stomach cancer find that diets high in salted, pickled or smoked foods (think pickled vegetables, herring, smoked salmon, etc.) and preserved or salt-cured meat (such as ham and bacon) significantly increase the risk of stomach cancer. These foods contain nitrites, which can form cancer-causing compounds, called nitrosamides, in the stomach.

Eat an orange a day Eating plenty of fresh fruit and vegetables can reduce your risk of stomach cancer, especially citrus fruits such as oranges. One review of 14 studies found that three or more serves of citrus fruit a week reduced the risk of stomach cancer by 28 per cent (though this may be a high estimate). Researchers suspect the anti-oxidant vitamin C and a carotenoid called beta-cryptoxanthin may protect stomach cells from cancer-causing damage.

Put the word whole in your diet If your diet is loaded with refined grains in the form of white bread, bagels and shop-bought baked goods, etc., and you avoid whole grains in the form of foods like barley and oats, you could be increasing your risk of stomach cancer by anywhere from 50 per cent to more than sevenfold. Conversely, the more fibre you eat, the lower your risk for stomach cancer, particularly for women.

Cut out the steaks and fatty takeaways A Mexican study of about 1000 people found that those who ate an average of 25 g of saturated fat a day were 3.3 times more likely to develop gastric cancer than those who kept their intake at 14 g or less. Another study found that every 100 g of meat eaten per day—no matter what type—increased the risk of stomach cancer nearly 2.5 times overall and more than five times in people infected with *H. pylori*.

Prevention boosters

Treat *H. pylori* infection early Infection with this bug is the leading cause of ulcers; now we also know that it's the leading cause of stomach cancer. Researchers think that inflammation related to *H. pylori* infection leads to changes in the stomach lining that make the stomach less acidic, encouraging the formation of cancer-causing nitrosamides.

Getting rid of the infection can lower your risk A Chinese study randomly assigned 1630 people infected with the bacteria to take either a placebo or therapy designed to eradicate the bacteria. After 7 $1/2$ years, six people in the placebo group had developed stomach cancer compared to none in the treatment group. The traditional treatment for *H. pylori* infection is 7 to 14 days of treatment with a proton-pump inhibitor such as omeprazole (Losec) or esomeprazole (Nexium) and the antibiotics clarithromycin and either amoxicillin or metronidazole. Ask your doctor if you should be tested for the bug.

Kick the habit The smoking habit, that is. As with so many other cancers, smoking increases your risk of stomach cancer; nearly one in five cases is related to smoking. Overall, European researchers found that people who had ever smoked had about a 40 per cent increased risk of stomach cancer; those still smoking had a risk 73 per cent (in men) to 87 per cent (in women) higher than that of people who never smoked.

Wash your hands thoroughly and often This is especially important before cooking and eating. Researchers suspect that one of the main ways *H. pylori* is transmitted is through person-to-person contact—such as inadvertently touching the vomit or stool of someone who has been infected by the bacteria. The other main transmission route may be well water, so if you have a well, stick to bottled water for drinking.

▶ WHAT CAUSES IT

The bacterium *Helicobacter pylori* causes the most common form of stomach cancer, non-cardia gastric cancer, or cancer anywhere in the stomach except the top 2.5 cm, where the stomach meets the oesophagus. Cancer in that area is called cardia gastric cancer. Ironically, the presence of *H. pylori* seems to reduce the risk of cardia cancer. Other risk factors include chronic gastritis, or inflammation of the stomach; age; being male; a diet high in salted, smoked or preserved foods and low in fresh fruit and vegetables; smoking; certain types of anaemia; and a family history of the disease.

▶ SYMPTOMS TO WATCH FOR

Internal bleeding; it may not be noticed unless you have a faecal occult blood test or the bleeding becomes extreme, causing anaemia. Symptoms of more advanced cancer include an uncomfortable feeling in your abdomen that antacids don't improve and that worsens when you eat; black, tarry stools; vomiting blood; vomiting after meals; weakness, fatigue and weight loss; and feeling full after meals even if you eat less than normal.

▶ LATEST THINKING

In the near future, we'll have a vaccine for *H. pylori*. It will have to be given early, however; studies have found children as young as seven who are infected with the bacteria.

Stomach ulcers

33% The reduction in ulcer risk if you eat seven serves of fruit and vegetables a day.

Eating bland food and taking stomach-coating antacids was once standard treatment for stomach ulcers, but now we know that the bacterium *Helicobacter pylori* is responsible for two-thirds of all stomach ulcers and duodenal ulcers (those in the beginning of the small intestine). Use of nonsteroidal anti-inflammatory drugs (NSAIDs) such as aspirin and ibuprofen causes almost all the rest, with a smaller proportion caused by steroid medications such as prednisone.

Key prevention strategies

Avoid common pain relievers If you regularly take low-dose aspirin for your heart or use ibuprofen or naproxen to help manage arthritis symptoms, you're raising your ulcer risk. These medications interfere with mechanisms that protect the stomach lining from corrosive acids. They thin the stomach's protective mucus coating, reduce production of an acid-neutralising chemical called bicarbonate and reduce blood flow, which helps stomach cells repair themselves. NSAIDs can also cause a bleeding ulcer to bleed more freely.

In one UK study of more than 3000 people, those who had taken NSAIDs were 2 to 30 times more likely to have bleeding ulcers than those who didn't take these pain relievers. What should you do? Experts suggest the following three strategies:

- **Switch to paracetamol for chronic pain relief** It's not an NSAID and won't harm the lining of your stomach. (To protect your liver, take no more than 4 g per day, and avoid alcohol when you take it or risk liver failure.)
- **Take the lowest possible dose of an NSAID, infrequently** If paracetamol doesn't help relieve your pain, then try taking this alternative.
- **Add another protective medication** Some experts recommend the prescription

Treat an ulcer right

If you're relying on antacids and a bland diet to control ulcer pain, it's time to update your strategy. The only way to prevent dangerous complications such as bleeding and stomach perforation: get tested to confirm a *Helicobacter pylori* infection, which causes most ulcers, then start treatment. A course of antibiotics, usually given along with an acid-reducing proton-pump inhibitor, is the only way to knock out the spiral-shaped germ, which burrows into the protective mucus layer lining the stomach wall, releasing toxins that burn holes in the stomach lining.

medications sucralfate (Carafate or Ulsanic) and misoprostol (Cytotec) to shield the stomach lining from damage if you must take an NSAID on a daily basis (in Australia, your doctor can tell you whether you're eligible for a PBS subsidy or whether you have to pay full price). However, if you are pregnant or planning to become pregnant, do not take misoprostol, which can cause miscarriage and birth defects.

Quit smoking Nicotine in tobacco increases the amount of acid in your stomach and makes it more concentrated. Studies show that smoking raises the ulcer risk seven times higher than normal. Some experts suspect that chemicals in tobacco smoke may somehow work with *H. pylori* to create stomach ulcers.

Cut down on or cut out alcohol Alcohol irritates and erodes your stomach lining and boosts acid production. While it may not cause ulcers on its own, scientists believe that it boosts risk in people with an *H. pylori* infection and those who use NSAIDs regularly. And since half of all adults are infected with this bacterium by the age of 60, holding back on alcohol sounds like a good idea.

Prevention boosters

Start the day with porridge and fresh fruit In a Harvard study of more than 47,000 men, those who ate seven serves of fruit and vegetables a day had a 33 per cent lower risk of developing ulcers than those who had less than three serves daily. Eating plenty of soluble fibre—the type found in legumes, barley, pears and porridge— cut risk by a huge 60 per cent. Experts aren't sure why these foods are protective. One possibility is that soluble fibre becomes a thick, smooth gel in your digestive system and may help protect the walls of your upper small intestine from damage by digestive juices.

Eat spinach and beetroot Vegetables such as spinach, lettuce, radishes and beetroot are rich in chemicals that raise levels of nitric oxide in the stomach, and Swedish researchers think that higher nitric oxide levels may strengthen the stomach's inner lining so it can better protect itself from digestive acids.

WHAT CAUSES IT
The bacterium *Helicobacter pylori*; regular use of non-steroidal anti-inflammatory drugs (NSAIDs), such as aspirin and ibuprofen; and regular use of steroids such as prednisone.

SYMPTOMS TO WATCH FOR
Burning pain in your abdomen that starts two to three hours after a meal, gets worse at night when your stomach is empty and eases when you eat something. An ulcer may also take away your appetite, cause weight loss, or make you feel nauseated. Get immediate help if you notice blood in your stool or in vomit; a bleeding ulcer can be a medical emergency.

LATEST THINKING
Three antibiotics are better than two against the ulcer bug. In a review of 10 studies involving more than 2800 people with ulcers, Italian researchers found that *H. pylori* was eliminated in 93 per cent of the volunteers when they used a 10-day therapy that involved three different antibiotics. In contrast, 77 per cent of those who got two antibiotics improved.

Stroke

42% The drop in stroke risk if you lower high blood pressure by just 5 points.

A tiny clot. A rip in a hair-thin blood vessel. The smallest things can trigger a stroke—a potentially life-altering event that shuts off the flow of blood and oxygen, destroying brain cells. Strokes kill at least five million people worldwide each year and disable millions more, yet most of us put it last on the list of our greatest health fears. The good news is that there's plenty you can do to prevent having a stroke.

Key prevention strategies

Lower your blood pressure If your blood pressure is above 120/80, your risk of having a stroke is dramatically higher than that of someone with lower blood pressure. Why? Blood moves faster through your arteries and veins, and this increased speed poses a triple threat. It damages blood vessels in your brain and in the carotid arteries in your neck that supply brain cells with life-giving oxygen. It can also create fragile 'bulges' in these arteries, which can rupture. And it can make arteries thicken to the point where they squeeze shut. Finally, it can damage the inner lining, allowing plaques to form; pieces of plaque can break off and travel in the bloodstream to the brain. Small wonder, then, that high blood pressure is the number one cause of stroke.

However, if your blood pressure is high, every 5-point drop can cut your stroke risk by 42 per cent or more. This strategy works whether you're 45 or ninety-five. In a UK study of nearly 3500 people over the age of 80 with high blood pressure, those who used medication to get their reading down to 150/80 cut their risk of stroke by 53 per cent compared to volunteers who received a placebo. That's higher than the healthy target (120/80) we mentioned above, but it illustrates the benefits of

Take TIAs seriously

Before a stroke, 30 to 40 per cent of people get a strange warning sign: a brief mini-stroke known to doctors as a transient ischaemic attack, or TIA. Symptoms can include loss of strength or sudden numbness in your face, arm or leg; feeling confused or unable to speak; loss of vision; and/or an unusual headache. They stop as swiftly as they start, but that doesn't mean the danger has passed. Your risk of having a full-blown stroke in the next two days is 1 in 20, and over the next three months, it's 1 in 10, unless you take action.

Call your doctor immediately and explain what happened. He or she may put you on medications to prevent blood clots, lower cholesterol and reduce blood pressure. In a British study, this combination cut the odds for a major stroke after a TIA by 80 per cent.

lowering high blood pressure. Ultimately, your own healthy blood pressure goal should be set by your doctor.

You may not even need medication to reach an optimal level. If your blood pressure's top number (systolic) is between 120 and 139, or your bottom number (diastolic) is between 80 and 89, you have prehypertension—and stand a good chance of reducing your pressure with weight loss, exercise and a healthy low-salt diet full of fruit, vegetables and low-fat dairy foods. If your reading stays above 140/90 despite lifestyle changes, your doctor may prescribe one or several medications to bring it down.

Reduce 'bad' LDL cholesterol Too much harmful LDL cholesterol in your bloodstream starts the process that leads to the thick, fatty streaks of plaque developing inside artery walls, including the carotid arteries supplying your brain. These blood vessels can eventually become so narrowed that the tiniest clot acts like a plug, blocking blood flow completely.

Reducing LDL with a low-fat diet plus a statin medication shrinks this plaque and protects the brain. In one study of 2531 men with slightly elevated LDL levels, those who took cholesterol-lowering medication cut their stroke risk by 31 per cent.

Start with a diet low in saturated fat and rich in fruit and vegetables, whole grains, and low-fat dairy foods. Avoid fatty red meats and full-fat dairy foods such as cheese. Lose weight if you need to and stay active. If your levels stay high (an ideal LDL reading is below 2.5 mmol/L if you have other risk factors for cardiovascular disease; higher levels may be safe if you don't have risk factors—your doctor can advise about a safe level for you), ask your doctor about taking a statin. If you've already had a stroke, taking one can cut your risk of a second stroke by 16 per cent.

Be physically active and snack on nuts Doing both these things can raise levels of HDL cholesterol—the type that removes LDL from the bloodstream. The minimum healthy HDL level is 1.0 mmol/L, but higher is better for your brain. In one study, people with the highest HDL cut their risk for the type of strokes caused by fatty plaque buildup by an incredible 80 per cent.

Avoid fatty takeaway foods and alcohol Until recently, experts didn't realise how dangerous triglycerides, another type of blood fat, were for brain health. But in one study, people with the highest

'If your blood pressure is high, every 5-point drop can cut your stroke risk by 42 per cent or more.'

levels tripled their stroke risk compared to those with the healthiest, lowest levels. A healthy triglyceride reading is below 8 mmol/L. You can manage high triglycerides by losing weight and skipping alcoholic beverages, having grilled or baked fish instead of burgers, and using canola and olive oil in place of butter. Cutting back on refined carbohydrates (found in white bread, sweets, snack foods and sugary drinks) is also important. Ask your doctor whether fish oil supplements could help (large doses may be needed.)

Stop smoking Smoking just 10 cigarettes a day increases stroke risk by 90 per cent—even if your cholesterol and blood pressure levels are low. Nicotine, carbon monoxide and a cocktail of other chemicals in burning tobacco stiffen arteries, pack more plaque onto artery walls and make blood stickier and more prone to clotting. Quit now, and stroke risk begins to fall immediately; within as few as five years your risk falls to that of someone who never smoked.

Fix a fluttering heart Atrial fibrillation (AF) occurs when the upper chambers of the heart quiver instead of beating strongly and steadily, and it quadruples stroke risk. It affects 1 in 25 people over the age of 65 and 1 in 10 over eighty. AF allows blood to pool in the heart and form clots; a strong heartbeat can then send a clot into your brain, resulting in a stroke.

If you're over 65, ask your doctor to assess you. Simply checking your pulse and listening to your heartbeat may be enough, or you may need a test called an electrocardiogram (ECG). The usual treatment for AF involves taking the blood thinning medication warfarin (Coumadin, Losec), which experts say could cut stroke risk by 69 per cent. Yet many people who would benefit from this lifesaving medication never get it, in part because doctors are cautious about giving it to older people who may bruise or bleed more easily if they have a fall.

Take a daily low-dose aspirin If you've already had a stroke or are a woman at high risk for a stroke, swallowing a 75-mg aspirin tablet daily could protect your brain. In one study, aspirin cut women's

Preventive stroke surgery

If the arteries in your neck are blocked by plaque, your stroke risk skyrockets, but surgically clearing them out could cut your odds by 50 to 75 per cent, according to studies. You may be a candidate if you've already had a stroke or mini-stroke or if X-rays using special dyes or other tests reveal that one of the arteries is 75 to 99 per cent blocked. (Warning signs of a blockage include blurred vision, slurred speech or weakness.) The main surgical technique for clearing the arteries supplying the brain—called carotid endarterectomy—involves making an incision in one or both arteries and scraping out the plaque.

stroke risk by 17 per cent (but didn't lower most men's risk). If you're at above-normal risk for stroke—due to high blood pressure, out-of-balance blood fats, atrial fibrillation or a family history of stroke—ask your doctor if low-dose aspirin therapy is appropriate for you.

Prevention boosters

Walk five days a week Taking a brisk hour-long walk five times a week cuts your odds of a stroke almost in half, and half an hour's walk reduces your odds by about 25 per cent. In fact, any vigorous physical activity that burns 4200 to 12,600 kilojoules per week will cut your risk, including swimming, cycling and most team sports.

Cultivate the fine art of resilience Breathe deeply, sing your favourite song, do yoga or dance. Learning to cope with anxiety and stress, in whatever way works for you, could cut your stroke risk by an extra 24 per cent.

Put fish on the menu Enjoying grilled or baked oily fish one to four times a week could cut your stroke risk by 27 per cent, possibly because healthy fats in fish can keep blood vessels flexible and discourage plaque. But don't eat greasy fish and chips: in a US study from Harvard Medical School, people who ate fried fish just once a week raised their stroke risk by as much as 44 per cent.

Enjoy alcohol in moderation One drink may lower your risk, but having too many raises it, according to Chinese researchers who followed 64,000 men for nine years. Their conclusion was that having one to six drinks per week lowers stroke risk by 8 per cent; having more than 21 standard drinks per week raises it by 22 per cent. And don't have all your drinks on one night; experts suggest two drinks on any one day and no more than four drinks on any single occasion.

Go for whole grains Opt for porridge, wholemeal bread and cereals, and brown rice. Women who ate the most whole grains had a 40 per cent lower risk of stroke than those who ate the fewest, according to a Harvard School of Public Health study.

▶ WHAT CAUSES IT

Nearly 90 per cent of strokes are the result of a clot breaking off or a bulging plaque that cuts off blood flow to part of the brain. The rest happen when a blood vessel in or near the brain ruptures, cutting off the supply of oxygen to surrounding brain cells.

▶ SYMPTOMS TO WATCH FOR

Classic signs are sudden numbness, weakness or paralysis of the face, arm or leg, usually on one side of the body; sudden difficulty talking or understanding speech; sudden blurred, double or reduced vision; sudden dizziness, imbalance or lack of coordination; sudden severe or unusual headache; confusion. Signs that may be unique to women include loss of consciousness or fainting; shortness of breath; falls; sudden pain in the face, chest, arms or legs; seizure; sudden hiccups, nausea, tiredness; or sudden pounding or racing heartbeat.

▶ LATEST THINKING

Your brain loves oranges, as well as strawberries, red capsicums and grapefruit—all foods rich in vitamin C. When UK scientists tracked 20,000 people for 10 years, they found that those with the highest blood levels of vitamin C had a 42 per cent lower risk of stroke compared to those with the lowest levels.

Thrush

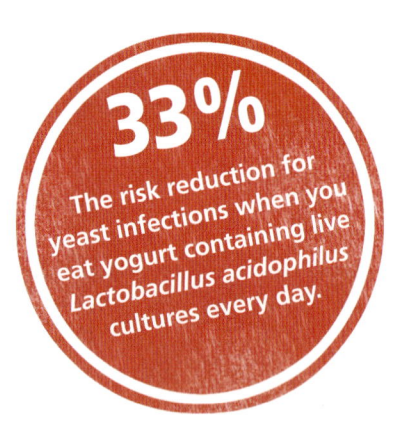

33% The risk reduction for yeast infections when you eat yogurt containing live *Lactobacillus acidophilus* cultures every day.

In essence, the vagina is a complex and delicate ecosystem, home to a variety of microscopic organisms—in this case, mostly bacteria (both 'good' and 'bad') including the yeast-like fungus *Candida* vulvovaginitis. Candida resides in the vagina trouble free in up to half of all women, but if the ecosystem is disrupted, and it overgrows, the result is itching, soreness and burning of this all-too-common yeast infection. Keep yourself infection free with this advice.

Key prevention strategies

Always opt for cotton underwear Skip that ubiquitous nylon lingerie in favour of old-fashioned cotton, which allows air to circulate and helps prevent yeast organisms from breeding. And always wear undies under pantihose.

Keep the area dry After a shower or bath, use a blow dryer on the coolest setting (be careful not to burn yourself) to dry the perineal area before getting dressed. And change out of a wet swimming costume as soon as possible. Yeast loves damp environments.

Wipe the right way After bowel movements, wipe from front to back, never back to front. One theory about yeast infections is that 'bad' bacteria get into the vagina from the rectum, disrupting the environment that normally keeps yeast in check.

Spoon up some yogurt Some studies suggest that eating 250 g a day of yogurt that contains live, active bacteria cultures helps maintain a healthy vaginal environment and could reduce the risk of recurrent yeast infections.

Check your blood sugar If you've ever made bread from scratch, you know that yeast needs sugar to grow. That's why women with diabetes are much more

DRUGS THAT PREVENT DISEASE

Up to 30 per cent of women taking antibiotics are prone to yeast infections. These medications can kill off beneficial bacteria that keep vaginal flora in balance. If you're taking antibiotics and you're prone to yeast infections keep some over-the-counter anti-yeast creams or suppositories (miconazole or clotrimazole) on hand and use them at the first sign of vaginal itching.

vulnerable to yeast infections. (See 'Diabetes', starting on page 164 for some prevention tips.)

Stick to regular sex Avoid engaging in oral sex for a while if you're susceptible to yeast infections, or at least cut back. Having your partner perform oral sex five or more times a month can increase your risk of yeast infections.

Prevention boosters

Avoid dyes and perfumes Skip coloured or perfumed toilet paper and scented sanitary pads and tampons, all of which can disrupt the normal vaginal environment.

Avoid most feminine hygiene products There's absolutely no need to use douches, powders or sprays; they can cause irritation.

Follow a low-GI diet Just as women with diabetes are more prone to yeast infections, so too are women with insulin resistance. This condition occurs when cells become resistant to insulin, the hormone that allows glucose into cells, leading to higher than normal blood sugar levels. Foods made with sugar, high-fructose corn syrup and white flour—most shop-bought baked goods as well as biscuits, crackers, chips and sweetened drinks—all contribute to insulin resistance because they spike blood sugar. White bread and white rice do the same. Instead, eat foods with a low glycaemic index (GI), which have less effect on blood sugar. These include most high-fibre foods such as vegetables, legumes and whole grains; 'good' fats from olives, nuts and avocados; and lean protein foods.

▶ WHAT CAUSES IT

Out-of-control growth of the yeast organisms that live on your skin, in your vagina and in your mouth. The growth occurs when the normally acidic vaginal environment loses its acidity. Numerous things can disrupt vaginal harmony, including menstruation, pregnancy, diabetes, antibiotics, oral contraceptives and steroids. Frequent sex, or anything that irritates the vagina, can trigger yeast growth.

▶ SYMPTOMS TO WATCH FOR

Itching and burning in the vagina and the surrounding area (the vulva), as well as vulval swelling; cottage cheese-like vaginal discharge; pain during intercourse.

▶ LATEST THINKING

A tablet designed to help maintain the normal acidity of the vagina could one day be used to prevent recurrent yeast infections. Such a tablet is currently under investigation.

Tinea

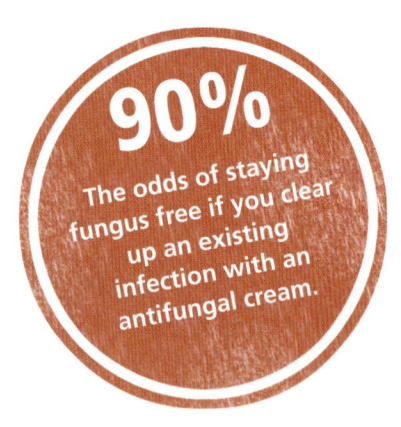

90% The odds of staying fungus free if you clear up an existing infection with an antifungal cream.

An itchy, scaly fungal rash between the toes, in the groin, under the breasts or elsewhere on your skin can be both embarrassing and very uncomfortable. Working up a sweat at the gym or pool, or even just mowing the lawn, is great for whole-body fitness, but if you aren't taking steps to protect sweat-moistened skin, you may end up with a fungal infection commonly known as tinea.

Key prevention strategies

Keep your feet dry Athlete's foot is a fungal infection. The fungus thrives wherever there is moisture and it's favourite food—keratin, a substance found in human skin. This means the insides of your joggers and socks are ideal breeding grounds. Change your footwear after exercise and when you come home from work or come in from gardening, and change your socks when they're damp. Don't wear the same shoes two days in a row, and when you're at home try to go barefoot or wear clean socks. In summer, it's a good idea to stick with wearing open sandals.

Wear thongs at the pool and gym Foot protection is the best way to avoid the fungi lurking on the floors of virtually all change rooms and public showers (they thrive in damp environments). When Japanese researchers swabbed the soles of 140 people taking swimming classes at the University of Tsukuba, they found that 64 per cent carried the tinea fungus.

Stand on a thick towel when in changing rooms It's nearly impossible to keep thongs on your feet while changing into your clothes, and socks may not offer enough protection. Researchers have found that foot fungus can easily travel between the fibres of cotton and nylon socks and attach itself to your skin; wool socks and extremely thick cotton socks do keep fungus off your feet, but you'll wind

Check your pets too

Dogs and cats can harbour hard-to-see fungal infections on their skin; you pick up an infection when you pat or groom them. In one study of 211 dogs, researchers found 89 fungal strains that can also infect humans—and 11 dog owners who had fungal infections of their feet or groin area. Look for areas of skin where fur is missing or ask your vet to check your dog or cat.

up 'infecting' your shoes. Take an extra towel to use as a floor mat, then wash it in hot water a washing machine.

Stay clean and dry Take a shower or bath every day. After a work-out, change out of sweaty clothes, including underwear, and shower as soon as you can. Carefully dry any moist areas, such as genitals, buttocks, inner thighs and under the breasts or any rolls of abdominal fat with a clean towel. Leaving skin damp gives the fungus a foothold, not only because moisture encourages the fungus to multiply but also because sweat and water dilute your natural oils, which contain fungus-fighting compounds.

Wash shorts, underwear and athletic gear after every use
They're not just a smelly turnoff; they may also carry fungus. Remember, they've gotten sweaty and chances are they've also hit the germy change room floor at some point. Get them out of your bag right away when you get home; fungus can breed in the bag's damp, dark interior. In fact, if your bag is wet, spray it with disinfectant spray, dry with a paper towel and then let it air in the sun for extra protection.

Use an antifungal preparation to prevent repeat infections
Once your skin is infected, it's hard to get rid of the fungus—and even harder to stay fungus free once the infection seems to clear up. That's because the fungus lies between the skin layers. If you get frequent infections, use an over-the-counter antifungal spray, powder or cream containing bifonazole, clotrimazole, econazole, ketoconazole, miconazole, terbinafine or tolnaftate.

If you are prone to fungal infections or will be spending lots of time wearing sweaty shoes or changing in public change rooms, using an antifungal product every day could help prevent infection.

Prevention boosters

Put hygiene first After you've washed, dry from head to foot, to avoid transferring the fungus to other parts of your body. Always disinfect the shower, bath and bathroom floor regularly, and avoid sharing towels.

Washing clothes and towels in hot water then drying them on high heat in a tumble-dryer also kills fungus; a regular cold wash isn't enough to do the job.

▶ WHAT CAUSES IT
The family of fungi called dermatophytes, which normally live on our skin. Tendrils growing into the top layer of the skin lead to increased cell production with thick, scaly, itchy skin.

▶ SYMPTOMS TO WATCH FOR
Burning, stinging or itching on your feet, groin, buttocks, inner thighs, below the breasts or underneath rolls of fat; peeling, cracking skin between your toes or on the bottoms of your feet; extremely dry skin on the bottoms or sides of your feet; crumbling, thickened and/or discoloured nails; a rash with slightly raised, brownish red patches of dry, scaly or bumpy skin.

▶ LATEST THINKING
The fungus that causes groin infections could be living on the seats of stationary bikes, weight machines and free-weight benches, warn experts from the Institute for Fungal Illness, Berlin, Germany. Before you sit down, clean equipment with disinfectant spray.

Tinnitus

40%
The reduction in severity of the condition after using a device that desensitises your brain to tinnitus.

Tinnitus—a buzzing, ringing or roaring sound in the ears—strikes 1 in 20 people. One theory links it to hearing loss, but for some, tinnitus can wreak havoc on their ability to lead normal lives. Whether you've never experienced it or it's just beginning to creep up on you, try to keep the worst at bay with these recommendations.

Key prevention strategies

Turn down the volume One common culprit in tinnitus is noise-related hearing loss, even if the loss isn't severe enough for you to notice. Even being in a noisy place like a restaurant can stimulate your hearing system and temporarily make tinnitus louder.

Don't use cotton buds Putting anything in your ears—including a finger or a cotton bud—can push wax against your eardrum, which can contribute to or worsen tinnitus. A better way to clear the wax is to put a drop or two of mineral oil in one ear and lie on the opposite side for an hour while the oil loosens the wax and brings it to the surface. When you turn over, have a serviette handy to catch the wax and oil.

Cut back on aspirin If you often take aspirin for headaches or pain, talk to your doctor about alternatives. Overuse can lead to tinnitus. If you're on daily low-dose aspirin therapy, though, don't worry; the amount isn't great enough to trigger tinnitus.

Relax your jaw Tinnitus is a common symptom of temporomandibular joint disease (TMJ), or more commonly known as jaw pain, in which the hinge that works the upper and lower jaw and the muscles and ligaments that support the jaw are stressed or misaligned. (See 'Jaw pain' on page 236 for prevention tips.)

Already have tinnitus?

Neuromonics uses an MP3-like device to deliver a pleasant, customised sound to people with tinnitus as part of an overall treatment approach that includes counselling and support. One study, sponsored by the device's manufacturer, found that, after six months, 86 per cent of people using the device improved at least 40 per cent, compared to just 47 per cent of people who were counselled and listened to other types of noise, and 23 per cent of those who received counselling only.

Watch your medications More than 200 medications are associated with tinnitus. If you're hearing ringing or buzzing, ask your doctor if one of your medications could be to blame and whether you can lower the dose or switch to another one. Some of the worst culprits are those that injure the inner ear, such as quinines (for malaria and rheumatoid arthritis); diuretics (for high blood pressure); certain antibiotics; and some chemotherapy drugs.

Control your blood pressure High blood pressure can lead to tinnitus. You're more likely to hear blood whooshing through blood vessels when the pressure of the flow is strong. You should also try to keep your cholesterol in check, since narrowed arteries can cause turbulent—and loud—blood flow.

Prevention boosters

Try to stay on top of things Depression, anxiety, stress and tinnitus seem to go hand in hand, although no one's sure which is the chicken and which is the egg. One study found that nearly half of people with disabling tinnitus also had major depression. People with tinnitus who take antidepressants or receive psychotherapy improve more than those who do neither.

Watch what you drink There's some evidence that drinking too much alcohol or too many soft drinks or cups of coffee or tea (the caffeine is the likely culprit) can lead to tinnitus.

Go easy on salt intake Consuming a lot of sodium can make tinnitus worse by increasing blood pressure. Using herbs and other nonsodium spices is one way to reduce sodium intake; the best way, however, is to stay away from processed foods.

Check your posture Holding your neck in a hyperextended position, such as when you ride a bicycle, can lead to tinnitus. Look in the mirror and ask yourself: Do I look like a bird pecking for worms? If the answer is yes, your neck is hyperextended. (Read more about proper neck posture in 'Neck pain' on page 256.)

Get a blood test Low blood levels of iron or thyroid hormones can sometimes be associated with tinnitus.

▶ WHAT CAUSES IT
Loud noises, noise- and age-related hearing loss, excess earwax, infections, medications, tumours, allergies, heart and blood vessel problems, issues with the jaw and neck.

▶ SYMPTOMS TO WATCH FOR
A ringing, buzzing, roaring, hissing or whistling noise in your ears. You may notice it only when you're in a quiet place.

▶ LATEST THINKING
Electrodes implanted in the part of the brain responsible for hearing and then electrically stimulated can suppress the phantom noises of tinnitus. One study of 12 people who underwent the implants showed a 97 per cent reduction in tinnitus.

Urinary tract infections

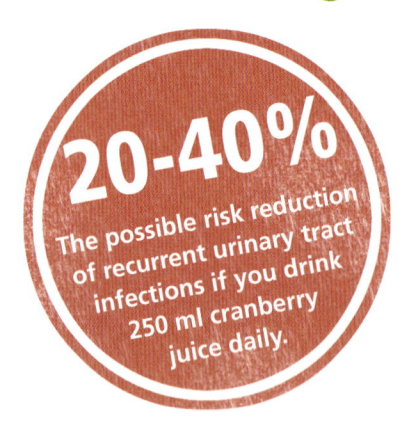

20-40% The possible risk reduction of recurrent urinary tract infections if you drink 250 ml cranberry juice daily.

Women are twice as likely as men to experience urinary tract infections (UTIs). The female urethra is much shorter, giving the bacteria responsible for these painful, often recurrent infections easier access. Plus, in women, that urethral opening is just a couple of centimetres from the rectum, making it far easier for bacteria from the bowel to slip in. About 6 out of 10 women will have at least one UTI, and about 2 out of 10 will experience them repeatedly.

Key prevention strategies

Practise good hygiene Prevent bacteria from getting in by wiping from front to back after a bowel movement—never from back to front. Use a clean cloth to wash the skin around your rectum (and especially between rectum and vagina) every day when taking a shower or bath.

Easy ways to eat more cranberries

Cranberry juice for urinary tract infections is one of those folk cures that may really work. An anti-oxidant compound in cranberries (and blueberries) prevents bacteria from adhering to bladder and urinary tract cells. Most studies on cranberries have been conducted with pure juice (buy unsweetened juice; if it's too tart, dilute with water or mineral water) or dried cranberry extract pills. Here are five other ways to get this important fruit into your diet.

1. Sprinkle dried cranberries over salads or yogurt, and mix them into pancake or muffin batter in place of raisins.

2. Use fresh cranberries with apples, blueberries, peaches or cherries in pies.

3. **Enjoy cranberry relish** Combine a bag of fresh cranberries, 1 cup sugar, the juice of one lemon and a cinnamon stick in a medium saucepan and cook over medium–low heat until the cranberries pop. Cool and use to top pork loin or chicken breasts or thighs.

4. **Whip up a cranberry smoothie** Blend together a banana, 1 cup low-fat mixed berry yogurt, 1 cup cranberry juice and 1 cup fresh or frozen blueberries.

5. **Make iceblocks** Mix equal amounts cranberry juice and mineral water, pour into iceblock trays, then freeze.

Drink up The more you drink, the more you urinate. The more you urinate, the more bacteria you flush out of your urinary tract. Any liquid will do, although unsweetened cranberry juice offers the best protection (see 'Easy ways to eat more cranberries', opposite). Blueberry juice and other berry juices are also good choices.

Visit the bathroom before and after sex Do two things: urinate to flush any bacteria from the urethra and then wash the area. Wet wipes designed for bathroom use are also handy for this. Although many experts continue to recommend this tactic, research has failed to confirm its effectiveness.

Wear 100 per cent cotton underpants Cotton breathes, keeping the area between the legs drier so it doesn't become a breeding ground for bacteria.

Don't use vaginal douches It's not necessary. All douches and vaginal sprays do is irritate the urethra and disrupt the natural balance of good and bad bacteria that keeps infections in check.

Prevention boosters

Ask about antibiotics If you're prone to UTIs, ask your doctor about prophylactic antibiotics—antibiotics taken to prevent infection. Whether taken daily, only after sex, or every few weeks, they work to prevent UTIs, according to studies.

Choose your contraceptive carefully Using a diaphragm and spermicide may increase the risk of UTIs in women with a history of repeated infections. Even condoms used with spermicide can up the risk. Skip the spermicide if you think it bothers you, or choose a contraceptive method that isn't inserted into the vagina, such as oral contraceptives, or contraceptive injections or implants.

Ration the intercourse The more often you have sex, and the more people with whom you have sex in a year, the higher your risk of UTIs.

▶ WHAT CAUSES IT
Usually, infection with *E. coli* bacteria, which tend to originate around the rectum and spread to the bladder opening in the vagina, then make their way to the bladder.

▶ SYMPTOMS TO WATCH FOR
Burning or pain during urination; feeling that you need to urinate more often than usual; feeling that you need to urinate but not being able to; leaking urine; cloudy, dark, smelly or blood-stained urine.

▶ LATEST THINKING
The bacteria that cause UTIs actually invade bladder cells, taking up residence there more or less permanently and leading to recurrent infections. This may be one reason that prophylactic (preventive) antibiotic therapy works so well. Previously, researchers didn't think the bacteria could get into bladder cells.

Varicose veins

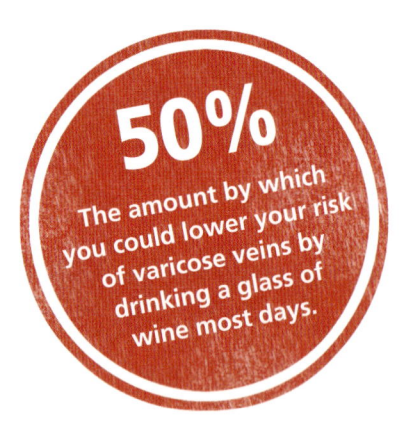

50% The amount by which you could lower your risk of varicose veins by drinking a glass of wine most days.

One-way valves in the leg veins prevent blood flowing backwards, but if the veins stretch out or the valves weaken—due to genetics, inactivity, a job that keeps you on your feet, pregnancy or other factors—blood can do just that, causing pooling that leads to twisted, bulging varicose veins and tired, achy, itchy, swollen legs. These steps can protect your legs and keep varicose veins from growing worse if you already have them.

Key prevention strategies

Don't stand when you can sit Standing for long periods every day raises your risk of varicose veins by 60 per cent, say researchers at Finland's Tampere University Hospital. Sitting down whenever possible helps by easing pressure on blood vessels. Keep your feet flat on the floor or cross your ankles when you sit; crossing your legs at the knees squeezes veins shut, further blocking blood flow.

Elevate your legs Raising your legs prevents blood from pooling. If you already have varicose veins or simply want to give your leg veins extra help, lie down at home and raise your legs higher than the level of your heart by propping them on pillows or even against a wall so that gravity works to move blood to your heart instead of having it pool in the veins of your legs and feet.

Lose any extra kilos you may have put on lately Being overweight puts extra pressure on the fragile veins just below the surface of the skin in your legs. And according to one large Scottish study, being overweight or obese raised the odds for varicose veins by as much as 58 per cent. By eating less and getting more

Rein in vein pain

Horse chestnut seed extract is one remedy for varicose vein discomfort that seems to really work. When Harvard Medical School doctors reviewed 16 well-designed studies of thousands of people with weak valves in their leg veins, they found that those who took the extract had four times less pain than those who got a placebo. Half saw a decrease in swelling, and 70 per cent had less itching. They also reported improvement in feelings of fatigue and heaviness in their legs. UK researchers say this safe botanical may be as effective as compression stockings. Escin, the active ingredient, has strengthened the walls of small blood vessels in lab studies.

The usual dose is 300 mg (containing 50 to 75 mg of escin per dose) every 12 hours for up to 12 weeks. A supplement is recommended because toxins found in horse chestnuts have been removed.

aerobic exercise, you'll lose weight and also reduce your risk of developing leg vein problems in the first place.

Keep your legs on the move Standing and even sitting still at a desk all day allows blood to pool. Push it back towards your heart as often as you can. How? If you're sitting, point and flex your feet to boost circulation. If you're on your feet, get the blood moving several times an hour by rising on your toes, shifting your weight from one foot to the other, bending your legs and walking in place.

Wear compression stockings These long elastic socks squeeze your legs so blood can't pool as much. They can ease aching and swelling if you have varicose veins and may help prevent them, too. When Japanese researchers measured the legs of 20 people with varicose veins, they found that all grades of compression stockings reduced swelling, but medium- and strong-grade stockings worked best. These are labelled '22 mmHg' or '30–40 mmHg'. UK researchers found that the stockings can reduce the amount of blood pooling in leg veins by about 20 per cent.

Wear flat shoes Stilettos may not cause varicose veins, but wearing them makes your calf muscles less effective at pumping blood back towards your heart when you walk, according to experts at Wake Forest University Baptist Medical Center in the US.

Prevention boosters

Stop straining Working too hard to have a bowel movement increases pressure on veins in the lower legs. Researchers at Scotland's University of Edinburgh report that this kind of pushing nearly doubled the risk of vein problems in men. To make bowel movements as easy and comfortable as possible, drink plenty of water during the day and increase your fibre intake.

Enjoy a glass of wine Spanish researchers who analysed the health records of 1778 people found that those who enjoyed a glass of wine every day had a 50 per cent lower risk of varicose veins than those who drank less—or more. Other research suggests that flavonoids and saponins in wine can help keep blood vessels flexible and healthy.

▶ WHAT CAUSES IT
Weakened valves in leg veins, which allow blood to pool instead of travelling back to your heart. Age, genetics, lack of exercise, standing for long periods, and extra pressure due to overweight or pregnancy can all make the valves malfunction.

▶ SYMPTOMS TO WATCH FOR
Enlarged, bulging veins; swelling in your legs and ankles; a 'heavy', painful, or crampy feeling in the legs; itching; discoloured skin.

▶ LATEST THINKING
Exercise your legs even if you wear compression stockings. Scientists in Hong Kong recently discovered a design flaw in the stockings: as study volunteers moved around, their stockings sometimes squeezed tighter at the point of the calves than at the ankles, which could actually promote blood pooling rather than prevent it. The researchers' conclusion was that compression stockings are still worth wearing if you're on your feet all day, but you should also attempt to exercise your calf muscles to help keep blood moving.

RECIPES FOR GOOD HEALTH

You'll increase your chances of living longer and better by eating well. Make delicious food at home with the help of these amazingly easy healthy dishes.

Eat well to live longer

The Disease Prevention Survey, based on advice from doctors specially trained in preventive medicine, outlined that the two best ways to avoid illness were to find ways to fit more exercise into your daily schedule and to eat healthier food. And these experts weren't shy about advising what 'ingredients' go into a healthy diet, either: plenty of fruit, vegetables, whole grains and healthy fats, especially the omega-3 fatty acids found in many types of fish. And it's not hard to translate those ingredients into delicious recipes that put taste first and health a close second. After all, eating good food is one of life's great pleasures, so why take that joy away?

The collection of easy-to-make, tasty recipes that follow on in this chapter are specifically designed to help you meet the following three goals central to disease prevention:

1. **Eat more fruit and vegetables**
2. **Eat more whole grains**
3. **Get more of your kilojoules from healthy fats.**

These goals are in line with advice that came up again and again in the survey. In their own words, the doctors polled told us that people should 'eat more plant-based foods', 'avoid refined and processed foods' and 'cut down on fatty red meat and foods high in saturated fat'. They also said that it's more important to limit simple carbohydrates than to have a low-fat diet.

The other notable goal mentioned in the survey was to eat less. Fortunately, thanks to sensible ratios of protein, healthy fats and whole grains, the recipes here will keep you feeling full longer, which is a great strategy for helping to control weight gain.

What you won't find is a lot of saturated fat, trans fat or refined carbs, which are all linked to an increased risk of disease.

About your goals

Achieving all three goals mentioned above will yield considerable health benefits. For starters, you'll be able to keep your blood sugar levels stable, improve your cholesterol ratio, lower your blood pressure and even decrease your risk of cancer and possibly dementia, too. Here's a bit more guidance to help you meet these goals.

What's a serve?

It's easier than you think to get seven serves of fruit and vegetables a day. You can knock off one serve just by starting your morning with fruit juice, and three or four more by having a big salad at lunch. Here's what one 'serve' actually amounts to:

Fruit

1 medium piece of fruit
2 smaller pieces of fruit
½ cup chopped, cooked or canned fruit
¼ cup dried fruit
½ cup (125 ml) 100 per cent fruit juice

Vegetables

1 cup raw leafy vegetables
½ cup chopped, cooked or canned vegetables
½ cup dried beans (measured after cooking)

Your fruit and vegetable goal: eat at least seven serves of fruit and vegetables a day.
Most doctors and dietitians agree that a plant-based diet—one full of fruit and vegetables, grains, and legumes—is the best way to prevent many major diseases. If you're eating these foods, you probably aren't eating as much unhealthy saturated fat or an overabundance of kilojoules. And you're getting adequate doses of vitamins, minerals and other plant nutrients, or phyto-nutrients, that fight against specific diseases. You're also realising an important target: getting at least 30 g of fibre per day.

Earlier in this book we recommended that you eat 'at least' seven serves of fruit and vegetables a day, based on the Disease Prevention Survey, but the simple truth is that getting more than those seven serves is going to be even better for your overall potential health outcome.

Your carbohydrate goal: get three of your daily grain serves from whole grains.
Eating refined carbohydrates (think: white rice, white bread and other foods made with white flour) can help to promote both weight gain and insulin resistance. Swapping these foods for slow-digesting whole grains (for instance, barley or burghul instead of rice) is one key to preventing many of the chronic diseases that plague us today, from obesity to heart disease.

One piece of advice from the survey was to 'stop and choose how you want to live life', which includes the way you eat. Each recipe in this section includes a box that shows what the recipe contributes towards your three dietary goals. And if your doctor has given you the OK to drink alcohol, enjoy having a glass of wine or beer with dinner, too.

Your fat goal: get about 25 per cent of daily kilojoules from healthy fats.
Leading nutrition experts now advocate getting 25 to 35 per cent of your kilojoules from fat. But most of that should be healthy monounsaturated fats (the kind found in nuts, avocados and canola and olive oils) and omega-3 fatty acids, found in foods such as salmon and linseeds. Less than 7 per cent of your kilojoules should come from saturated fat (the kind found in fatty meat, butter and full-fat cheese), which promotes insulin resistance and heart disease. We also recommend limiting fat from corn, safflower and sunflower oils, as these may promote inflammation. See 'Daily fat targets', below, to find out how many grams of fat these recommendations amount to.

Daily fat targets

DAILY KILOJOULES	DAILY GOOD FAT GOAL	DAILY SATURATED FAT GOAL
6000	41 g	Less than 12 g
7000	47 g	Less than 14 g
8000	54 g	Less than 16 g
9000	61 g	Less than 17 g
10,000	68 g	Less than 19 g
11,000	74 g	Less than 21 g

Breakfast

Fruity bircher muesli

Cooking healthy, tasty grains takes something that's often in short supply—time. Now you can wake up to fragrant wholegrain oats that have 'cooked'—almost magically—overnight. Rolled oats, nuts, fruit juice and dried fruit all provide a healthy dose of fibre.

1 Grate the apples (without peeling them) and toss well with the freshly squeezed lemon juice.

2 Mix in the oats, cranberries or other dried fruit, nuts, cinnamon, apple or orange juice and honey. Leave to stand in a glass or ceramic container, covered, overnight so that the grains soften and the flavours merge.

3 Before serving, stir in the yogurt.

Tip Don't buy the quick-cooking porridge oats often found in the cereal section of supermarkets to use in this recipe as they aren't as nutritious. Look for old-fashioned rolled oats. And if you aren't a big fan of yogurt, try adding a little soy milk before eating; it adds a wonderful flavour and is a great source of phyto-oestrogens, which are especially good for women's health.

MEETING YOUR GOALS
Each portion provides:
1.3 serves fruit
1 serve whole grains
10 g good fat

SERVES 4

PREPARATION 10 minutes, plus overnight soaking

2 large apples, cored

Juice of 1 lemon

½ cup (50 g) rolled oats

½ cup (65 g) dried cranberries or other dried fruit such as sultanas, cherries, chopped apricots, chopped figs or chopped pitted prunes

½ cup (70 g) nuts (almonds, macadamias, walnuts or whatever you choose), chopped

1 teaspoon ground cinnamon

1 cup (250 ml) unsweetened apple or orange juice

2 tablespoons honey

½ cup (125 g) low-fat plain yogurt

NUTRITION • *Per serving*
1410 kilojoules, 7 g protein,
53 g carbohydrate, 6 g fibre,
11 g total fat, 1 g saturated fat,
2 mg cholesterol, 34 mg sodium

Breakfast

Ricotta hotcakes with lime cardamom fruit salad

These ricotta hotcakes make a warming and delicious breakfast that is both healthy and satisfying. Double the recipe and make them on weekends for your friends and family. For added anti-oxidant power, use fresh or frozen berries in the fruit salad.

1 Toss the fruit in lime juice to prevent browning. In a small saucepan, heat the apple juice with cardamom seeds and lime zest, then simmer for 10 minutes. Allow to cool then stir through the chopped fruit.

2 For the hotcakes, beat the ricotta until smooth, then add the milk, oil and eggs and beat well. Fold in the flour, bicarbonate of soda and sugar. Let stand for a few minutes. Add a little more milk if the batter is too thick.

3 Spray or brush a large non-stick frying pan with oil and spread 1/4-cup circles of batter into the pan. Cook until golden on both sides. Repeat with the remaining batter.

MEETING YOUR GOALS
Each portion provides:
1.3 serves fruit
8 g good fat

SERVES 4
PREPARATION 10 minutes
COOKING 25 minutes

FRUIT SALAD

2 cups (about 350 g) chopped fresh fruit (whatever is in season)

Juice and zest of 1 lime

1/2 cup (125 ml) unsweetened apple juice

1 teaspoon cardamom seeds, crushed

HOTCAKES

1 cup (250 g) low-fat ricotta

1/2 cup (125 ml) low-fat milk

1 tablespoon canola oil

2 eggs

3/4 cup (110 g) wholemeal self-raising flour

1 teaspoon bicarbonate of soda

2 tablespoons sugar

Olive oil cooking spray

NUTRITION • *Per serving*
1430 kilojoules, 15 g protein,
41 g carbohydrate, 5 g fibre,
13 g total fat, 5 g saturated fat,
121 mg cholesterol, 697 mg sodium

Recipes for good health

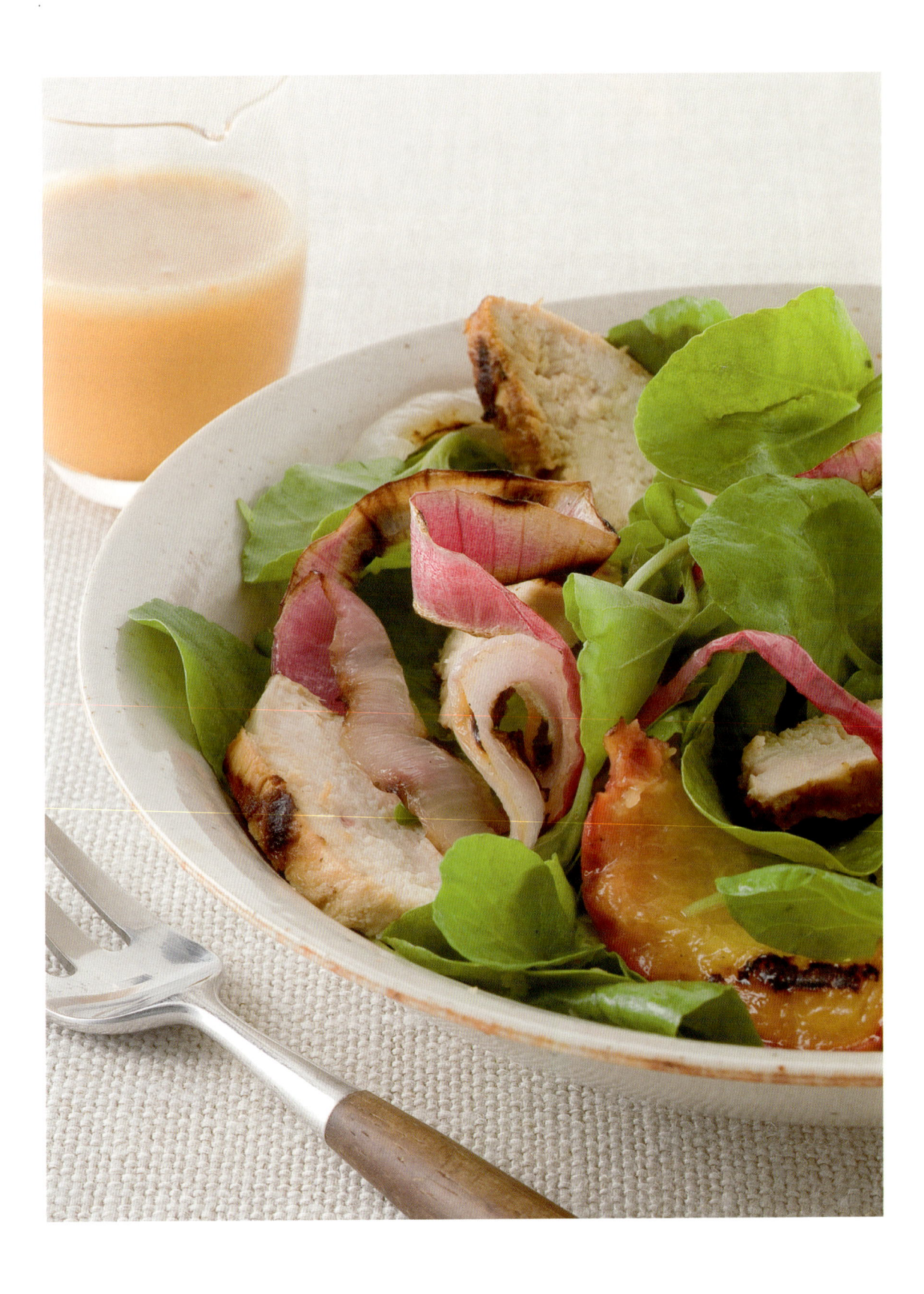

Salads

Barbecued chicken and peach salad

This main-dish salad is perfect for a summer's evening. The fruity dressing balances the peppery bite of watercress—a cancer-fighting cruciferous vegetable rich in beta-carotene and vitamin C—and infuses the chicken with flavour. And the ginger helps to ward against inflammation.

1 To make the marinade and dressing, blend together the peach or apricot nectar, oil, vinegar, soy sauce, ginger and garlic. Continue blending until smooth.

2 To marinate the chicken, place the chicken breasts in a zip-lock bag, add ¼ cup (60 ml) of the juice mixture, seal the bag and turn the chicken to coat. Refrigerate for at least 30 minutes or up to a day. (Reserve the remaining marinade, covered, in the refrigerator, for dressing the salad.)

3 Preheat a lightly oiled ridged stovetop grill pan to medium. Remove the chicken from the bag and remove the excess. Brush the peaches and onion with oil and place on the pan, along with the chicken. Cook, turning once halfway through cooking, until the chicken is browned and cooked through and the onion and peaches are lightly browned, about 10 to 12 minutes.

4 Cut the chicken into thin slices and the peaches into wedges. Separate the onion rings. In a large bowl, combine the watercress, chicken, peaches and onion. Add the reserved dressing and toss to coat well.

Tip Look for unsweetened peach or apricot nectar in the natural foods section of your supermarket or in a health food shop.

SERVES 4
PREPARATION 25 minutes
MARINATING 30 minutes to 1 day
COOKING 15 minutes

MARINADE AND DRESSING

⅓ cup (80 ml) unsweetened peach or apricot nectar (see Tip) or juice

¼ cup (60 ml) canola oil

1 tablespoon rice vinegar

2 teaspoons salt-reduced soy sauce

2 slices fresh ginger, peeled and crushed

1 clove garlic, crushed and peeled

CHICKEN AND SALAD

500 g boneless skinless chicken breasts, trimmed

2 teaspoons canola oil

2 peaches, peeled, stoned and halved

1 small red onion, cut into medium slices

6 cups (180 g) trimmed watercress sprigs, washed and dried

NUTRITION • *Per serving*
517 kilojoules, 10 g protein, 3 g carbohydrate, 1 g fibre, 8 g total fat, 1 g saturated fat, 28 mg cholesterol, 64 mg sodium

MEETING YOUR GOALS
Each portion provides:
1 serve fruit
1.7 serves vegetables
7 g good fat

Salads

Pear and walnut salad

Including fresh fruit in a green salad is a great way to make it more interesting. And a topping of nuts—rich in healthy fats—is a much healthier option than croutons. Here, the nuts are toasted with a honey glaze for added sweetness.

1 To prepare the walnuts, preheat the oven to 180°C. Coat a small baking dish with cooking spray. In a small bowl, combine the walnuts, oil and honey and stir to coat. Spread the mixture evenly in the baking dish. Bake, stirring occasionally, until fragrant, about 12 to 15 minutes. Allow to cool.

2 To make the dressing, combine the walnut oil, shallot, vinegar, mustard and pepper in a jar with a tight-fitting lid or in a small bowl. Shake or whisk to blend.

3 To make the salad, just before serving, combine the greens, witlof, pear and grapes in a large bowl. Add the dressing and toss to coat well. Divide the salad among four plates and top each serving with 2 tablespoons walnuts.

Tip Walnut oil's delicate, nutty flavour makes it an excellent choice for dressing salads, especially when paired with nuts or strong-tasting cheeses. It's also a good source of heart-healthy omega-3 fatty acids. You can find it in most large supermarkets and in specialty food stores. The oil is expensive, but a little goes a long way in distinguishing your salad. Refrigerate the bottle after opening.

SERVES 4
PREPARATION 25 minutes
COOKING 15 minutes

WALNUTS
¼ cup (25 g) walnut halves
1 teaspoon olive oil
1 teaspoon honey

DRESSING
¼ cup (60 ml) walnut oil (see Tip) or extra-virgin olive oil
2 tablespoons finely chopped French shallot
1 tablespoon balsamic vinegar
1 teaspoon dijon mustard
Freshly ground black pepper

SALAD
4 cups (180 g) mixed baby salad greens (mesclun), washed and dried
1 witlof (Belgian endive), cored and cut crosswise into medium slices
1 ripe but firm red pear, peeled, cored and thinly sliced
1 cup (180 g) red seedless grapes, washed, patted dry and halved

NUTRITION • *Per serving*
1002 kilojoules, 2 g protein,
17 g carbohydrate, 2 g fibre,
18 g total fat, 2 g saturated fat,
0 mg cholesterol, 53 mg sodium

MEETING YOUR GOALS	Each portion provides: 0.8 serve fruit 1.2 serves vegetables 16 g good fat

Salads

Thai-style beef salad

Tangy Asian-flavoured marinade turns lean, budget-friendly skirt steak into a tender cooked meat, while also doubling as a dressing. If you're short on time, use a strip loin steak and marinate it for just 20 minutes before cooking.

1 To make the marinade and dressing, whisk together the lime juice, vinegar, fish sauce, sugar, ginger, chilli and garlic in a bowl until the sugar dissolves.

2 To marinate the beef, place the steak in a zip-lock bag, add ¼ cup (60 ml) of the dressing, seal the bag and turn the steak to coat. Refrigerate for at least 6 hours or overnight. (Reserve the remaining marinade, covered, in the refrigerator, for dressing the salad.)

3 Preheat the barbecue or a ridged stovetop grill pan to medium–high. Remove the steak from the marinade and discard the excess. If barbecuing, lightly oil the grill, then cook the steak until it's done to your liking, about 5 to 6 minutes per side for medium–rare. Transfer to a clean cutting board and leave to stand for 5 minutes. Carve across the grain into thin slices.

4 In a large bowl, combine the lettuce, capsicum, cucumber, mint and spring onion. Add the steak and reserved dressing and toss to coat. Top with coriander and bean sprouts. Sprinkle each serving with peanuts.

MEETING YOUR GOALS
Each portion provides:
0.2 serve fruit
4 serves vegetables
9 g good fat

SERVES 2
PREPARATION 30 minutes
MARINATING 6 hours or overnight
COOKING 15 minutes

MARINADE AND DRESSING

¼ cup (60 ml) fresh lime juice

2 tablespoons rice vinegar

1 tablespoon fish sauce

1 tablespoon grated palm sugar or dark brown sugar

2 teaspoons grated fresh ginger

2 teaspoons chopped red chilli

1 large clove garlic, crushed

STEAK AND SALAD

250 g skirt steak, trimmed

3 cups sliced cos lettuce (1 small head)

1 cup (155 g) diced red capsicum

1 cup (175 g) sliced Lebanese cucumber

½ cup (10 g) fresh mint leaves, cut into thin slivers

¼ cup (30 g) chopped spring onions

¼ cup (7 g) fresh coriander leaves

½ cup (45 g) mung bean sprouts

2 tablespoons unsalted roasted peanuts, coarsely chopped

NUTRITION • *Per serving*
1394 kilojoules, 34 g protein,
20 g carbohydrate, 7 g fibre,
12 g total fat, 3 g saturated fat,
74 mg cholesterol, 1028 mg sodium

Salads

Quinoa salad with corn and lime dressing

Grain salads are ideal for picnics and backyard entertaining. While quinoa (pronounced keen-wa) isn't technically a grain, it's used as one and is a great source of fibre and protein. This salad is perfect with grilled pork, chicken or fish.

1 In a saucepan, combine the quinoa with 1^1/$_2$ cups (375 ml) water. Bring to a simmer, then cover and cook over low heat until the quinoa is tender and most of the liquid has been absorbed, about 12 to 15 minutes. Remove from the heat and let stand for 5 minutes. Fluff with a fork, transfer to a large bowl and cool.

2 Bring 2 or 3 cm of water to the boil in a large pot. Add the corn, cover and cook until tender, about 5 minutes. Refresh under cold running water. Cut the kernels off the cobs (you should have about 1 cup [200 g] in total).

3 Meanwhile, in a small bowl, whisk together ^{1}/$_4$ cup (60 ml) lime juice with the chilli, garlic, cumin and pepper. Gradually whisk in the canola oil.

4 Add the tomatoes, spring onions, coriander and corn to the quinoa. Add the dressing and toss to coat well. The salad will keep, covered, in the refrigerator for up to two days. Just before serving, dice the avocados and toss with the remaining 1 tablespoon lime juice in a small bowl and garnish the salad with avocados.

SERVES 6

PREPARATION 30 minutes
COOKING 20 minutes

^{3}/$_4$ cup (150 g) quinoa, rinsed thoroughly

2 corncobs, husked

^{1}/$_4$ cup (60 ml) plus 1 tablespoon fresh lime juice

1 red chilli, seeded and finely chopped

1 small clove garlic, crushed

1 teaspoon ground cumin

Freshly ground black pepper

^{1}/$_4$ cup (60 ml) canola oil

2 cups (300 g) cherry or grape tomatoes, halved

^{1}/$_2$ cup (60 g) chopped spring onions

^{1}/$_2$ cup (15 g) chopped fresh coriander leaves

2 avocados

NUTRITION • *Per serving*
1702 kilojoules, 8 g protein,
29 g carbohydrate, 6 g fibre,
30 g total fat, 5 g saturated fat,
0 mg cholesterol, 11 mg sodium

MEETING YOUR GOALS

Each portion provides:
1.2 serves fruit
1.1 serves vegetables
0.7 serve whole grains
25 g good fat

Salads | 329

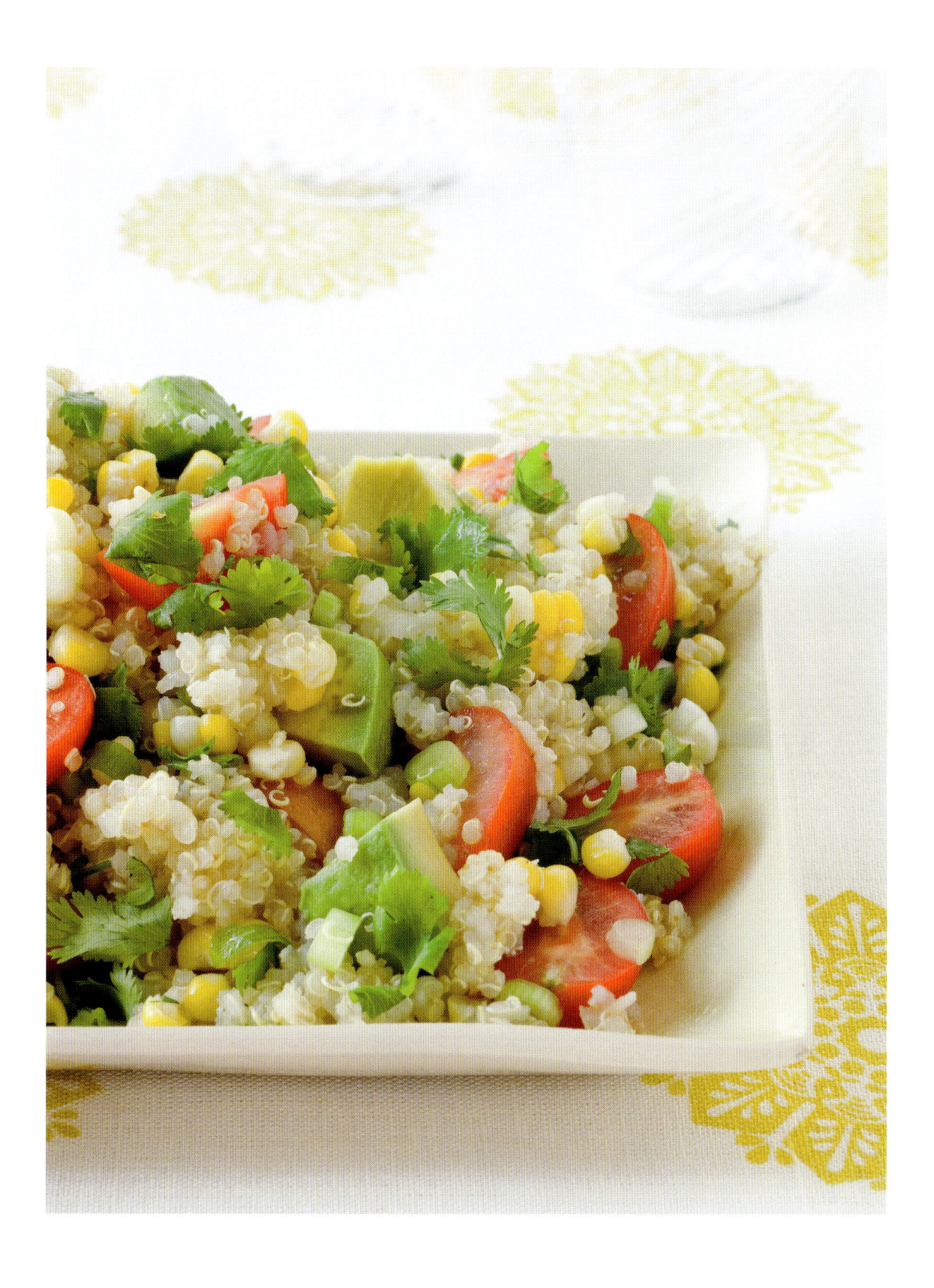

Salads

Burghul salad with dried apricots and mint

This fruity version of tabouleh features dried fruit, colourful red capsicum and sweet mint in a lightly spiced citrus dressing. Burghul is one of the most convenient whole grains, and it doesn't need to be cooked, just soaked. It's also a great low-GI food choice, meaning it doesn't raise blood glucose levels as much as rice does.

1 Bring about 2½ cups (625 ml) water to the boil in a small saucepan. Place the burghul and apricots in a large bowl and add enough boiling water to cover. Let stand for 20 minutes, then drain and press out excess water.

2 Meanwhile, toast the pine nuts in a dry frying pan over medium–low heat, stirring constantly, until golden and fragrant, about 2 to 3 minutes. Transfer to a plate to cool.

3 In a large bowl, whisk the orange juice, vinegar, garlic, cumin, coriander and pepper. Gradually whisk in the oil. Add the burghul, apricots, capsicum, spring onions and mint and toss to coat well. The salad will keep, covered, in the refrigerator for up to two days. Sprinkle with pine nuts before serving.

MEETING YOUR GOALS

Each portion provides:
0.5 serve fruit
0.7 serve vegetables
0.6 serve whole grains
21 g good fat

SERVES 4

PREPARATION 25 minutes, plus 20 minutes standing
COOKING 5 minutes

¾ cup (130 g) burghul, rinsed
½ cup (90 g) dried apricots, diced
⅓ cup (50 g) pine nuts
⅓ cup (80 ml) unsweetened orange juice
¼ cup (60 ml) cider vinegar
1 small clove garlic, crushed
½ teaspoon ground cumin
¼ teaspoon ground coriander
Freshly ground black pepper
¼ cup (60 ml) extra-virgin olive oil
1 small red capsicum, seeded and diced
½ cup (60 g) chopped spring onions
½ cup (25 g) chopped fresh mint

NUTRITION • *Per serving*
1551 kilojoules, 7 g protein,
34 g carbohydrate, 9 g fibre,
23 g total fat, 2 g saturated fat,
0 mg cholesterol, 16 mg sodium

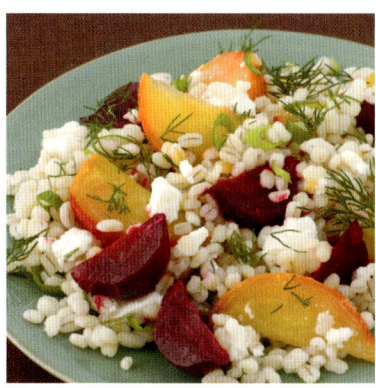

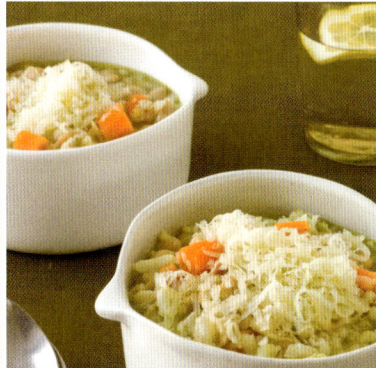

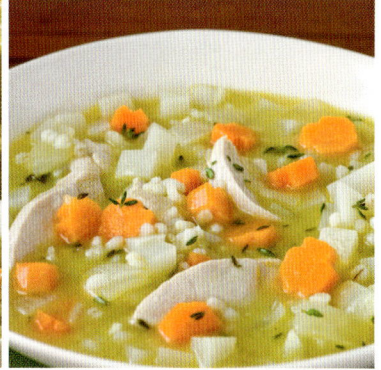

Three great ways to eat barley

With a deliciously nutty flavour, barley is great in soups, pilafs and salads, and it won't raise your blood glucose levels the way most rice does. It's also high in soluble fibre to help lower cholesterol.

Barley and beetroot salad

Serves 5

½ cup (110 g) pearl barley

⅓ cup (80 ml) extra-virgin olive oil

¼ cup (60 ml) balsamic vinegar

Freshly ground black pepper

1½ cups (300 g) diced cooked beetroot

½ cup (60 g) chopped spring onions

½ cup (75 g) crumbled feta

¼ cup (15 g) chopped fresh dill

In a small saucepan, combine 2½ cups (625 ml) water and the barley. Cover and simmer over medium–low heat until tender, 40 to 45 minutes. Transfer to a large bowl to cool. In a small bowl, whisk the oil, vinegar and pepper. Add to the barley along with the beetroot, spring onions, feta and dill. Toss to coat.

Bean and barley soup

Serves 10

2 x 400-g cans cannellini beans, drained and rinsed

1 tablespoon olive oil

1 medium onion, chopped

2 medium carrots, diced

30 g prosciutto, diced

4 cups (300 g) shredded green cabbage

4 cloves garlic, crushed

4 cups (1 litre) salt-reduced chicken stock

½ cup (110 g) quick-cooking barley

1¼ cups (165 g) grated reduced-fat Swiss or Jarlsberg cheese

Mash 1½ cups of beans. Heat the oil in a large pot, add the onion, carrots and prosciutto and cook until golden. Add the cabbage and garlic and cook until the cabbage wilts. Add the stock, 1½ cups (375 ml) water, barley, and all the beans. Simmer 8 to 10 minutes. Top each serving with cheese.

Chicken soup with barley and root vegetables

Serves 8

1 large onion, chopped

3 cloves garlic, crushed

1 tablespoon canola oil

5 cups (1.25 litres) salt-reduced chicken stock

½ cup (110 g) pearl barley

350 g boneless skinless chicken breast, sliced

2 cups (310 g) diced root vegetables, such as carrots and parsnips

2 tablespoons fresh lemon juice

Freshly ground black pepper

Fresh dill or parsley sprigs

In a large pot, cook the onion and garlic in the oil until softened. Add the stock and barley, cover and simmer for 25 minutes. Add the chicken and vegetables. Simmer, covered, for about 20 minutes. Season with the lemon juice and pepper. Garnish with the dill or parsley.

Soups

Spring vegetable soup

Take advantage of the arrival of tender spring vegetables by making this fresh, simple and delicious potage (a type of rustic French soup). It has a delicate, velvety consistency without the need to add cream.

1 Heat the oil in a large saucepan over medium–high heat. Add the onion and cook, stirring often, until softened, about 2 to 3 minutes, then add the potato and garlic. Cook, stirring, for 20 to 30 seconds. Add the stock and bring to a simmer. Reduce the heat to medium–low, cover and simmer for 15 minutes.

2 Add the asparagus and increase the heat to medium. Cover and cook until tender, 4 to 5 minutes. Stir in the spinach and cook just until it starts to wilt, 30 to 60 seconds.

3 Working in batches, puree the soup in a blender or food processor. (Take care when blending hot liquids: do not fill the blender more than half full, always cover the lid with a tea towel and hold it securely in place.) Return the soup to the pot and heat through before stirring in lemon juice and pepper. In a small bowl, whisk the yogurt and milk together until smooth. Ladle the soup into bowls and add small dollops of yogurt mixture into each, then draw the tip of a knife or toothpick through the yogurt to make decorative swirls. Sprinkle with tarragon.

MEETING YOUR GOALS
Each portion provides:
1.8 serves vegetables
0.4 serve whole grains
4 g good fat

SERVES 6

PREPARATION 20 minutes
COOKING 25 minutes

1 tablespoon olive oil

1 medium red onion, sliced

1 medium all-purpose potato, peeled and sliced

1 clove garlic, crushed

4 cups (1 litre) salt-reduced chicken or vegetable stock

700 g (about 3 cups) asparagus, trimmed and cut into medium lengths

4 cups (200 g) baby English spinach, washed and dried

1 tablespoon fresh lemon juice

Freshly ground black pepper

$^1/_3$ cup (90 g) low-fat plain yogurt

2 tablespoons low-fat milk

A few sprigs fresh tarragon or 1 tablespoon snipped fresh chives

NUTRITION • *Per serving*
423 kilojoules, 8 g protein,
9 g carbohydrate, 3 g fibre,
4 g total fat, 0 g saturated fat,
1 mg cholesterol, 459 mg sodium

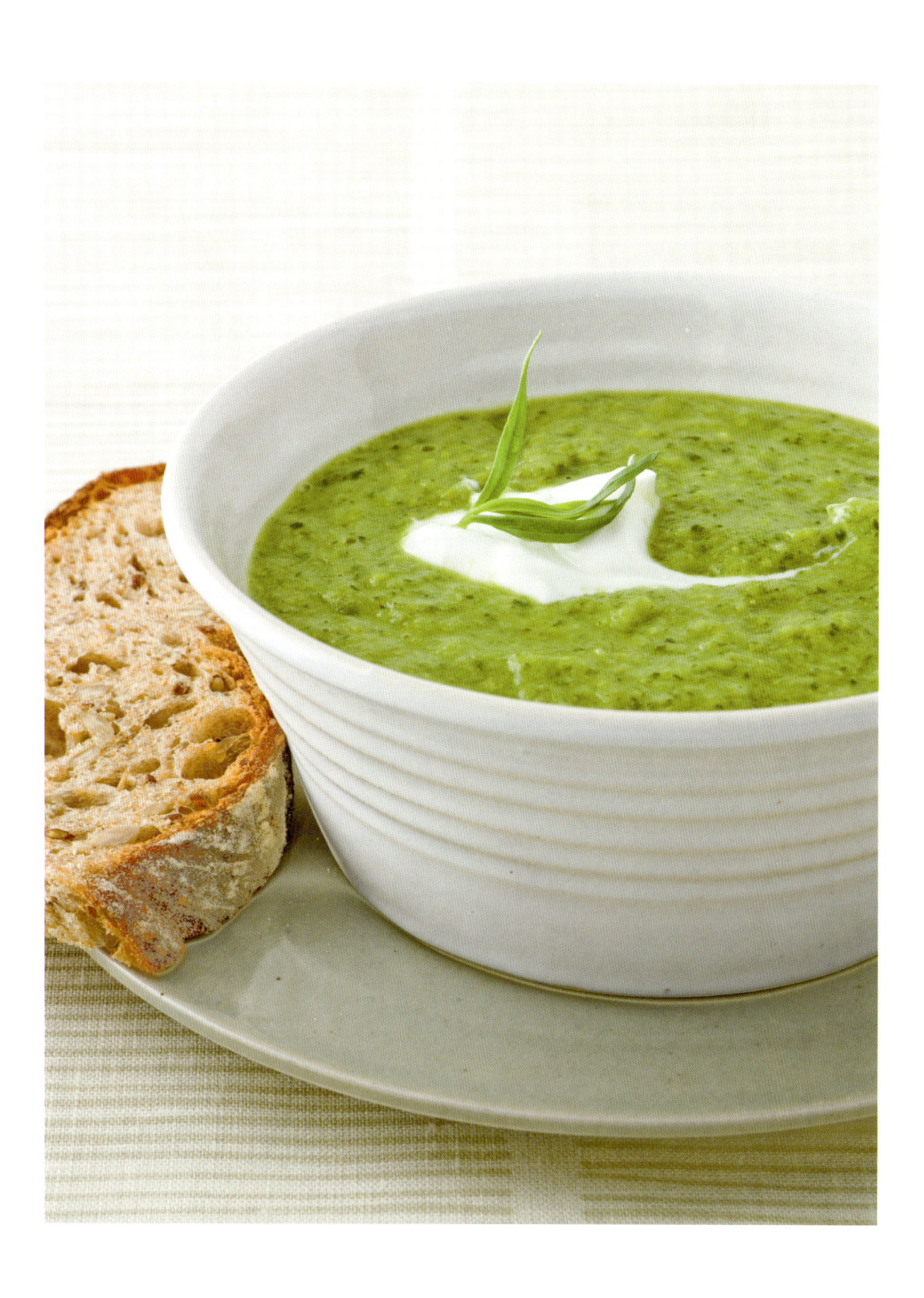

Soups

Minestrone with basil pesto

There's nothing like farm-fresh produce to motivate you to eat more vegetables. Simmer them into this delicious soup and you'll get more than two serves in one hit.

1 Bring the stock to the boil in a large saucepan and add the garlic. Partially cover the saucepan and simmer over medium–low heat for 15 minutes to deepen the flavours. Pour the stock through a strainer into a large bowl, pressing the cooked garlic through the strainer.

2 Heat the oil in a large pot over medium heat. Add the leeks and onion, then cook, stirring often, until softened but not browned, about 2 to 4 minutes. Add the stock, carrots, cauliflower, tomatoes and pasta. Partially cover and simmer over medium heat for about 10 minutes.

3 Meanwhile, make the basil pesto (see recipe below) or use shop-bought pesto if you're short on time.

4 Add the beans and zucchini to the soup. Partially cover and cook until the vegetables are tender, about 5 minutes. Ladle into bowls and stir about 1 tablespoon pesto into each. The soup will keep, covered, in the refrigerator for up to two days. (You can add a little water if the soup seems too thick.)

Basil pesto Toast 1/3 cup (50 g) pine nuts in a frying pan over medium–low heat, stirring constantly, until golden and fragrant, about 2 to 4 minutes, then cool. In a food processor, combine 3 cups (90 g) lightly packed basil leaves, 2 cloves crushed garlic, freshly ground black pepper and the pine nuts, and process to a coarse consistency. With the motor running, gradually add 1/4 cup (60 ml) olive oil in a thin stream until the mixture begins to form a loosely liquid paste. Add 1/2 cup (50 g) grated parmesan cheese and pulse until blended. The pesto will keep, covered with plastic wrap (to prevent it turning brown), in the refrigerator for up to two days or you can freeze it for up to 6 months.

SERVES 10

PREPARATION 50 minutes (including the pesto)
COOKING 45 minutes

8 cups (2 litres) salt-reduced chicken stock

8 cloves garlic, crushed

2 tablespoons olive oil

2 medium leeks, white and pale green parts, washed and sliced

1 medium onion, chopped

4 medium carrots, peeled, halved lengthwise and sliced

2 cups (250 g) cauliflower florets, cut into small pieces

1 x 410-g can diced tomatoes

1 cup (90 g) small wholemeal pasta shells

1 cup (125 g) sliced green beans

1 small zucchini, quartered lengthwise and sliced

3/4 cup (185 g) basil pesto (see recipe at left)

NUTRITION • *Per serving*
954 kilojoules, 8 g protein,
13 g carbohydrate, 4 g fibre,
16 g total fat, 2 g saturated fat,
3 mg cholesterol, 606 mg sodium

MEETING YOUR GOALS

Each portion provides:
2.2 serves vegetables
14 g good fat

Chicken

Brown rice paella

This colourful dish is a complete, wholesome meal. Opt for short- or medium-grain brown rice as it cooks up into the creamy consistency characteristic of a great paella.

1 In a small saucepan, bring the stock and saffron to a simmer. Remove from the heat, cover and set aside.

2 Heat 2 teaspoons of the oil in a large non-stick frying pan over medium–high heat. Add the sausage and cook, turning once, until browned, about 2 to 3 minutes. Transfer to a plate. Add the chicken and cook, turning occasionally, until browned, about 3 to 5 minutes. Transfer to the plate with the sausage.

3 Add the remaining 2 teaspoons of oil to the frying pan along with the onion. Cook, stirring often, until softened and starting to brown, about 3 to 4 minutes. Add the garlic, capsicums and paprika and cook, stirring, until fragrant, about 20 to 30 seconds. Add the tomatoes and bring to a simmer. Cook, stirring, until most of the liquid has evaporated.

4 Add the rice and stir to coat well. Add the stock, sausage and chicken and bring to a simmer. Reduce the heat to low, cover and cook for 45 minutes. If the paella seems dry, add a little extra stock or water.

5 Stir in the prawns and peas. Cover and cook until the rice is tender, the prawns are pink and most of the liquid has been absorbed. Remove from heat and let stand, covered, for 5 minutes. Serve with lemon wedges.

SERVES 6
PREPARATION 30 minutes
COOKING 1 hour 10 minutes

3¼ cups (810 ml) salt-reduced chicken stock

¼ teaspoon saffron threads, crumbled

1 tablespoon olive oil

100 g cooked chicken sausage, sliced into medium pieces

300 g boneless skinless chicken thighs, cut into chunks

1 medium onion, chopped

2 cloves garlic, crushed

1 small red capsicum, seeded and sliced

1 small green capsicum, seeded and sliced

1 teaspoon paprika

1 x 410-g can diced tomatoes

1 cup (200 g) short- or medium-grain brown rice (see Tip)

350 g raw prawns, peeled and deveined

1 cup (155 g) frozen peas, rinsed under cold running water to thaw

Lemon wedges

MEETING YOUR GOALS
Each portion provides:
2 serves vegetables
1.2 serves whole grains
6 g good fat

NUTRITION • *Per serving*
1256 kilojoules, 22 g protein, 34 g carbohydrate, 3 g fibre, 8 g total fat, 2 g saturated fat, 10 mg cholesterol, 547 mg sodium

Chicken

Glazed chicken with root vegetables

Autumn is when earthy-tasting root vegetables are usually at their best. A tasty maple glaze acts as a faux skin for this chicken, giving it a delicious crust and keeping the flesh moist and juicy—without the saturated fat found in skin.

1 Preheat the oven to 200°C. Coat a large roasting pan with cooking spray.

2 Place the vegetables in the pan and toss with the oil, salt and half the pepper. Push the vegetables towards the outside of the pan. Sprinkle the chicken with the rest of the pepper and place, skin side down, in the centre of the roasting pan. Bake, uncovered, for 15 minutes.

3 Meanwhile, in a small bowl, combine the mustard, maple syrup and thyme.

4 Stir the vegetables and turn the chicken pieces. Brush the chicken with the mustard mixture. Bake, stirring the vegetables occasionally until they are glazed and tender and the chicken is cooked through (an instant-read thermometer should register 80°C), about 30 to 40 minutes. (If either the chicken or vegetables are done first, remove and keep warm.) Transfer to a platter or individual plates. Add the apple cider and stock to the roasting pan, place on the stovetop, and bring to the boil over a medium–high heat. Boil for 2 to 3 minutes. Drizzle the sauce over the chicken and vegetables.

SERVES 4

PREPARATION 30 minutes
COOKING 55 minutes

4 cups (about 600 g) assorted diced peeled root vegetables, such as carrots, parsnips, celeriac, kohlrabi and/or turnips

1 tablespoon olive oil

¼ teaspoon salt

½ teaspoon freshly ground black pepper

1 kg bone-in chicken thighs and/or drumsticks, skin removed and fat trimmed

1 tablespoon dijon mustard

1 tablespoon maple syrup

2 teaspoons chopped fresh thyme or ¾ teaspoon dried thyme

½ cup (125 ml) apple cider

½ cup (125 ml) salt-reduced chicken stock

NUTRITION • *Per serving*
1902 kilojoules, 49 g protein, 19 g carbohydrate, 3 g fibre, 21 g total fat, 5 g saturated fat, 252 mg cholesterol, 674 mg sodium

MEETING YOUR GOALS
Each portion provides:
0.2 serve fruit
2 serves vegetables
16 g good fat

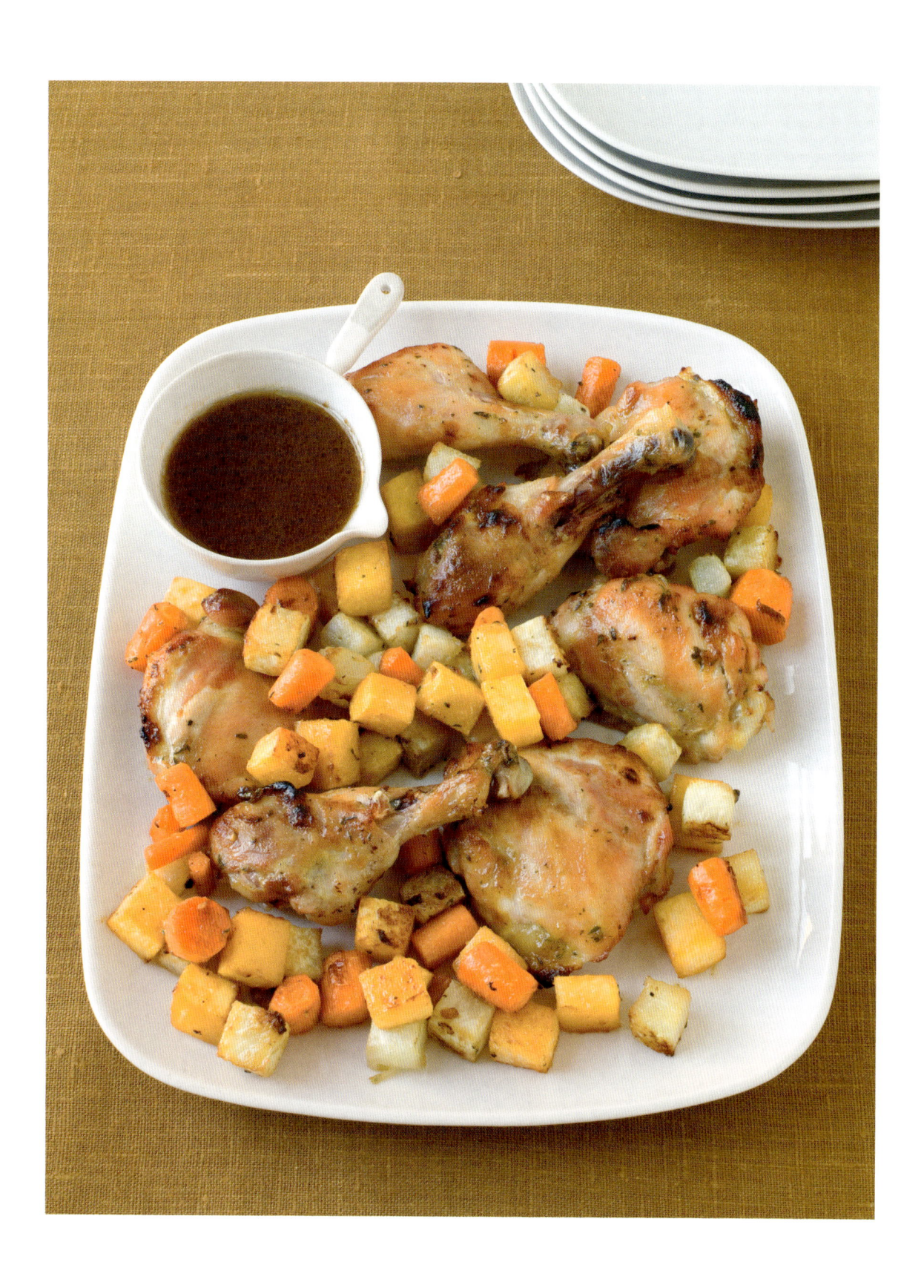

Chicken

Chicken

Chicken and white bean cassoulet

Cabbage is a nutritional superstar, with cancer-fighting powers and an impressive roster of vitamins and minerals. This dish will convince even the most reluctant greens-eaters just how delicious cabbage can be.

1 Preheat the oven to 220°C. Lightly coat a baking dish with cooking spray.

2 Process bread until coarse crumbs form. Transfer to a bowl, add 2 teaspoons of the oil and stir to coat.

3 Bring 2.5 cm of water to a boil in a large pot. Add the cabbage and stir to submerge. Cook, uncovered, until just tender, about 4 to 5 minutes. Drain and refresh under cold running water, then press out excess water.

4 Cook the sausages in a large non-stick frying pan over medium–high heat, breaking it up into chunks, until browned, about 3 to 4 minutes. Drain on paper towel.

5 Add the remaining 1 teaspoon oil to the frying pan. Add the onion and cook over medium–high heat, stirring often, until softened, 2 to 3 minutes. Add the garlic and cook, stirring, until fragrant, 20 to 30 seconds. Add the wine, bring to a simmer and cook for 1 minute. Remove from the heat and add the beans, tomatoes, stock, pepper, cabbage and sausage. Stir to mix well. Transfer to the baking dish and sprinkle with parmesan, then the breadcrumb mixture.

6 Bake the casserole until bubbly and the top is browned, about 25 to 35 minutes.

SERVES 6

PREPARATION 35 minutes
COOKING 50 minutes

2 slices wholemeal bread, crusts trimmed, torn into pieces

3 teaspoons olive oil

350 g savoy cabbage or cavolo nero, stems trimmed, leaves washed and coarsely chopped

250 g chicken sausages

1 medium onion, chopped

4 cloves garlic, crushed

½ cup (125 ml) dry white wine

2 x 400-g cans cannellini beans, drained and rinsed

1 x 410-g can diced tomatoes

½ cup (125 ml) salt-reduced chicken stock

Freshly ground black pepper

½ cup (50 g) freshly grated parmesan

NUTRITION • *Per serving*
1276 kilojoules, 17 g protein, 20 g carbohydrates, 11 g fibre, 16 g total fat, 5 g saturated fat, 29 mg cholesterol, 762 mg sodium

MEETING YOUR GOALS
Each portion provides:
1.4 serves vegetables
0.3 serve whole grains
11 g good fat

Meat

Kangaroo meatloaf with Asian flavours

The secret ingredient in this meatloaf is sweet potato, one of the most nutritious of all vegetables. Kangaroo mince is a much healthier alternative to beef mince, and it can be found in many supermarkets in Australia. Substitute turkey or low-fat beef mince if kangaroo mince is not available.

1 Preheat the oven to 180°C. Line a loaf tin with aluminium foil, leaving a short overhang along the two long sides. Coat the insides with cooking spray to prevent sticking.

2 In a large bowl, combine the mince, sweet potato, onion, breadcrumbs, egg, eggwhites, 2 tablespoons of the stir-fry sauce, the ginger, garlic and pepper, and mix well. Transfer to the prepared tin and press into a loaf. Spread 1 tablespoon stir-fry sauce over the top.

3 Place the tin on a baking tray and bake for 1 hour. Drain off any fat, then bake until firm and an instant-read thermometer inserted in the centre registers 80°C, about 10 to 20 minutes. Drain off any fat and let stand for 5 minutes.

4 In a small microwavable bowl, whisk the remaining ¼ cup (60 ml) stir-fry sauce and ¼ cup (60 ml) water. Cover with baking paper and microwave on *High* until properly heated through, about a minute.

5 Use the foil overhang to lift the meatloaf out of the loaf tin and transfer it to a cutting board, then slice. Drizzle a little sauce over each slice. The leftovers will keep, covered in the refrigerator, for up to two days.

Tip To make fresh wholemeal breadcrumbs, trim the crusts from three slices wholemeal bread. Tear the bread into pieces and process in a food processor until coarse crumbs form. Makes about 1 cup.

SERVES 8
PREPARATION 30 minutes
COOKING 1 hour 20 minutes

500 g kangaroo mince

2 cups (250 g) grated sweet potato

1 cup (155 g) chopped onion

¾ cup (60 g) fresh wholemeal breadcrumbs (see Tip)

1 large egg, lightly beaten

2 large eggwhites, lightly beaten

6 tablespoons Asian-style stir-fry sauce

1 tablespoon grated fresh ginger

1 clove garlic, crushed

½ teaspoon freshly ground black pepper

NUTRITION • *Per serving*
651 kilojoules, 18 g protein,
13 g carbohydrate, 2 g fibre,
4 g total fat, 1 g saturated fat,
28 mg cholesterol, 195 mg sodium

MEETING YOUR GOALS
Each portion provides:
0.5 serve vegetables
0.2 serve whole grains
3 g good fat

Recipes for good health

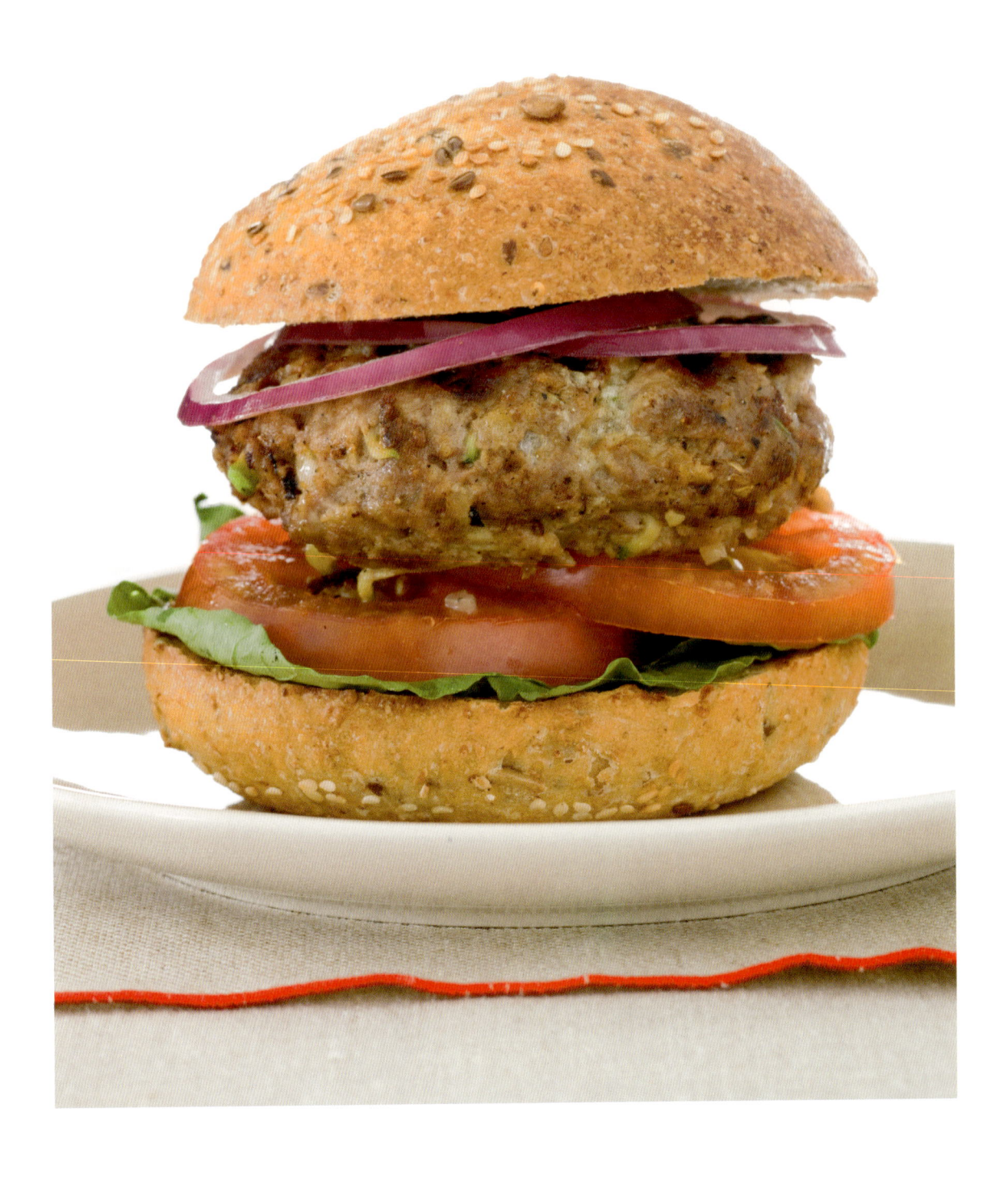

Meat

Lean beef burgers

Hamburgers as part of a healthy diet? The trick is to stretch the meat with a few different grated vegetables and then top the burger with plenty of tomato and greens.

1. To make the patties, mix the mince, eggwhite, zucchini, onion, breadcrumbs, worcestershire sauce, mustard and pepper together in a large bowl. Form into four 1-cm-thick patties.

2. Put the sliced onion in a medium bowl, cover with iced water and soak for about 10 to 20 minutes. Drain.

3. Preheat a lightly oiled ridged stovetop grill pan to medium–high, then cook the patties until browned and cooked through (an instant-read thermometer inserted in the center should register 80°C), about 5 minutes per side. About 1 minute before the patties are done, place the bread rolls, cut side down, on the grill until lightly toasted, about 30 to 60 seconds.

4. To assemble, divide the spinach, cheese and tomato slices among the bread roll bottoms. Add the patties and top with the onion slices. Replace the bread roll tops.

MEETING YOUR GOALS
Each portion provides:
2.3 serves vegetables
2.8 serves whole grains
6 g good fat

SERVES 4

PREPARATION 15 minutes, plus 10 to 20 minutes soaking
COOKING 10 minutes

PATTIES

250 g lean beef mince

1 eggwhite, lightly beaten

1 cup (135 g) grated zucchini

1/3 cup (50 g) finely chopped onion

2/3 cup (55 g) fresh wholemeal breadcrumbs (see Tip on page 339)

1 tablespoon worcestershire sauce

2 teaspoons dijon mustard

Freshly ground black pepper

ROLLS AND GARNISH

1 cup (155 g) thinly sliced sweet, white onion or red onion

2 cups (100 g) baby English spinach or rocket, washed and dried

4 slices low-fat cheese

1 medium tomato, sliced

4 large wholemeal rolls or burger buns, split crosswise

NUTRITION • *Per serving*
1722 kilojoules, 32 g protein, 49 g carbohydrate, 7 g fibre, 9 g total fat, 3 g saturated fat, 39 mg cholesterol, 823 mg sodium

Meat

Roasted pork with pomegranate sauce

Lean pork tenderloin and delicious roasted vegetables are a natural pairing with anti-oxidant-rich pomegranate syrup.

1 Preheat the oven to 220°C. Coat a large roasting pan with cooking spray.

2 In a bowl, combine the pumpkin, shallots or onions, 1 tablespoon of the oil and ¼ teaspoon pepper and toss to coat. Spread out the vegetables in the pan and bake for 15 minutes.

3 Meanwhile, in a small bowl, mix the cumin, brown sugar, coriander, chilli and the remaining pepper. Using a paper towel pat the pork dry then rub with the spice mixture.

4 Heat the remaining 2 teaspoons oil in a large non-stick frying pan over medium–high heat. Add the pork and cook, turning occasionally, until browned on all sides, about 4 minutes.

5 Stir the vegetables and push them to the outside of the pan, placing the pork in the centre. Bake, stirring the vegetables occasionally, until the pork is just cooked through (an instant-read thermometer inserted in the centre should register 70°C; the temperature will rise to 75°C during resting) and the vegetables are tender, about 20 to 25 minutes.

6 Meanwhile, add the pomegranate juice to the frying pan and bring to the boil. Continue to boil until reduced to ⅔ cup (165 ml), about 10 minutes. In a small bowl, mix the stock with cornflour, then add to the frying pan sauce and cook, stirring, until slightly thickened, about 1 minute.

7 Transfer the vegetables to a bowl and the pork to a cutting board. Let the pork rest for 5 minutes before carving. Cut into medium slices and serve with the vegetables and sauce.

SERVES 4
PREPARATION 10 minutes
COOKING 45 minutes

4 cups (about 600 g) cubed peeled butternut pumpkin

2 cups (270 g) whole French shallots, pickling onions or small brown onions, peeled

1½ tablespoons olive oil

½ teaspoon freshly ground black pepper

1 teaspoon ground cumin

1 teaspoon soft brown sugar

½ teaspoon ground coriander

¼ teaspoon chilli powder or cayenne pepper

500 g pork tenderloin, trimmed

¾ cup (185 ml) unsweetened pomegranate juice

¾ cup (185 ml) salt-reduced chicken stock

1 teaspoon cornflour

NUTRITION • *Per serving*
1349 kilojoules, 30 g protein, 30 g carbohydrate, 4 g fibre, 10 g total fat, 2 g saturated fat, 81 mg cholesterol, 261 mg sodium

MEETING YOUR GOALS

Each portion provides:
0.3 serve fruit
1.4 serves vegetables
8 g good fat

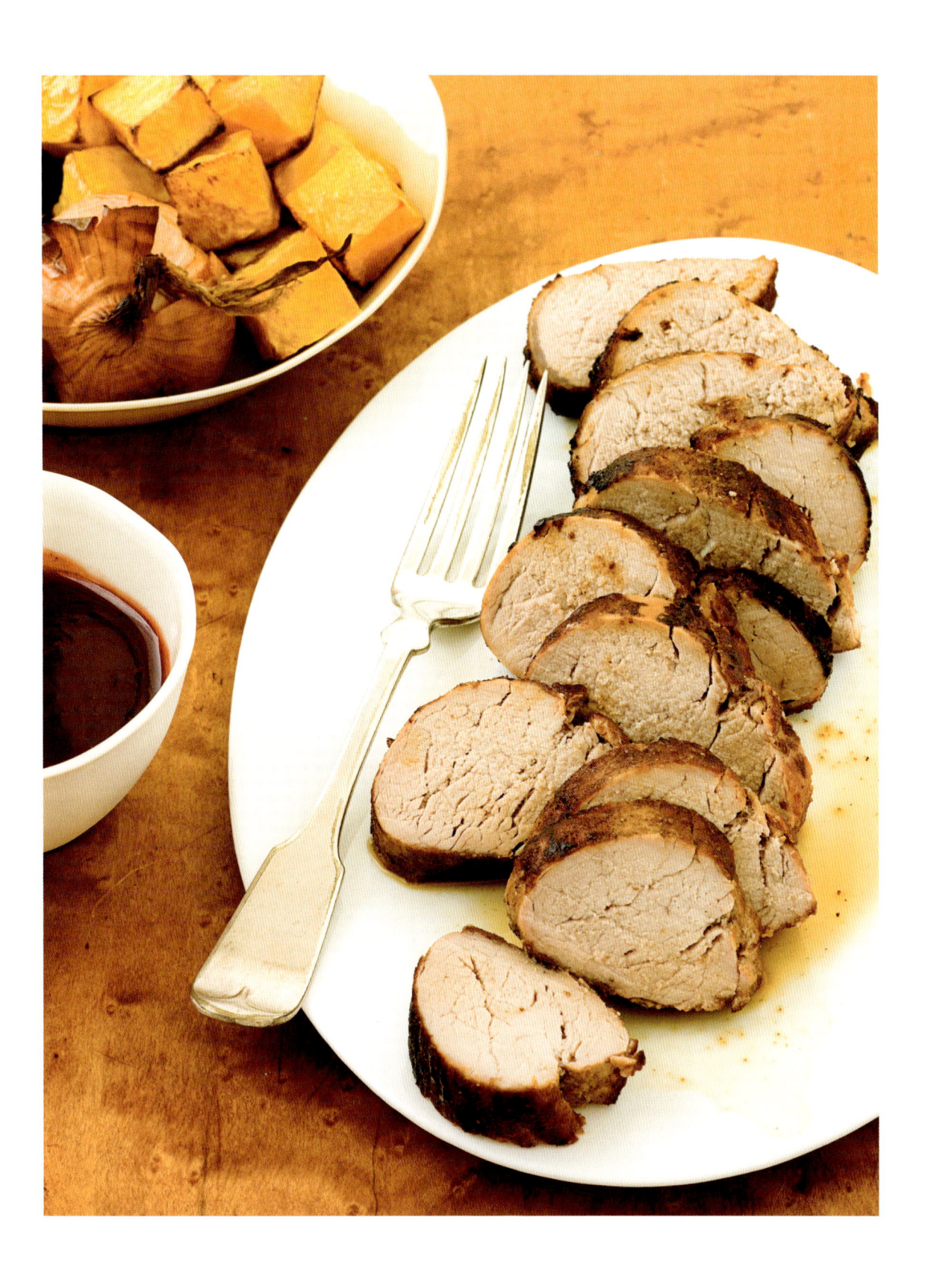

Fish and seafood

Hoisin-glazed salmon with stir-fried bok choy

This sophisticated yet easy dinner combines nature's best source of omega-3 fatty acids with bok choy, a fibre-rich cancer-fighting member of the cabbage family. Hoisin sauce makes the perfect base for a full-flavoured glaze.

1 Preheat the oven to 220°C. Line a small roasting pan with aluminium foil and coat with cooking spray.

2 To make the salmon and glaze, whisk together the hoisin sauce, soy sauce, vinegar, ginger, garlic and sweet chilli sauce in a small bowl. Place the salmon, skin side down, in the roasting pan and spoon or brush the sauce over the salmon. Bake until the flesh is opaque and flakes when prodded with the tip of a knife or a fork, about 15 to 20 minutes, depending on thickness.

3 Meanwhile, for the bok choy, toast the sesame seeds in a small frying pan over medium–low heat, stirring constantly, until golden and fragrant, about 1 to 2 minutes. Transfer to a small bowl to cool.

4 Heat the oil in a large non-stick frying pan or wok over medium–high heat. Add the ginger and garlic and stir-fry until fragrant, 10 to 20 seconds. Add the bok choy and stir-fry for 1 minute. Add 1/3 cup (80 ml) water, cover and cook until crisp-tender, about 4 to 5 minutes. Add the soy sauce and sesame oil and stir to coat. Divide the bok choy between two plates. Place a piece of salmon over each portion. (If the salmon skin sticks to the foil, just lift the fillets.) Sprinkle with sesame seeds and serve with lemon wedges.

MEETING YOUR GOALS
Each portion provides:
1.6 serves vegetables
15 g good fat

SERVES 2
PREPARATION 15 minutes
COOKING 25 minutes

SALMON AND GLAZE
1 tablespoon hoisin sauce
1½ teaspoons salt-reduced soy sauce
1 teaspoon rice vinegar
2 teaspoons grated fresh ginger
1 small clove garlic, crushed
1 teaspoon sweet chilli sauce
250 g salmon fillet, cut into two portions

BOK CHOY
2 teaspoons sesame seeds
2 teaspoons canola oil or peanut oil
1 teaspoon grated fresh ginger
1 small clove garlic, crushed
250 g baby bok choy, rinsed, stem ends trimmed and halved or quartered lengthwise
1 teaspoon salt-reduced soy sauce
1 teaspoon sesame oil
Lemon wedges

NUTRITION • *Per serving*
1299 kilojoules, 27 g protein,
9 g carbohydrate, 4 g fibre,
18 g total fat, 3 g saturated fat,
65 mg cholesterol, 504 mg sodium

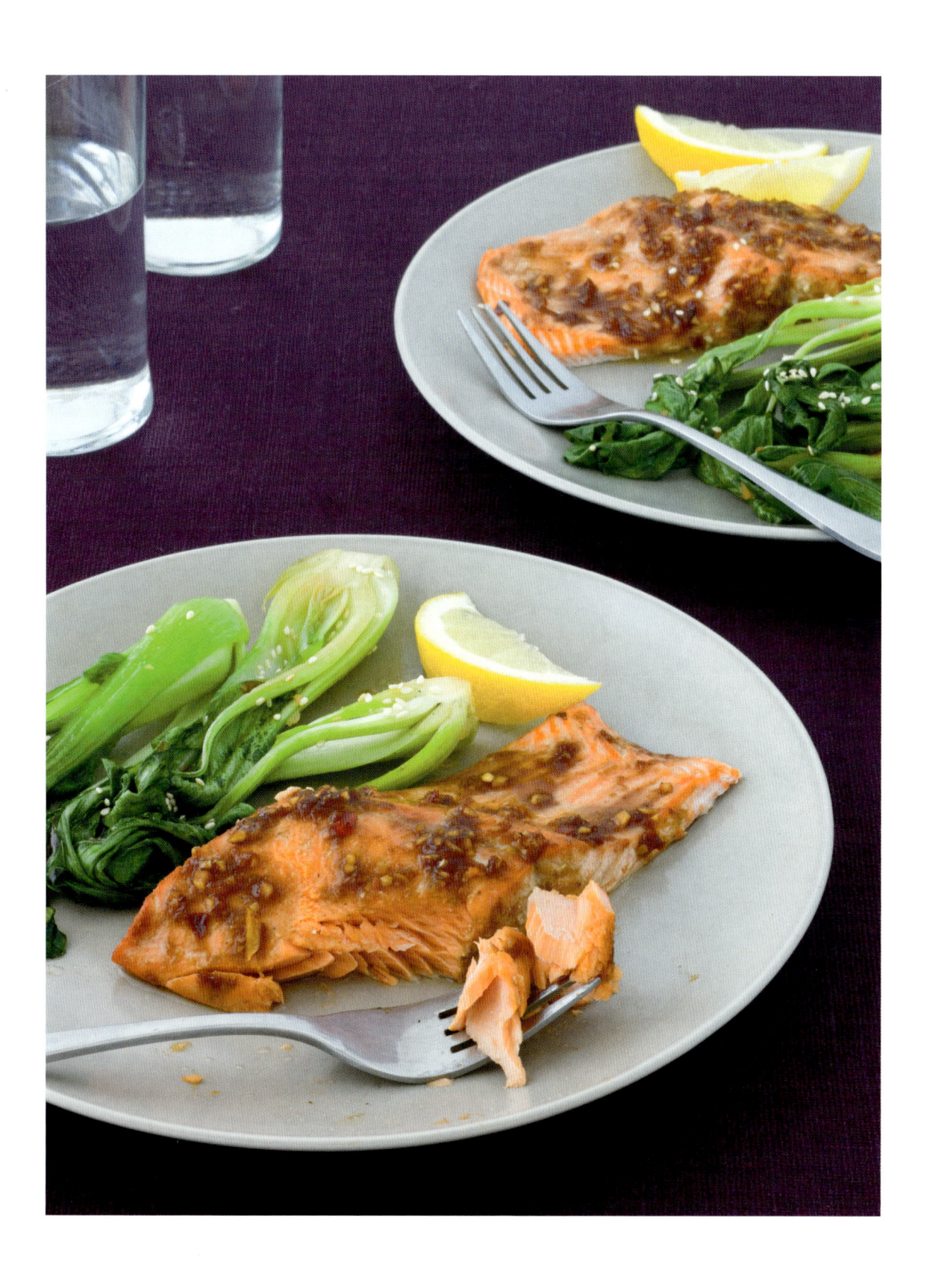

Fish and seafood

Fish and seafood

Coriander prawns with mango salad

Prawns were once thought to be too high in cholesterol, so had to be limited as part of a balanced diet, but that's no longer current thinking. In fact, some of the other sterols found in prawns may have beneficial health effects.

1 Soak 16 bamboo skewers in water for 30 minutes so that they don't burn on contact with heat. Thread one prawn lengthwise onto each skewer.

2 To make the marinade, combine the coriander, 1/3 cup (80 ml) of the lime juice, the green chilli, sesame oil, cumin seeds and garlic in a small bowl. Brush the marinade thoroughly over the prawns and put aside for 10 minutes.

3 Meanwhile, combine the mangoes, spring onions, red chillies, palm sugar, mint leaves, snow pea sprouts and the remaining lime juice in a serving bowl.

4 Preheat the barbecue or a ridged stovetop grill pan. Cook the prawns for 1 minute on each side or until properly cooked through. Serve with bowls of the salad.

MEETING YOUR GOALS
Each portion provides:
0.5 serve vegetables
3 g good fat

SERVES 4
PREPARATION 15 minutes
MARINATING 10 minutes
COOKING 5 minutes

16 large raw prawns (about 750 g), peeled with tails intact

1/4 cup (15 g) chopped fresh coriander leaves

1/2 cup (125 ml) lime juice

1 green chilli, seeded and finely chopped

2 teaspoons sesame oil

1 teaspoon cumin seeds

1 clove garlic, crushed

2 medium green mangoes, thinly sliced

4 spring onions, sliced

2 red chillies, seeded and sliced

2 teaspoons palm sugar or dark brown sugar

1/2 cup (10 g) fresh mint leaves

1/2 cup (45 g) snow pea sprouts

NUTRITION • *Per serving*
1161 kilojoules, 41 g protein,
19 g carbohydrate, 3 g fibre,
4 g total fat, 1 g saturated fat,
279 mg cholesterol, 662 mg sodium

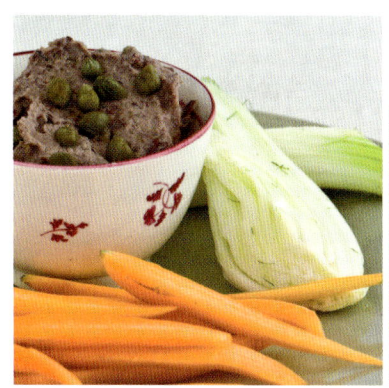

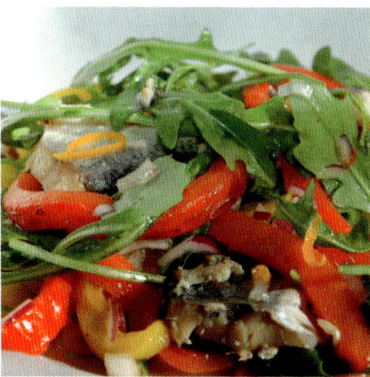

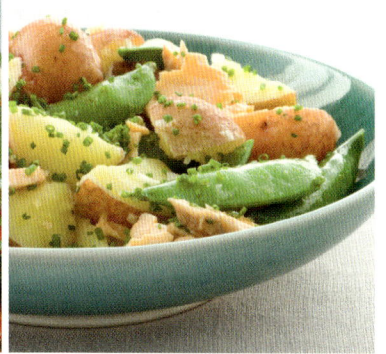

Three ways to use canned fish

Both the Australian National Heart Foundation and the New Zealand Heart Foundation recommend eating fish at least twice a week. For those times when you can't get fresh fish, look to canned to meet your weekly goal.

Tuna tapenade

Serves 4

1 x 180-g can tuna in spring water, drained
¼ cup (30 g) pitted black olives
¼ cup (60 ml) fresh lemon juice
2 tablespoons capers, drained and rinsed
1 teaspoon dijon mustard
½ teaspoon anchovy paste
2 tablespoons extra-virgin olive oil

In a food processor, combine the tuna, olives, lemon juice, capers, mustard and anchovy paste and process until pureed. With the motor running, gradually add the olive oil through the feeder tube. Transfer to a small bowl. Serve with raw vegetable sticks or use as a spread with wholemeal or wholegrain crackers or toast or as sandwich filling.

Greens with sardines and orange dressing

Serves 2

Juice and zest of 1 orange
Freshly ground black pepper
2 tablespoons extra-virgin olive oil
½ small red onion, thinly sliced
4 cups (180 g) mixed salad greens, baby spinach or rocket
2 x 200-g cans sardines in oil
1 medium red capsicum
1 medium yellow capsicum

In a bowl, whisk together the orange juice, zest and pepper. Gradually add the oil, then the onion and greens and toss to coat. With a knife split the sardines lengthwise and remove the backbones. Cut the capsicums into flat sections then place under a hot grill until their skins blacken. Cool, then peel the skins off and slice into long strips. Stir the capsicums and sardines into the salad.

Potato salad with salmon

Serves 4

500 g small red potatoes (such as desiree), scrubbed and quartered
1 teaspoon grated lemon zest
¼ cup (60 ml) fresh lemon juice
1 medium French shallot, finely chopped
Freshly ground black pepper
¼ cup (60 ml) extra-virgin olive oil
2 cups (200 g) sugar snap or snow peas, strings removed
1 x 210-g can salmon, drained and flaked
2 tablespoons snipped chives

Cook the potatoes until tender. In a bowl, whisk together the lemon zest, lemon juice, shallot and pepper. Gradually whisk in the olive oil. Drain the potatoes and toss with the dressing. Cool. Steam the peas 2 to 4 minutes. Refresh under cold water. Add to the potatoes along with the salmon and chives and toss.

Fish and seafood

Tuna-bean cakes with green salad

Together, canned tuna and cannellini beans create delicious fish cakes, and this recipe has a beautifully crisp crust without using too much oil. Add a salad, and dinner's done.

1 Preheat the oven to 220°C. Coat a large baking tray with cooking spray.

2 Heat 1 teaspoon of the oil in a large non-stick frying pan over medium–high heat. Add the onion and celery and cook, stirring frequently, until softened, about 3 to 5 minutes.

3 In a large bowl, mash the beans. Add the tuna, 1 eggwhite, ½ cup (50 g) of the breadcrumbs, the dill, lemon juice, pepper and the onion mixture. Mix together well.

4 Place the remaining 1 cup (100 g) breadcrumbs in a shallow bowl and the remaining eggwhite in another one. Using a generous ¼ cup per cake, form the bean mixture into eight cakes. Coat each with eggwhite, then dredge in breadcrumbs.

5 Heat 1 teaspoon of the oil in a large non-stick frying pan over medium–high heat. Add the tuna cakes and cook until the undersides are browned, about 2 to 3 minutes. Flip the cakes over onto the baking tray and bake until browned and hot in the centre, about 20 minutes.

6 To make the salad and dressing whisk together the lemon juice, garlic and pepper, then gradually whisk in the oil. In a large bowl, toss the rocket and tomatoes with ¼ cup (60 ml) of the dressing. Whisk the mayonnaise into the remaining dressing and stir in the capers.

7 Divide the salad among four plates. Top each serving with two cakes and spoon a little dressing over each.

MEETING YOUR GOALS
Each portion provides:
2.8 serves vegetables
0.6 serve whole grains
18 g good fat

SERVES 4
PREPARATION 45 minutes
COOKING 25 minutes

TUNA CAKES
2 teaspoons olive oil
1 medium onion, chopped
2 stalks celery, chopped
1 x 400-g can cannellini beans, drained and rinsed
1 x 425-g can tuna in spring water, drained
2 large eggwhites, lightly beaten
1½ cups (150 g) dry wholemeal breadcrumbs
2 tablespoons chopped fresh dill or 1½ teaspoons dried dill
1 tablespoon fresh lemon juice
Freshly ground black pepper

SALAD AND DRESSING
¼ cup (60 ml) lemon juice
1 clove garlic, crushed
Freshly ground black pepper
¼ cup (60 ml) olive oil
6 cups (210 g) lettuce leaves, washed and dried
1 cup (150 g) cherry or grape tomatoes, halved
1 tablespoon reduced-fat mayonnaise
2 teaspoons capers, drained, rinsed and chopped

NUTRITION • *Per serving*
2086 kilojoules, 34 g protein, 41 g carbohydrate, 12 g fibre, 21 g total fat, 3 g saturated fat, 37 mg cholesterol, 740 mg sodium

Fish and seafood

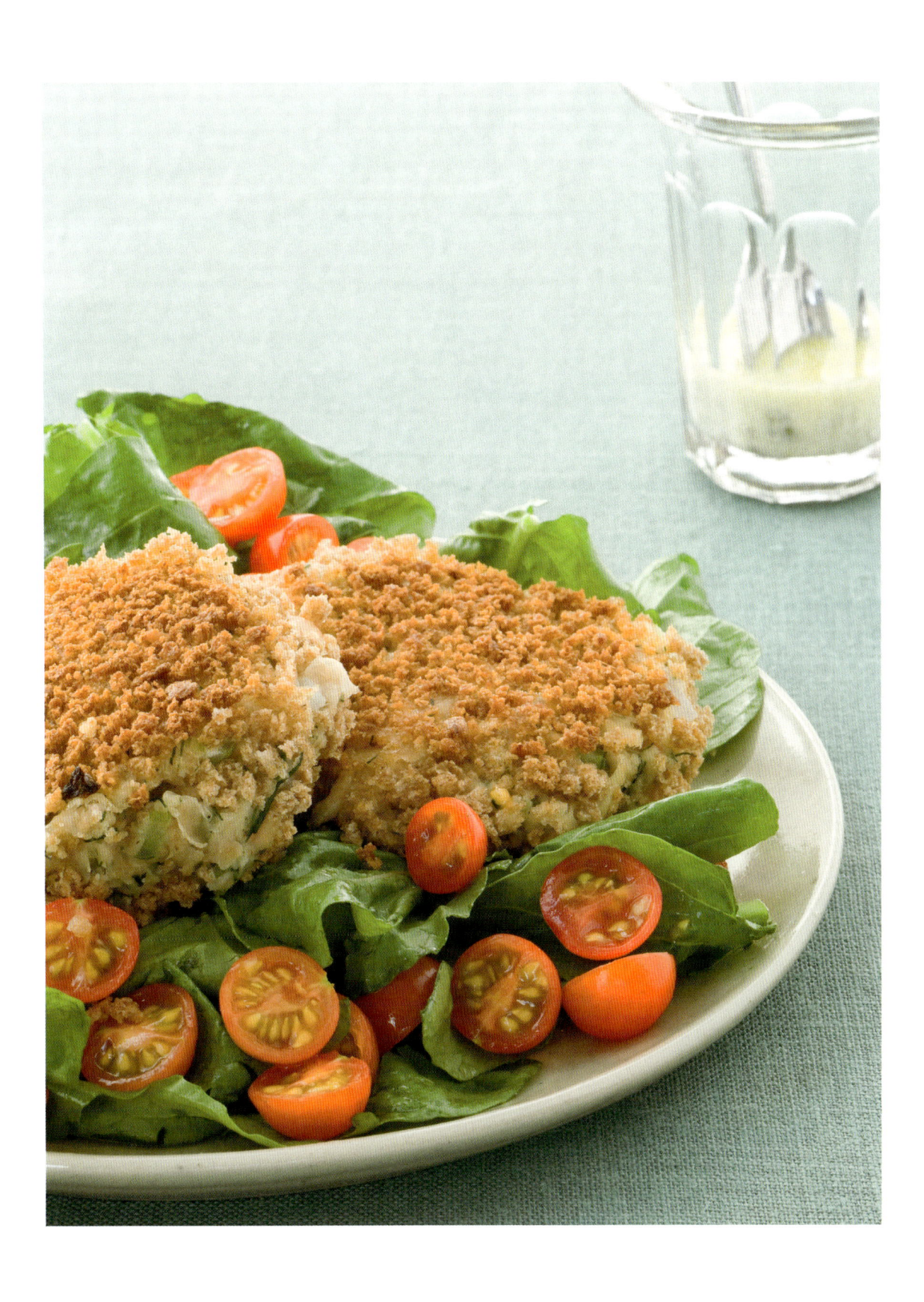

Recipes for good health

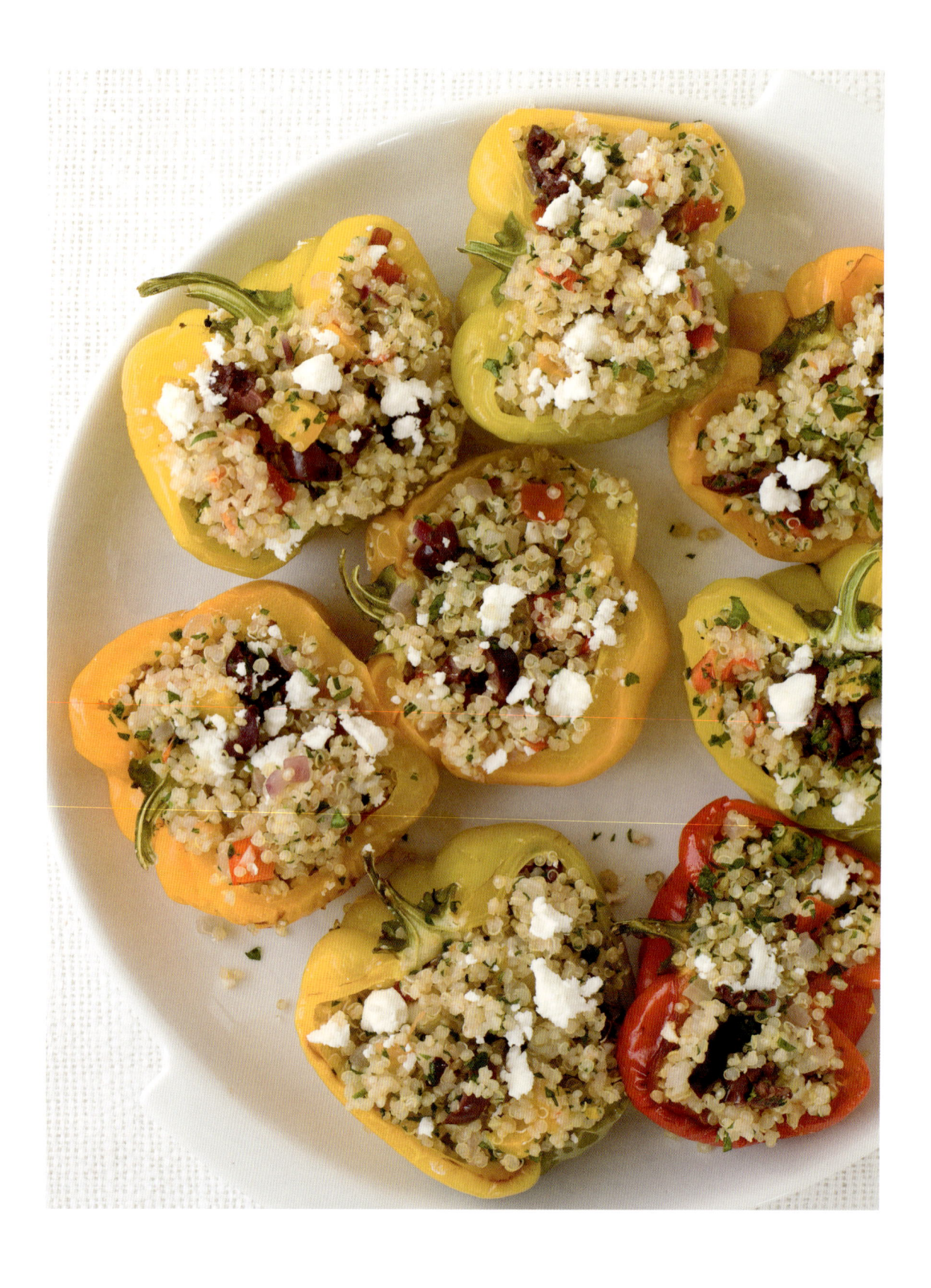

Meatless mains

Quinoa-stuffed capsicums

This recipe features high-protein quinoa enlivened with the flavours of a Greek salad. Serve as a vegetarian main meal or a side dish with chicken, pork or fish.

1 Preheat the oven to 220°C. Coat a large baking tray with cooking spray. Place the capsicum halves, cut side down, on the baking tray and bake just until tender, about 12 to 15 minutes. When cool enough to handle, discard the stems from two of the halves and coarsely chop the capsicum flesh. Set aside. Reduce the oven temperature to 175°C.

2 Meanwhile, in a saucepan, combine the quinoa and 1½ cups (375 ml) water. Bring to a simmer, cover and cook over low heat until the quinoa is tender and most of the liquid has been absorbed, about 12 to 15 minutes. Leave to stand for 5 minutes, then fluff the grains using a fork.

3 Heat the oil in a large non-stick frying pan over medium–high heat. Add the onion and cook, stirring frequently, until softened. Add the garlic and oregano and cook, stirring, until fragrant. Stir in the tomato and cook for 3 minutes. Remove from the heat. Stir in the quinoa, reserved chopped capsicums, feta, olives, parsley and pepper and mix well.

4 Using about ⅔ cup per capsicum shell, divide the quinoa mixture among the remaining eight capsicum halves. Place in a medium baking dish. (If you're making this meal ahead of time, you can cover and refrigerate for up to two days.)

5 Add 2 tablespoons water to the baking dish and cover with foil. Bake until the filling is heated through, about 30 to 40 minutes. Serve two halves for a main meal; one half as a side.

SERVES 4
PREPARATION 40 minutes
COOKING 1 hour

4 large red, yellow and/or orange capsicums, halved lengthwise (leave stems intact) and seeded

¾ cup (150 g) quinoa, rinsed well

2 teaspoons olive oil

1 cup (155 g) chopped red onion

3 cloves garlic, crushed

1 teaspoon dried oregano

1 medium tomato, seeded and diced

1 cup (150 g) crumbled feta

⅓ cup (40 g) pitted black olives, chopped

⅓ cup (20 g) chopped fresh parsley

Freshly ground black pepper

NUTRITION • *Per main-dish serving*
1406 kilojoules, 15 g protein, 35 g carbohydrate, 5 g fibre, 16 g total fat, 7 g saturated fat, 26 mg cholesterol, 543 mg sodium

MEETING YOUR GOALS
Each main-dish portion provides:
3.8 serves vegetables
1.1 serves whole grains
9 g good fat

Meatless mains

Penne with parsley-walnut pesto and green beans

Two time-honoured pairings—green beans and walnuts, and pasta and pesto—come together in this simple dish. Using walnuts instead of the traditional pine nuts in pesto is an easy way to boost your intake of omega-3 fatty acids.

1 Bring a large pot of water to the boil. Meanwhile, toast the walnuts in a small dry frying pan over medium–low heat, stirring constantly, until fragrant, about 2 to 3 minutes. Transfer to a plate and leave to cool.

2 In a food processor, combine the parsley, garlic, pepper and ¼ cup (25 g) of the walnuts. Process until the walnuts are ground. With the motor running, gradually add the oil through the feeder tube. Add the cheese and pulse until mixed in thoroughly.

3 Add the penne to the boiling water and cook for about 6 minutes. Add the beans and cook until penne is al dente (almost tender) and the beans are crisp-tender, about 5 minutes. Reserve ½ cup (125 ml) of the cooking water, then drain the penne and beans and place in a large bowl. Add the pesto and reserved cooking water and toss to coat well. Sprinkle with the remaining toasted walnuts.

SERVES 3
PREPARATION 20 minutes
COOKING 15 minutes

⅓ cup (35 g) walnut halves, coarsely chopped

¼ cup (15 g) lightly packed fresh parsley leaves, washed and dried

1 clove garlic, crushed

Freshly ground black pepper

2 tablespoons extra-virgin olive oil

¼ cup (25 g) freshly grated parmesan

1½ cups (135 g) wholemeal penne or rigatoni pasta

2 cups (250 g) trimmed and halved green beans

NUTRITION • *Per serving*
1610 kilojoules, 12 g protein, 30 g carbohydrate, 8 g fibre, 24 g total fat, 4 g saturated fat, 8 mg cholesterol, 130 mg sodium

MEETING YOUR GOALS
Each portion provides:
1 serve vegetables
1.7 serves whole grains
20 g good fat

Meatless mains | 353

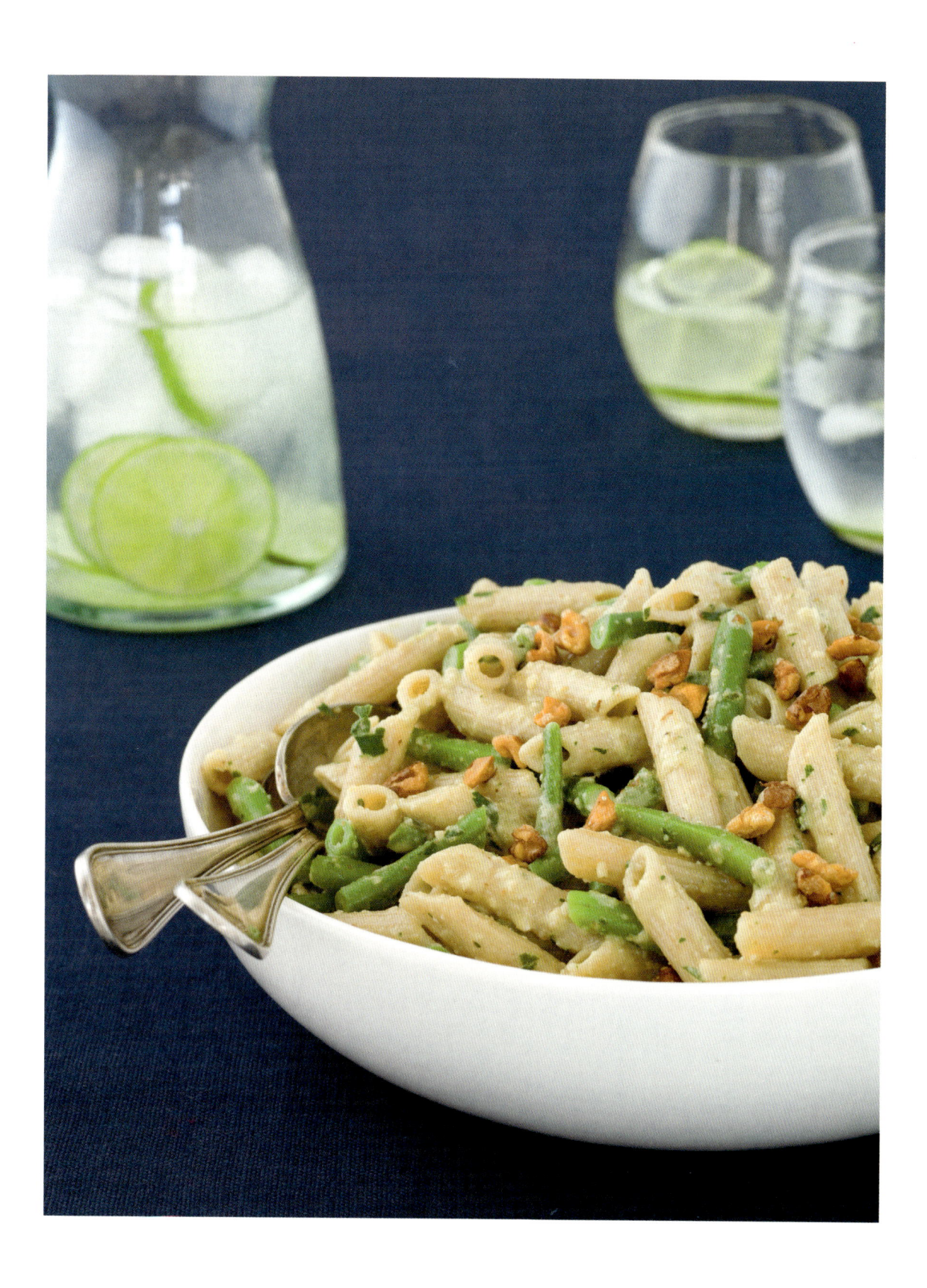

Meatless mains

Wholemeal lasagne with mushrooms and silverbeet

To give crowd-pleasing lasagne a healthy update, we've used wholemeal lasagne and layers of vegetables rather than fatty mince. And instead of silverbeet, you can use spinach, cooked according to the instructions for silverbeet, below.

1 Preheat the oven to 200°C. Bring about 2 cm of water to the boil in a large pot. Separate the stems from the silverbeet leaves (see Tip on opposite page). Wash the stems and leaves thoroughly. Cut the stems into medium lengths and the leaves into medium pieces. Add the stems to the boiling water, cover and cook for 3 minutes. Add the leaves to the pot, cover and cook until wilted and tender. Drain, refresh under cold running water, then press out excess water.

2 Heat 2 teaspoons of the oil in a large non-stick frying pan over medium–high heat. Add half of the mushrooms and cook, turning occasionally, until browned and tender, about 4 to 6 minutes. Transfer to a large bowl. Add another 2 teaspoons oil to the frying pan, sauté the remaining mushrooms then transfer to the bowl.

3 Add the remaining 2 teaspoons oil to the frying pan, along with the garlic and oregano, and stir until fragrant. Add the silverbeet and turn to coat. Transfer to the bowl with the mushrooms. Season with pepper and toss to mix.

4 In a bowl, whisk together the egg, ricotta, 1/3 cup (35 g) of the parmesan and the remaining pepper.

5 To assemble the lasagne, coat a large baking dish with cooking spray. Spread about 1/2 cup (125 g) of the pasta sauce in the baking dish and arrange three lasagne sheets over the sauce. Spread about 2/3 cup (160 g) of the ricotta mixture over the lasagne sheets and scatter about 1 1/3 cups vegetables on the ricotta. Spoon another 1/2 cup (125 g) pasta sauce over the vegetables and sprinkle with 1/2 cup (75 g) mozzarella. Add another layer of lasagne sheets and repeat the layering with the ricotta, vegetables,

SERVES 9
PREPARATION 1 hour
COOKING 1 hour 10 minutes

1 bunch silverbeet

1 1/2 tablespoons olive oil

5 cups assorted mushrooms, such as Swiss browns, shiitake (discard stems) and/or oyster mushrooms, wiped clean and quartered

3 cloves garlic, crushed

1/2 teaspoon dried oregano

Freshly ground black pepper

1 large egg

2 cups (500 g) reduced-fat ricotta

2/3 cup (65 g) freshly grated parmesan

3 cups (750 g) prepared tomato pasta sauce

12 wholemeal instant lasagne sheets

2 cups (300 g) grated reduced-fat mozzarella

NUTRITION • *Per serving*
1547 kilojoules, 26 g protein, 22 g carbohydrate, 4 g fibre, 18 g total fat, 9 g saturated fat, 80 mg cholesterol, 495 mg sodium

pasta sauce, mozzarella and lasagne sheets two more times. Spread the remaining sauce evenly over the final layer of lasagne. (Reserve the remaining parmesan and mozzarella.) Cover with a sheet of baking paper and then aluminium foil. (If making ahead, cover and refrigerate for up to two days.)

6 Bake, covered, for about 35 minutes. Sprinkle with the remaining $1/3$ cup (35 g) parmesan and $1/2$ cup (75 g) mozzarella. Bake, uncovered, until the pasta sheets are tender and the lasagne is bubbly, about 15 minutes. Let stand for at least 5 minutes before serving.

Tip To prepare silverbeet, fold each leaf in half lengthwise. Place a large knife at a slight angle to the stem and cut off the stem, including the thicker portion in the leaf area. Wash the stems and greens in several changes of water. Trim the ragged ends of the stems, then cut the stems as desired. Stack several leaves, then roll. Using a sharp knife, cut the leaves into ribbons, then turn the ribbons and cut again.

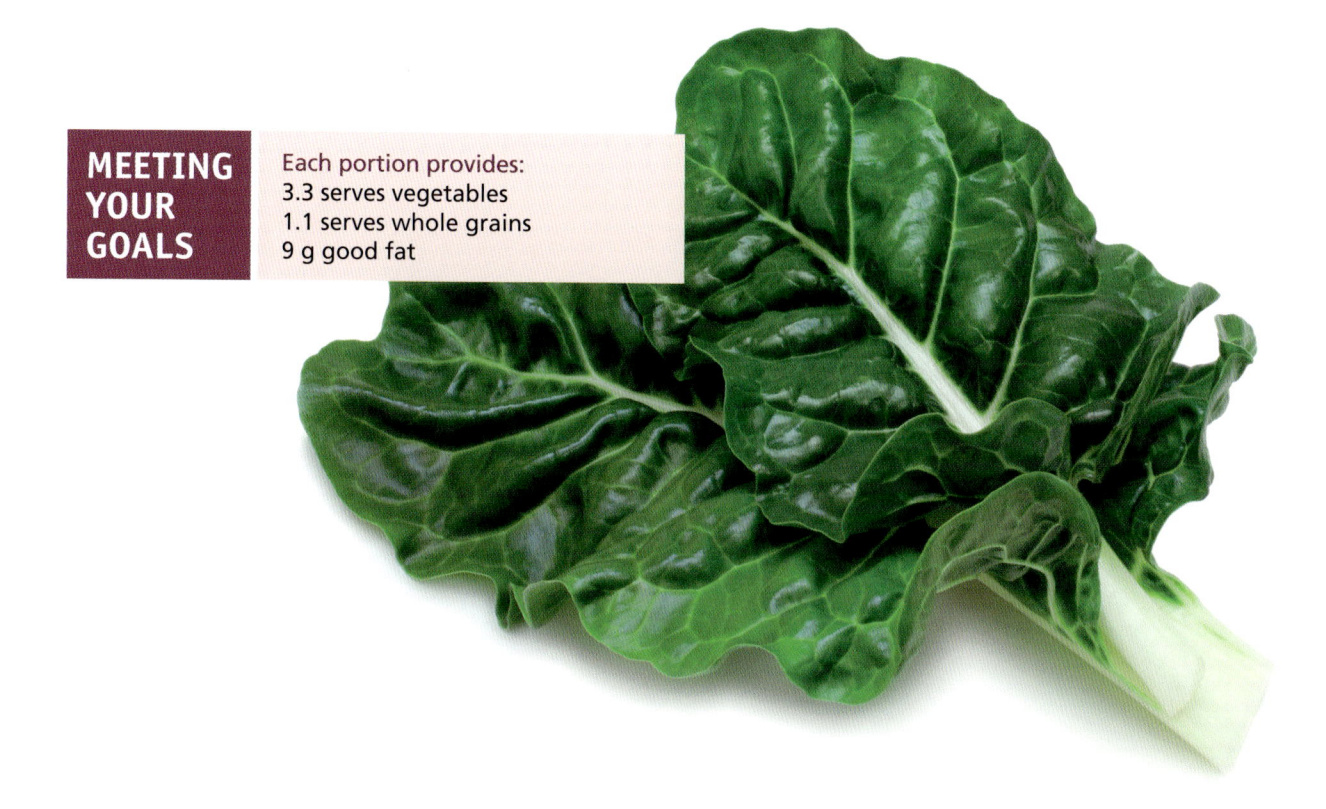

MEETING YOUR GOALS

Each portion provides:
3.3 serves vegetables
1.1 serves whole grains
9 g good fat

Meatless mains

Lentil and spinach ragout

This warm, hearty ragout features cholesterol-lowering lentils and nearly two serves of vegetables per portion. A drizzle of olive oil gives this comforting dish a delicious finish; use good-quality olive oil for heightened flavour.

1 Heat 1 tablespoon of the oil in a large pot over medium heat. Add the onions and carrots and cook, stirring frequently, until softened, about 4 to 6 minutes. Add the garlic and cook, stirring, for 30 seconds. Add the lentils and thyme and stir to coat. Add the stock and bay leaf and bring to a simmer. Reduce the heat to low, cover and simmer for 20 minutes.

2 Add the pasta shells and simmer, covered, stirring occasionally, until the pasta and lentils are almost tender, about 10 to 15 minutes.

3 Add the tomatoes and simmer, covered, until the lentils and pasta shells are tender and the mixture has thickened, about 5 to 10 minutes. Discard the bay leaf. Add the spinach and cook, stirring, just until wilted, about a minute. Stir in the lemon juice and season with pepper. The ragout will keep, covered, in the refrigerator for up to two days. Top each serving with a drizzle of the remaining oil.

MEETING YOUR GOALS
Each portion provides:
1.8 serves vegetables
0.3 serve whole grains
7 g good fat

SERVES 10
PREPARATION 20 minutes
COOKING 50 minutes

1/3 cup (80 ml) extra-virgin olive oil

2 medium onions, chopped

1 cup (155 g) diced carrots

6 cloves garlic, crushed

1 1/4 cups (230 g) brown lentils, rinsed and picked over

1 teaspoon dried thyme

6 cups (1.5 litres) salt-reduced chicken or vegetable stock

1 bay leaf

1 1/4 cups (115 g) wholemeal pasta shells

1 x 410-g can diced tomatoes

8 cups (400 g) baby English spinach, washed and dried

2 tablespoons fresh lemon juice

Freshly ground black pepper

NUTRITION • *Per serving*
850 kilojoules, 11 g protein, 22 g carbohydrate, 6 g fibre, 8 g total fat, 1 g saturated fat, 0 mg cholesterol, 435 mg sodium

Meatless mains

Macaroni cheese with vegetables

This is a refreshingly healthy version of an old classic. A generous quantity of vegetables cooks alongside wholemeal pasta, while the calcium-rich sauce is made in the same pot, making this a one-pot family favourite. Just add a salad.

1 Bring a large pot of water to the boil. In a small frying pan, combine the breadcrumbs and oil. Cook over medium–low heat, stirring constantly, until golden and crisp, about 2 to 3 minutes. Transfer to a small bowl to cool. In a small bowl, combine the cornflour, mustard and chilli.

2 Add the cauliflower and macaroni to the boiling water and cook just until tender, about 7 minutes (the macaroni will continue to cook while you make the sauce). Add the spinach and stir to submerge, then drain immediately.

3 Return the macaroni and vegetables to the pot. Add the cornflour mixture and stir to coat well, then stir in the milk. Cook over medium–high heat, stirring, until the milk starts to bubble and thicken. Remove from the heat, add the cheese and stir until melted and smooth, then season with pepper. Sprinkle each serving with 1 tablespoon toasted breadcrumbs.

MEETING YOUR GOALS
Each portion provides:
2.1 serves vegetables
1.7 serves whole grains
4 g good fat

SERVES 5
PREPARATION 15 minutes
COOKING 10 minutes

¼ cup (25 g) dry wholemeal breadcrumbs

1 teaspoon olive oil

2 tablespoons cornflour

1¼ teaspoons mustard powder

⅛ teaspoon chilli powder

3 cups (375 g) cauliflower florets

2 cups (about 300 g) wholemeal macaroni

6 cups (about 300 g) baby English spinach, washed and dried

1½ cups (375 ml) low-fat milk

1½ cups (185 g) grated reduced-fat cheese, such as cheddar

Freshly ground black pepper

NUTRITION • *Per serving*
1565 kilojoules, 27 g protein,
52 g carbohydrate, 8 g fibre,
6 g total fat, 2 g saturated fat,
15 mg cholesterol, 363 mg sodium

Meatless mains

Tofu in peanut sauce with sweet potatoes and spinach

If you're looking for ways to turn yourself and your family on to tofu, this recipe is the way to do it. Peanut butter lends a richness to the sauce, while sweet potato and spinach add colour and powerful nutrients.

1 In a large saucepan, combine the rice and 3 ¾ cups (935 ml) water. Bring to a simmer, then reduce the heat to low, cover and simmer until the rice is tender and most of the liquid has been absorbed, 45 to 50 minutes.

2 Meanwhile, heat the oil in a large pot over medium–high heat. Add the onion and cook, stirring often, until softened, 2 to 3 minutes. Add garlic, chillies and curry powder, then cook, stirring, until fragrant, about 20 seconds. Add the tofu and stir to coat. Add the stock, tomatoes and sweet potato. Bring to a simmer, then reduce the heat to low, cover and simmer until the sweet potato is tender, about 20 to 25 minutes.

3 Add the peanut butter and stir until blended, then gradually add the spinach, stirring until it has wilted. Stir in the lime juice. Spoon the stew over rice then sprinkle a tablespoon of peanuts over each portion. Serve with lime wedges and Tabasco sauce. The stew will keep, covered, in the refrigerator for up to two days.

SERVES 10
PREPARATION 30 minutes
COOKING 50 minutes

1½ cups (300 g) brown rice
1 tablespoon canola oil
1 medium onion, chopped
3 cloves garlic, crushed
2 long red chillies, seeded and finely chopped
1 tablespoon curry powder
800 g firm tofu, drained, patted dry and cut into small cubes
2½ cups (625 ml) vegetable or salt-reduced chicken stock
1 x 410-g can diced tomatoes
1 medium sweet potato, peeled and cut into medium pieces
½ cup (125 g) natural peanut butter
12 cups (600 g) baby English spinach, washed and dried
2 tablespoons lime juice
⅔ cup (110 g) unsalted roasted peanuts, coarsely chopped
Lime wedges
Tabasco sauce

NUTRITION • *Per serving*
1246 kilojoules, 11 g protein,
31 g carbohydrate, 5 g fibre,
15 g total fat, 2 g saturated fat,
0 mg cholesterol, 340 mg sodium

MEETING YOUR GOALS
Each portion provides:
2 serves vegetables
1.1 serves whole grains
13 g good fat

Meatless mains

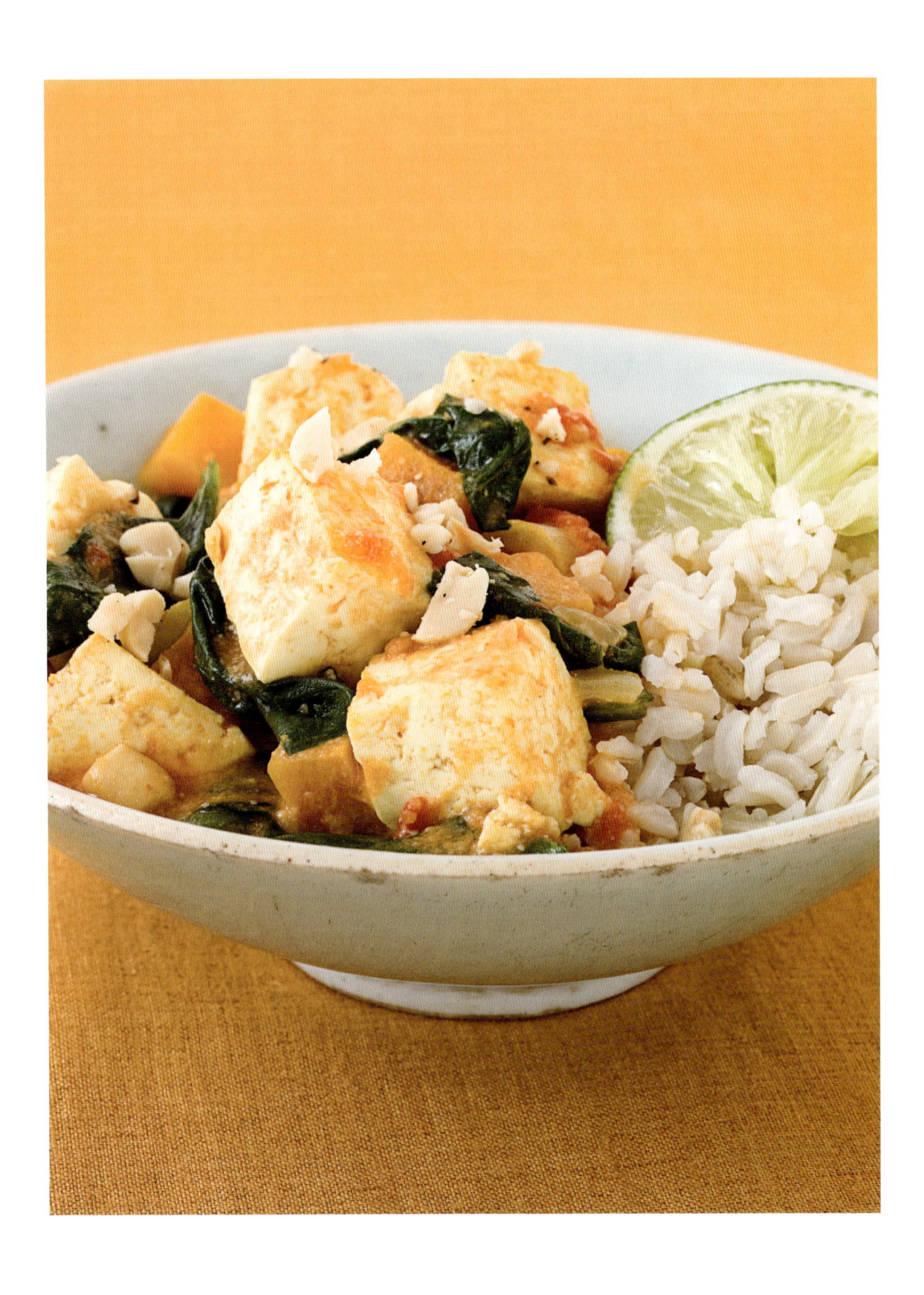

Sides

Coleslaw with gado gado

With its delicate flavour and crisp texture, Chinese cabbage (also known as wombok) makes an appealing alternative to traditional green cabbage in a coleslaw. Instead of a saturated fat-laden mayonnaise, this coleslaw is dressed with a spicy peanut dressing that is rich in good fat.

1 Place the peanut butter in a large bowl and gradually whisk in the hot tea. Add the soy sauce, vinegar, palm sugar, Tabasco and garlic and whisk until smooth.

2 Add the cabbage, carrots and spring onions and toss to coat well. Sprinkle with peanuts.

Tip This coleslaw gets watery as it sits, so toss it with the dressing just before serving. However, you can prepare the vegetables and dressing up to a day ahead and store them in separate covered containers in the refrigerator.

MEETING YOUR GOALS

Each portion provides:
2 serves vegetables
1.1 serves whole grains
10 g good fat

SERVES 6
PREPARATION 20 minutes

⅓ cup (90 g) natural peanut butter

¼ cup (60 ml) hot brewed black or green tea

1 tablespoon salt-reduced soy sauce

1 tablespoon rice vinegar

1½ teaspoons palm sugar or dark brown sugar

1 teaspoon Tabasco sauce

1 clove garlic, crushed

4 cups (180 g) thinly sliced Chinese cabbage (wombok)

1 cup (155 g) grated carrot

½ cup (60 g) chopped spring onions

⅓ cup (50 g) unsalted roasted peanuts

NUTRITION • *Per serving*
652 kilojoules, 7 g protein,
5 g carbohydrate, 4 g fibre,
12 g total fat, 2 g saturated fat,
0 mg cholesterol, 183 mg sodium

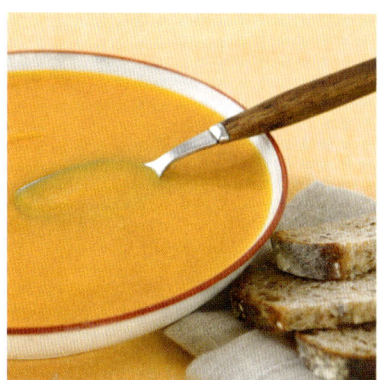

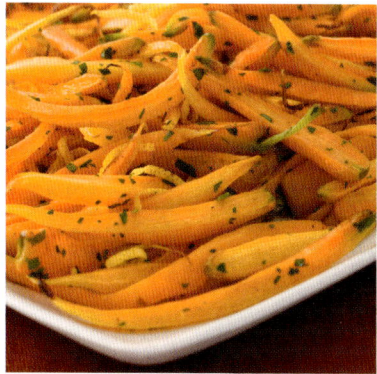

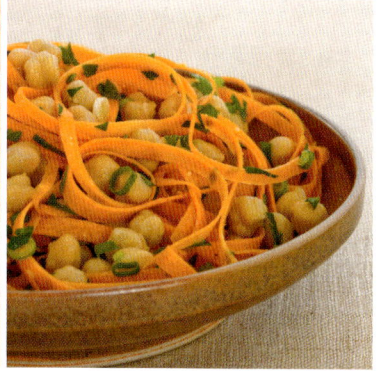

Three great ways to eat carrots

Sturdy carrots are great keepers, so stock up. They're a superb source of beta-carotene—an anti-cancer agent that also guards against diseases such as macular degeneration, cataracts and even arthritis. These simple recipes demonstrate how delicious and versatile the common carrot can be.

Carrot-ginger soup

Serves 5

4 cups (1 litre) salt-reduced chicken stock
12 baby carrots, peeled
1 cup (155 g) chopped onion
2 tablespoons grated fresh ginger
1 clove garlic, crushed
¼ teaspoon ground turmeric
¼ teaspoon curry powder
⅓ cup (80 ml) orange juice

In a large saucepan over medium–low heat, simmer the stock, carrots, onion, ginger, garlic, turmeric and curry powder until very tender, 25 to 35 minutes. Remove from the heat and allow the mixture to cool a little. Working in two batches, puree the soup in a blender. Return to the pan, reheat if necessary, and stir in the orange juice.

Lemony roasted carrots

Serves 2

3 cups (270 g) carrot sticks
2 teaspoons olive oil
Freshly ground black pepper
1 tablespoon chopped fresh parsley
1 teaspoon grated lemon zest
1 tablespoon fresh lemon juice

Preheat the oven to 220°C. Lightly oil a rimmed baking tray. In a medium bowl, toss the carrots with the oil and pepper. Spread on the baking tray and bake, stirring once or twice, until tender and lightly browned, about 20 minutes. Toss with the parsley, lemon zest and lemon juice.

Carrot and chickpea salad

Serves 4

¼ cup (60 ml) olive oil
2 tablespoons fresh lemon juice
1 small clove garlic, crushed
1 teaspoon ground cumin
Freshly ground black pepper
2 cups (180 g) shredded carrots
1 x 200-g can chickpeas, drained and rinsed
2 tablespoons chopped fresh parsley
2 tablespoons chopped spring onions

In a medium bowl, whisk the oil, lemon juice, garlic, cumin and pepper. Add the carrots, chickpeas, parsley and spring onions and toss to coat.

Recipes for good health

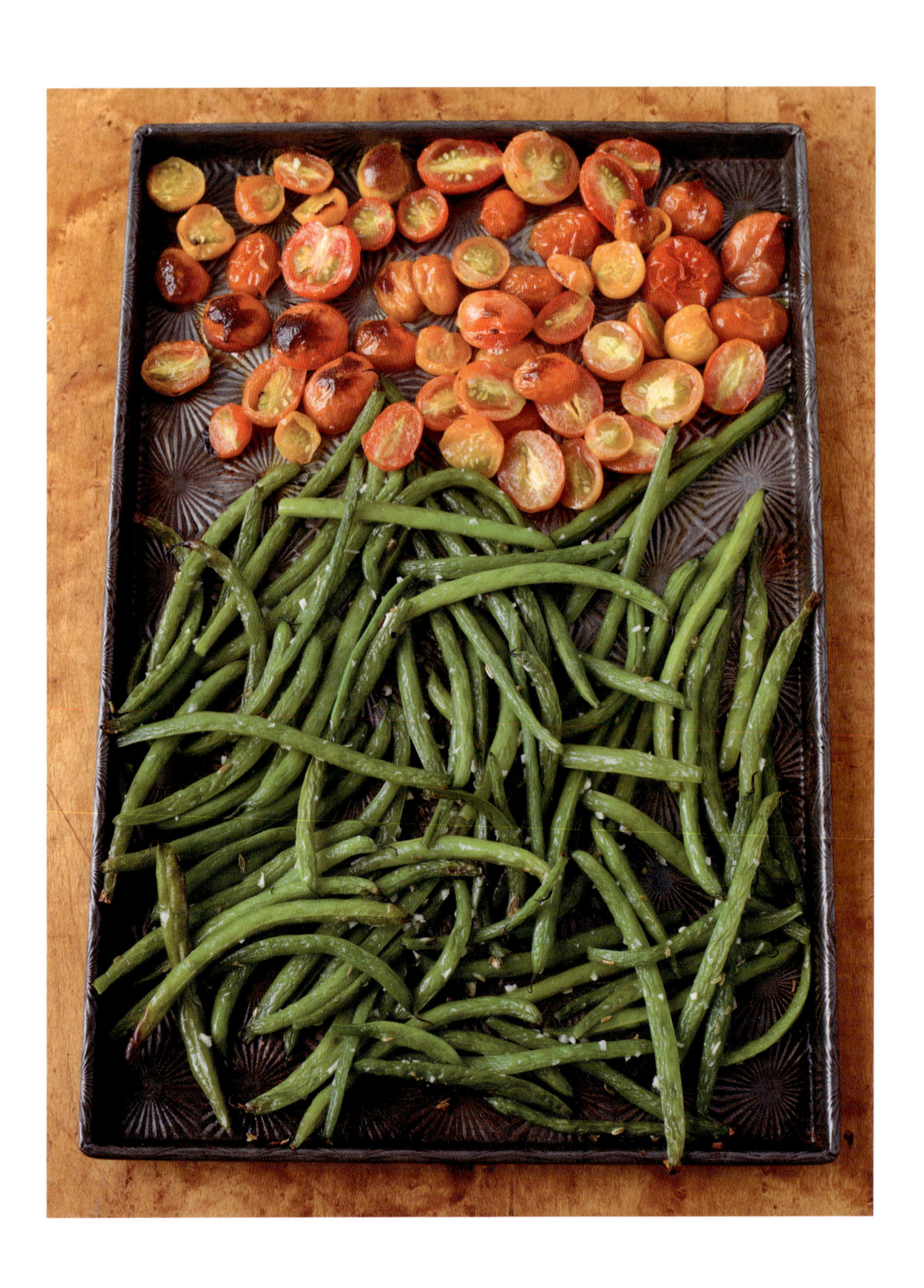

Sides

Roasted green beans and cherry tomatoes

Roasting vegetables in a hot oven is an excellent way to bring out their inherent sweetness. Green beans are delicious when roasted, but to become tender, they must be blanched before roasting. The tomatoes roasted alongside form a light but flavourful sauce for the garlicky beans.

1 Bring a large pot of water to the boil. Preheat the oven to 220°C. Coat a large rimmed baking tray with cooking spray.

2 Cook the beans in the boiling water until crisp-tender, about 3 to 4 minutes, then drain and refresh under cold running water to halt the cooking process.

3 Using the bottom of a saucepan, crush the fennel seeds on a cutting board to bring out their fragrance. Transfer to a bowl and add garlic, 2 teaspoons of the oil and the beans, then toss to coat. Spread the beans on one end of the baking tray. In the same bowl, combine the tomatoes, the remaining 2 teaspoons oil, brown sugar, balsamic vinegar and pepper. Toss to coat. Spread on the other end of the baking tray.

4 Bake the vegetables until the beans are tender and browned in spots, and the tomatoes start to collapse, about 20 to 25 minutes. Toss the beans and tomatoes together.

SERVES 4
PREPARATION 20 minutes
COOKING 30 minutes

400 g green beans, trimmed
2 teaspoons fennel seeds
1 clove garlic, crushed
1 tablespoon olive oil
1 2/3 cups (260 g) cherry or grape tomatoes
1 tablespoon soft brown sugar
1 tablespoon balsamic vinegar
Freshly ground black pepper

NUTRITION • *Per serving*
388 kilojoules, 3 g protein,
9 g carbohydrate, 4 g fibre,
5 g total fat, 1 g saturated fat,
0 mg cholesterol, 12 mg sodium

MEETING YOUR GOALS
Each portion provides:
1.9 serves vegetables
4 g good fat

Baked goods
Oat and apricot choc-chip cookies

The secret ingredient in these oat cookies is canned beans. They do a superb job of standing in for butter, and no one will notice the difference. Dried apricots contrast beautifully with dark chocolate, while toasted nuts add healthy fat.

1 Preheat the oven to 180°C. Line several baking trays with baking paper or coat with cooking spray.

2 In a small bowl, combine the apricots and orange juice. Cover loosely with plastic wrap and microwave on *High* for 1 minute. Set aside to plump and cool.

3 Spread the almonds in a small baking dish and bake until fragrant, 10 to 12 minutes. Transfer to a plate and let cool. In a large bowl, whisk the flour and bicarbonate of soda.

4 Puree the beans in a food processor. Add the egg, eggwhites, brown sugar, sugar, oil and vanilla. Process until smooth, stopping once or twice to scrape down the sides of the bowl. Scrape into the flour mixture and mix with a spatula. Stir in the oats, chocolate chips, ginger, apricots and almonds.

5 Drop the batter by tablespoon 5 cm apart on the baking trays. Bake one batch at a time until the edges of the cookies are golden, about 14 to 16 minutes. Let cool on the baking tray for 2 minutes. Transfer to a wire rack to cool completely.

MAKES 50
PREPARATION 25 minutes
COOKING 30 minutes

1 cup (180 g) dried apricots, coarsely chopped

¼ cup (60 ml) orange juice

½ cup (80 g) almonds, coarsely chopped

1 cup (150 g) white wholemeal plain flour

½ teaspoon bicarbonate of soda

1 cup (200 g) drained canned cannellini beans, rinsed

1 large egg

2 large eggwhites

⅔ cup (155 g) firmly packed soft brown sugar

⅔ cup (140 g) sugar

½ cup (125 ml) canola oil or light olive oil

2 teaspoons vanilla extract

2 cups (200 g) rolled oats

1 cup (170 g) dark chocolate chips

¼ cup (55 g) glacé ginger, finely chopped

NUTRITION • *Per serving*
982 kilojoules, 4 g protein, 32 g carbohydrate, 3 g fibre, 10 g total fat, 2 g saturated fat, 9 mg cholesterol, 77 mg sodium

MEETING YOUR GOALS
Each portion provides:
0.2 serve fruit
0.3 serve whole grains
8 g good fat

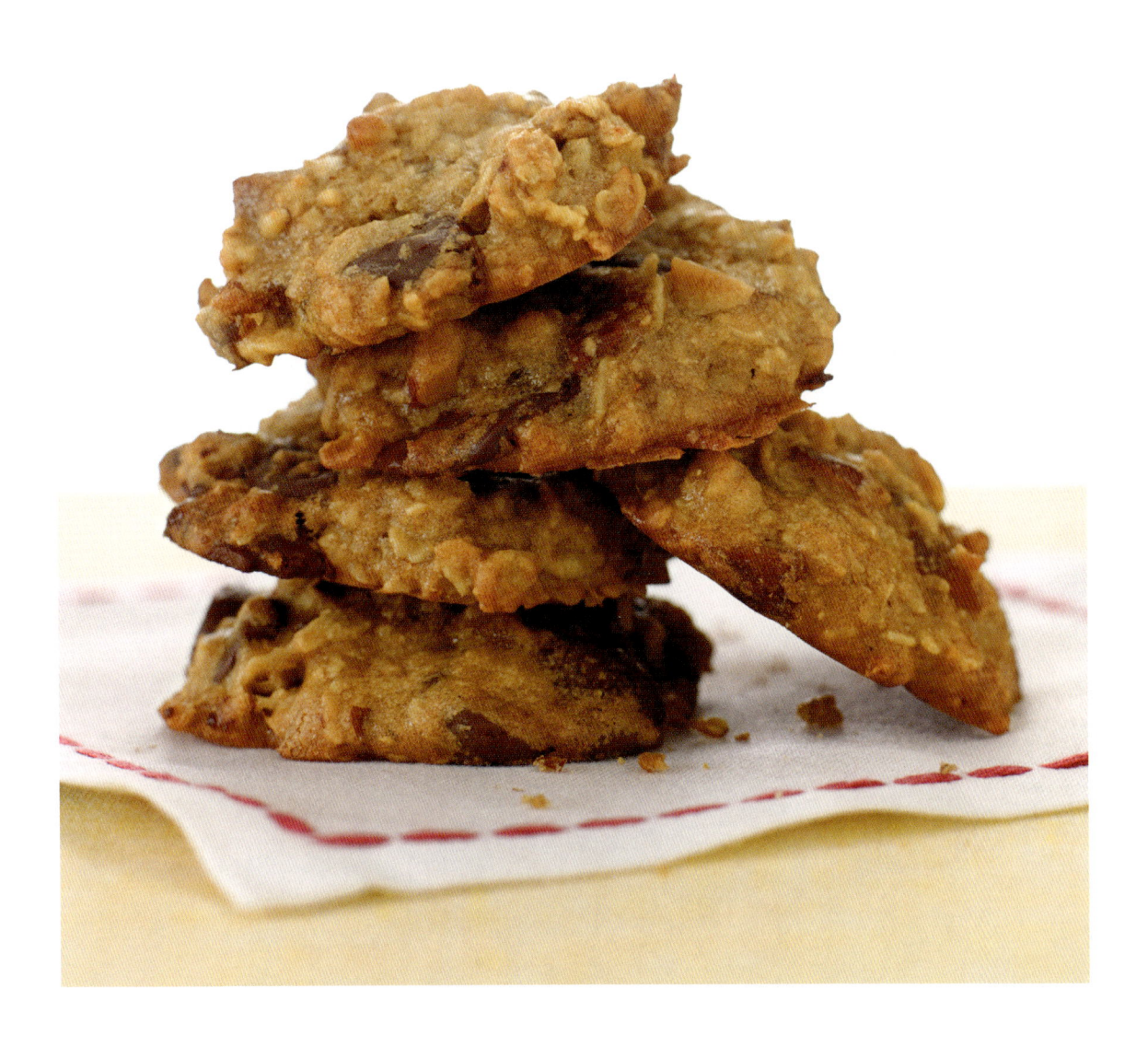

Recipes for good health

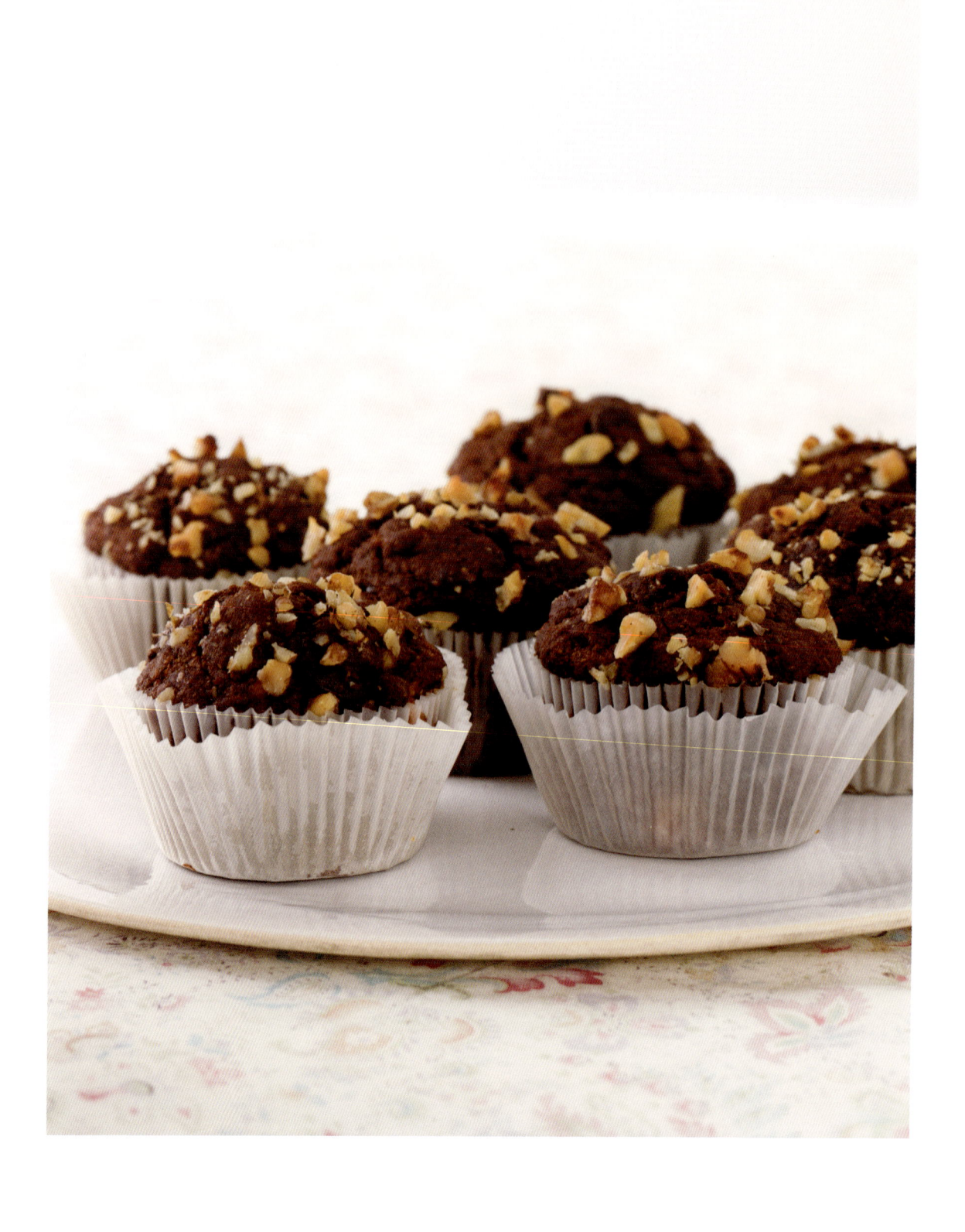

Baked goods

Banana-chocolate muffins

The cocoa and dark chocolate chips in these tasty muffins contribute a wonderful flavour as well as anti-oxidant health benefits. These muffins are tender and moist, thanks to the canola oil and mashed banana.

1 Preheat the oven to 200°C. Coat a 12-hole standard size muffin tray with cooking spray.

2 Spread ¼ cup (25 g) walnuts in a small baking tray. Toast in the oven until fragrant, about 6 to 8 minutes, then cool.

3 Sift the cocoa into a large bowl and add the flour and bicarbonate of soda, then whisk to blend. In a bowl, whisk the egg, sugar, buttermilk, banana, oil and vanilla. Add to the flour mixture and mix with a spatula just until the dry ingredients are moistened. Stir in the chocolate chips and toasted walnuts. Scoop the batter into the muffin tin and sprinkle with the remaining ¼ cup walnuts.

4 Bake until the tops of the muffins spring back when touched lightly, about 20 to 25 minutes. Let cool in the tin on a rack for 5 minutes. Loosen the edges of the muffins and turn out onto a wire rack to cool.

Tip If you don't have buttermilk, substitute ¾ cup (185 ml) low-fat milk plus 3 teaspoons lemon juice or white vinegar.

SERVES 12

PREPARATION 25 minutes
COOKING 25 minutes

½ cup (50 g) walnut halves or pecans, chopped

⅓ cup (40 g) unsweetened 'natural' cocoa powder (not Dutch-process)

1½ cups (225 g) wholemeal plain flour

1 teaspoon bicarbonate of soda

1 large egg

½ cup (110 g) sugar

¾ cup (185 ml) buttermilk (see Tip)

¾ cup (180 g) mashed banana (2–3 very ripe bananas)

⅓ cup (80 ml) canola oil

2 teaspoons vanilla extract

½ cup (85 g) dark chocolate chips

NUTRITION • *Per serving*
1064 kilojoules, 5 g protein,
30 g carbohydrate, 3 g fibre,
13 g total fat, 3 g saturated fat,
20 mg cholesterol, 140 mg sodium

MEETING YOUR GOALS
Each main-dish portion provides:
0.1 serve fruit
0.8 serve whole grains
10 g good fat

Baked goods
Wholemeal oat and fruit scones

The oversized scones often encountered in cafés are usually loaded with butter or shortening and refined carbohydrate. These are a better size, and are made with 100 per cent whole grains, fruit and healthy fats such as canola oil and nuts. Serve with a little honey or sugarfree fruit spread.

1 Preheat the oven to 200°C. Line a large baking tray with baking paper, or coat with cooking spray.

2 In a large bowl, whisk the flour, 1/4 cup (55 g) of the sugar, cinnamon, bicarbonate of soda and baking powder. In a measuring jug, put the yogurt, apple juice and egg and mix with a fork until blended.

3 Add the cream cheese to the flour mixture and blend with a pastry blender or your fingers until it forms small balls the size of peas. Add the oil and toss with a fork to coat. Stir in the apple, cranberries and oats. Add the yogurt mixture to the flour mixture and stir with a fork until a soft dough forms. Using a 1/2-cup measure, drop the dough onto the baking tray, leaving about 5 cm between scoops. Sprinkle with nuts, pressing lightly so they adhere, then sprinkle with the remaining 1 teaspoon sugar.

4 Bake until golden and firm, about 20 to 25 minutes. Transfer to a rack to cool slightly before serving.

MEETING YOUR GOALS
Each portion provides:
1.2 serves fruit
1.2 serves whole grains
7 g good fat

SERVES 10

PREPARATION 20 minutes
COOKING 25 minutes

1½ cups (225 g) wholemeal plain flour

¼ cup (55 g) plus 1 teaspoon sugar

1 teaspoon ground cinnamon

½ teaspoon bicarbonate of soda

¼ teaspoon baking powder

⅓ cup (90 g) low-fat plain yogurt

⅓ cup (80 ml) unsweetened apple juice

1 large egg, lightly beaten

¼ cup (60 g) reduced-fat cream cheese, cut into pieces

2 tablespoons canola oil

1 small apple, such as granny smith or golden delicious, peeled and diced

¾ cup (90 g) dried cranberries

½ cup (50 g) rolled oats

⅓ cup (40 g) chopped walnuts or pecans

NUTRITION • *Per serving*
971 kilojoules, 6 g protein,
33 g carbohydrate, 4 g fibre,
9 g total fat, 2 g saturated fat,
26 mg cholesterol, 120 mg sodium

Desserts

Burghul pudding with sultanas and pistachios

Creamy and comforting, this Middle Eastern-inspired pudding is simply a wholemeal version of rice pudding. It has a delicate perfume of cardamom, an accent of fresh lemon zest and a crowning touch of pistachios.

1 In a saucepan, combine the burghul, cardamom and 2 cups (500 ml) water. Bring to a simmer over medium–high heat. Immediately remove from the heat, cover and let stand until the burghul is tender, about 20 minutes. Drain and press out excess water. Return the burghul to the pan.

2 Add the milk, sultanas, cinnamon and sugar and bring to a simmer, stirring often, over medium–high heat. Reduce the heat to medium–low and cook, stirring, for 2 minutes.

3 Whisk the egg in a bowl. Gradually stir in the burghul mixture. Return to the pan and cook, stirring, over medium–low heat, until slightly thickened, 1 to 2 minutes. (Do not boil. You can use an instant-read thermometer to gauge readiness; the pudding should reach a temperature of 70°C.) Transfer to a clean bowl and stir in lemon zest and vanilla. Allow to cool slightly, then cover and refrigerate until chilled. Sprinkle each serve with 1 tablespoon pistachios. The pudding will keep, covered, in the refrigerator for up to two days.

Tip For a more fragrant effect, add a few drops of rosewater to the pudding with the egg. Rosewater is available from supermarkets.

SERVES 6
PREPARATION 10 minutes
COOKING 25 minutes
(including soaking time)

1/3 cup (60 g) fine or medium burghul, rinsed
1/4 teaspoon ground cardamom
1 1/4 cups (310 ml) low-fat milk
2/3 cup (85 g) sultanas
1/4 teaspoon ground cinnamon
1/4 cup (55 g) sugar
1 large egg
2 teaspoons freshly grated lemon zest
1/2 teaspoon vanilla extract
1/3 cup (40 g) chopped pistachios or slivered almonds

NUTRITION • *Per serving*
786 kilojoules, 7 g protein,
30 g carbohydrate, 3 g fibre,
5 g total fat, 1 g saturated fat,
39 mg cholesterol, 50 mg sodium

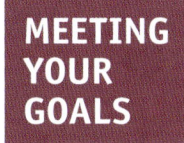

MEETING YOUR GOALS
Each portion provides:
0.9 serve fruit
0.3 serve whole grains
4 g good fat

Desserts

No-bake wholegrain treats

These bars are perfect energy-boosting snacks, and much healthier than the ones you'll find in supermarkets. With this easy homemade version you get the goodness of whole grains, fruit and healthy fats—without hydrogenated oils.

1 Line a baking dish with aluminium foil, leaving a small overhang on each long side. Coat with cooking spray.

2 Toast the oats in a frying pan over medium–low heat, stirring constantly, until aromatic and golden, about 3 to 4 minutes. Transfer to a large bowl. Toast the linseeds in the frying pan over medium–low heat until aromatic and starting to pop, 2 to 3 minutes. Transfer to a small bowl to cool. Grind the linseeds into a coarse meal in a spice grinder (such as a clean coffee grinder) or blender. Add to the oats. Add the puffed rice or wheat, blueberries or cranberries, peanuts, almonds and powdered milk and stir to mix.

3 In a small saucepan, combine the peanut butter and honey. Cook, stirring, over low heat until blended and smooth. Stir in the vanilla. Add to the oat mixture, mix well and transfer to the baking dish. Use a piece of plastic wrap to press the mixture firmly into an even layer. Cover with plastic wrap and refrigerate until firm, about 30 minutes. Using the foil overhang, lift the bars and transfer to a cutting board, then cut into 24 squares. Store the bars, covered or individually wrapped, in the refrigerator for up to 2 weeks.

Tip Toasting rolled oats brings out their nutty flavour. Make extra and have some on hand to sprinkle over fruit and yogurt. After cooling, store in a zip-lock bag for up to 2 weeks. If you prefer, toast the oats in a small baking dish in a 180°C oven for 10 to 15 minutes.

SERVES 24

PREPARATION 25 minutes, plus 30 minutes refrigeration
COOKING 5 to 10 minutes

1 cup (100 g) rolled oats
¼ cup (40 g) whole linseeds
1 cup (30 g) wholegrain puffed rice or puffed wheat
1 cup (130 g) dried blueberries or cranberries
½ cup (80 g) unsalted roasted peanuts
½ cup (80 g) almonds, coarsely chopped
½ cup (50 g) skim powdered milk
¾ cup (185 g) natural peanut, almond or cashew nut butter
⅔ cup (235 g) honey
1 teaspoon vanilla extract

NUTRITION • *Per serving*
715 kilojoules, 5 g protein,
20 g carbohydrate, 2 g fibre,
9 g total fat, 1 g saturated fat,
1 mg cholesterol, 11 mg sodium

MEETING YOUR GOALS
Each portion provides:
0.3 serve fruit
0.2 serve whole grains
8 g good fat

Desserts | 371

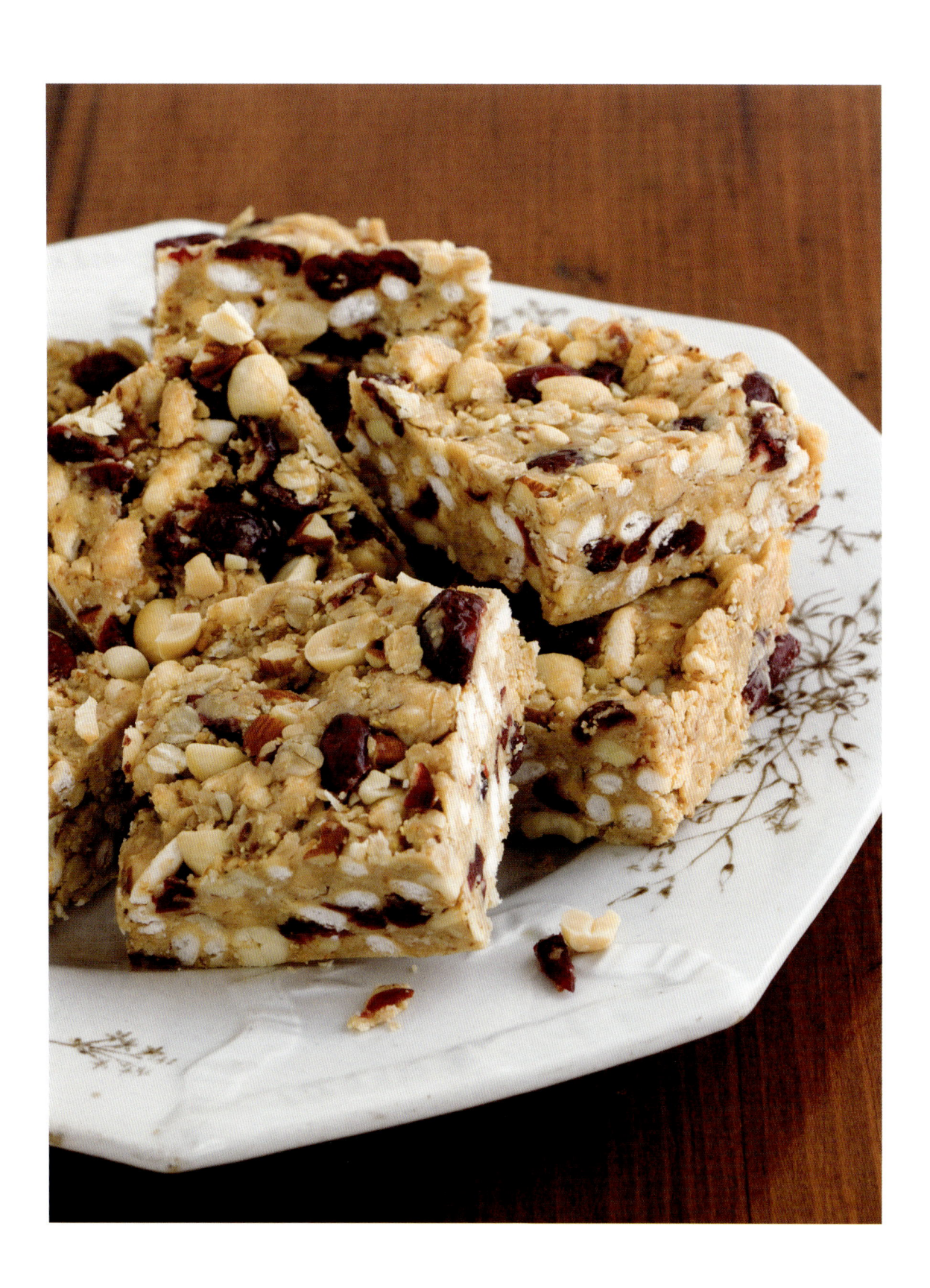

Desserts

Old-fashioned fruit cobbler

A cobbler is like a crumble with a tender biscuit topping, and is great for showcasing seasonal fruits. Instead of butter, the topping is a mixture of low-fat cream cheese and canola oil. The linseeds boost fibre and healthy fat.

1 Preheat the oven to 200°C. Coat a 20 x 20-cm baking dish with cooking spray.

2 To make the filling, combine the rhubarb, strawberries, sugar, cornflour and orange zest in a large bowl and toss to mix, then spread into the baking dish.

3 To make the topping, grind the linseeds into a coarse meal in a clean spice grinder or blender. Transfer to a large bowl. Add the flour, 1/4 cup sugar, bicarb and baking powder and whisk to blend. Add the cream cheese and blend, using your fingers, until the mixture resembles coarse crumbs. Add the oil and toss with a fork. Gradually add the buttermilk, stirring with a fork until the dough clumps. Transfer to a lightly floured surface and knead several times. Pat into a 1-cm-thick square and cut into nine pieces. Arrange the pieces over the fruit, leaving a little space between them. Sprinkle with the almonds and remaining 1 teaspoon sugar.

4 Bake until the fruit is bubbly and the biscuit is golden and firm, about 35 to 40 minutes. Let cool slightly. Serve warm.

Tips If you don't have buttermilk, substitute 1/4 cup (60 ml) low-fat milk plus 1 teaspoon lemon juice or white vinegar. You can serve this in individual ramekins: cut the topping into 12 rounds and place three in each ramekin.

MEETING YOUR GOALS
Each portion provides:
1.2 to 1.6 serves fruit
0.25 serve whole grains
9 g good fat

SERVES 8
PREPARATION 30 minutes
COOKING 40 minutes

FILLING
3 cups (about 1 large bunch) chopped rhubarb
2 cups (300 g) halved strawberries
1/4 cup (55 g) sugar
1/4 cup (30 g) cornflour
1 1/2 teaspoons grated orange zest

TOPPING
1/4 cup (40 g) whole linseeds
1/3 cup (50 g) wholemeal plain flour
1/3 cup (50 g) plain flour
1/4 cup (55 g) plus 1 teaspoon sugar
1 teaspoon bicarbonate of soda
1/2 teaspoon baking powder
1/4 cup (55 g) reduced-fat cream cheese
2 tablespoons canola oil
1/4 cup (60 ml) buttermilk (see Tips)
1/4 cup (25 g) flaked almonds

NUTRITION • *Per serving*
871 kilojoules, 5 g protein,
26 g carbohydrate, 4 g fibre,
10 g total fat, 1 g saturated fat,
4 mg cholesterol, 254 mg sodium

Desserts | 373

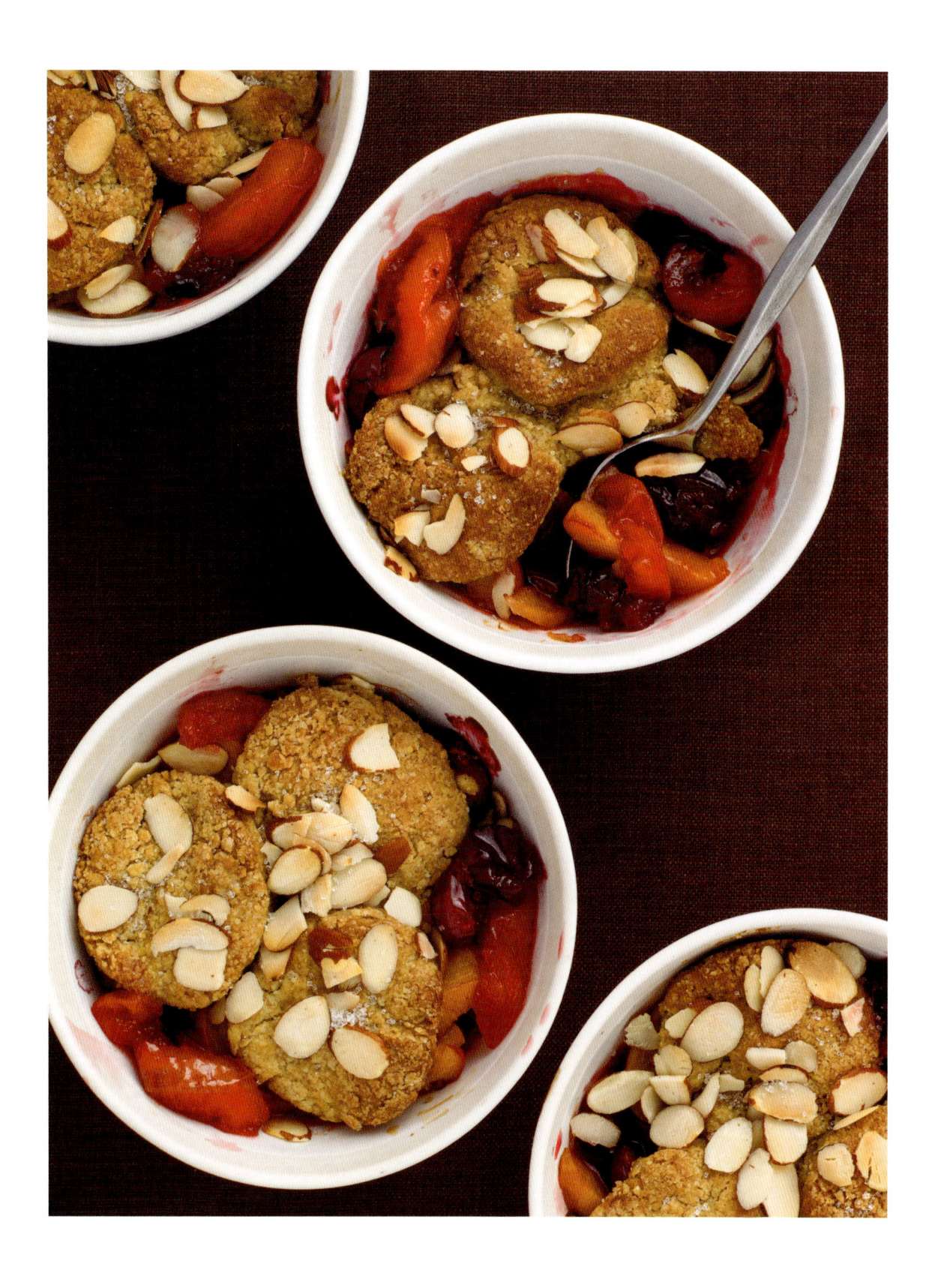

Desserts

Apple and pear compote

The goodness of apples and pears are further complemented by their wonderfully smooth texture. Serve this compote with yogurt as a delicious dessert in itself or enjoy it as a healthy topping on breakfast cereal or warm porridge.

1. In a large saucepan, add the apples, pears, sugar, lemon juice, lemon zest and ginger and toss to mix well. Cover and cook until the fruit is very tender and almost translucent but not pureed. Discard the lemon zest. Gently stir in the vanilla. Transfer to a bowl and let cool slightly. Cover and refrigerate until chilled. The compote will keep, covered, in the refrigerator for up to four days or in the freezer for up to four months.

2. Meanwhile, toast the almonds in a small frying pan over medium–low heat, stirring constantly, until golden and fragrant, about 3 to 4 minutes.

3. Top each serving with a dollop of yogurt and sprinkle with almonds.

MEETING YOUR GOALS

Each portion provides:
1 serve fruit
2 g good fat

SERVES 8
PREPARATION 25 minutes
COOKING about 1 hour

1 kg firm cooking apples, such as granny smith or golden delicious

2½ cups (about 45 g) peeled, cored and sliced ripe but firm pears, such as Beurre Bosc or Anjou

¼ cup (55 g) sugar

1 tablespoon fresh lemon juice

2 strips lemon zest

1 teaspoon grated fresh ginger

1 teaspoon vanilla extract

¼ cup (30 g) slivered almonds

½ cup (125 g) low-fat plain or vanilla yogurt

NUTRITION • *Per serving*
504 kilojoules, 2 g protein,
23 g carbohydrate, 3 g fibre,
2 g total fat, 0 g saturated fat,
1 mg cholesterol, 14 mg sodium

Desserts

Chocolate truffles with almonds and figs

Instead of a cream filling high in saturated fat, these truffles get their rich flavour from almonds and dark chocolate, both of which offer health benefits. Dried figs provide the sweetness, along with valuable dietary fibre.

1 Preheat the oven to 180°C. Spread the almonds in a small baking dish and toast in the oven until fragrant, about 10 to 15 minutes. Transfer to a plate to cool.

2 Melt the chocolate in the top half of a double boiler over hot (not simmering) water, stirring often.

3 Place the almonds and cinnamon in a food processor and pulse until coarsely chopped. Add the figs and pulse until the figs and almonds are finely chopped. Add to the chocolate and mix with a wooden spoon, adding a few drops of water if necessary to make the mixture adhere together.

4 Place the cocoa in a shallow dish. Form the chocolate mixture into 2.5-cm balls and roll in cocoa until coated all over. The truffles will keep, in a covered container in the refrigerator, for up to two weeks.

SERVES 20

PREPARATION 15 minutes
COOKING 15 minutes

¾ cup (115 g) almonds

85 g dark chocolate (70% cacao), coarsely chopped

¼ teaspoon ground cinnamon

¾ cup (140 g) dried figs or dates

2 tablespoons cocoa powder

NUTRITION • *Per serving*
312 kilojoules, 2 g protein,
6 g carbohydrate, 2 g fibre,
5 g total fat, 1 g saturated fat,
0 mg cholesterol, 7 mg sodium

MEETING YOUR GOALS
Each portion provides:
0.3 serve fruit
4 g good fat

Desserts

Rich dark chocolate cake with raspberries

This cake has the intense chocolate flavour and fudge-like texture of a rich flourless chocolate cake, but it contains a fraction of the saturated fat. And don't worry, you can't taste the red kidney or black beans, but the fibre and protein from the beans helps to balance the carbohydrate.

1 Preheat the oven to 180°C. Coat an 18-cm round layer cake tin with cooking spray. Line the bottom with a circle of baking paper.

2 Melt the chocolate in a plastic or glass bowl in the microwave on *High*, about 1 to 2 minutes.

3 Puree the beans in a food processor. Add the eggs, sugar, baking powder and vanilla. Process until smooth and creamy, stopping several times to scrape down the sides of the bowl. Add the chocolate and pulse several times until thoroughly blended. Scrape the batter into the cake tin.

4 Bake until the top springs back when touched lightly, 35 to 45 minutes. (The cake will look cracked.) Cool in the tin on a wire rack for 5 minutes, then loosen the edges, invert the cake onto the rack and peel off the baking paper. Let cool. Dust with icing sugar. Serve slightly warm or at room temperature for the fudgiest texture, accompanied by raspberries.

Tip For a special presentation, place a paper doily over the cake before dusting with the icing sugar. You can also create your own stencil using strips of waxed paper.

SERVES 8
PREPARATION 20 minutes
COOKING 45 minutes

120 g dark chocolate (70% cacao), chopped

1 x 400-g can red kidney beans or black beans, rinsed and drained

2 large eggs, lightly beaten

½ cup (110 g) sugar

¼ teaspoon baking powder

2 teaspoons vanilla extract

Icing sugar

4 cups (500 g) fresh raspberries, rinsed, or sliced strawberries

NUTRITION • *Per serving*
867 kilojoules, 6 g protein,
27 g carbohydrate, 5 g fibre,
8 g total fat, 4 g saturated fat,
55 mg cholesterol, 149 mg sodium

MEETING YOUR GOALS

Each portion provides:
1 serve fruit
0.25 serve vegetables
4 g good fat

Desserts | 377

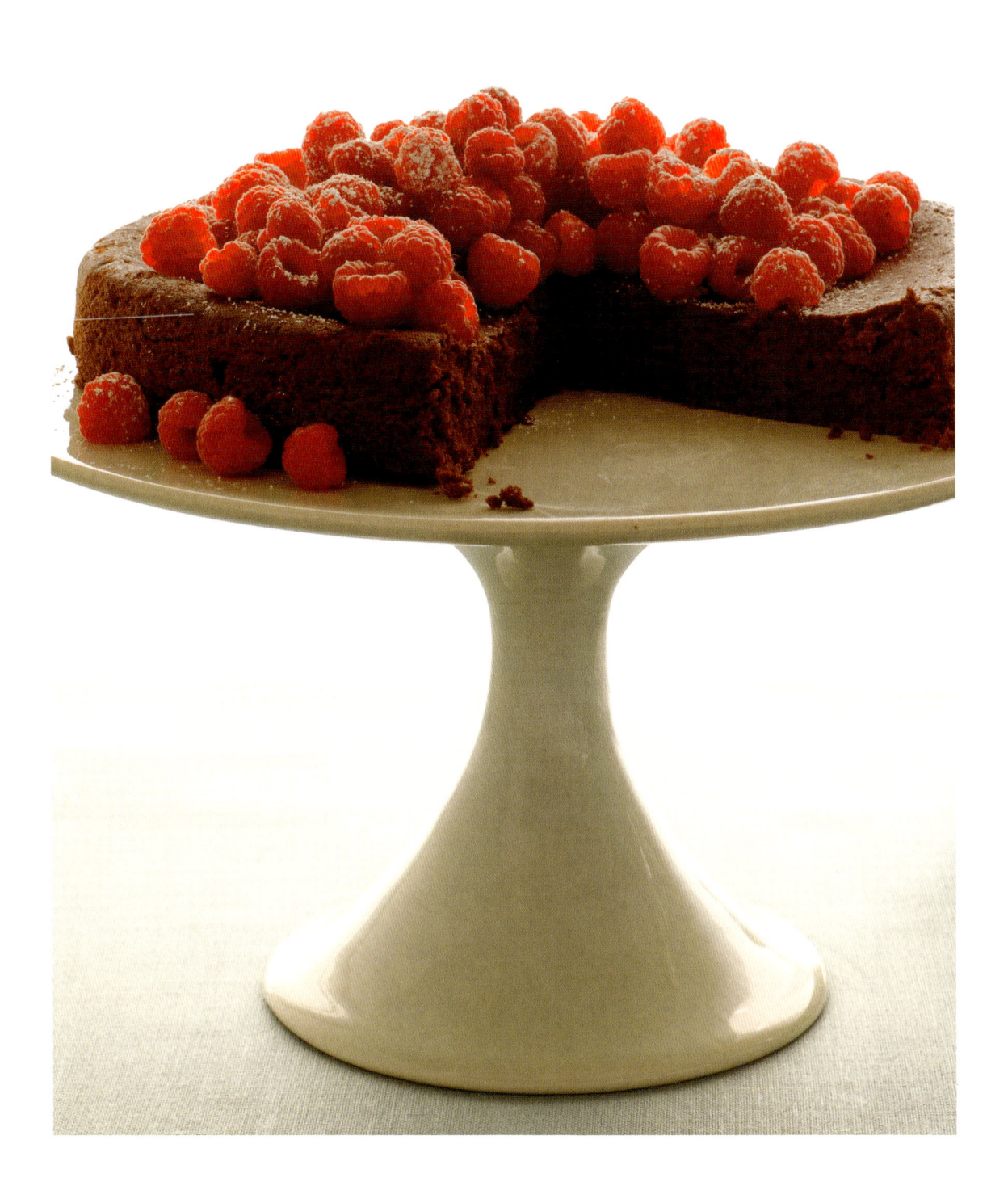

Index

Page numbers in **bold** print refer to main entries

A

abdominal aortic aneurism, 35
abdominal fat, 26, 164, 166, 168, 241
　see also intra-abdominal fat
abdominal pain, **34–5**, 42, 50, 51, 56, 57, 151, 171, 184, 227, 233, 235, 241, 251, 270, 271
absolute risk reduction, 61
absorptive hypercalciuria, 240
accidental deaths, 15
accidents
　confusion and memory loss after, 41
　nausea and vomiting after, 50
　numbness and tingling after, 52
　stress and, 77
　travel and, **88**
　vision loss after, 58
ACE inhibitors, 40, **153**, 238
acetaldehyde, 150
acetylcysteine, 178
achilles tendonitis, 135
aciclovir, 208, 287
acid reflux *see* heartburn
acne, 55, 57, **94–5**
acromegaly, 136
ACTH, 26
acupuncture, 205
acute angle-closure glaucoma, 191
adalimumab, 281
adapalene, 95
adenitis, 255
adenosine, 183
adiponectin, 24
adrenaline, 76, 104, 183
adult acne, 94
adult-onset allergies, 96

aerobic exercise, 21, 65, 162, 166, 192, 216, 242, 317
African descent
　glaucoma and, 190
　prostate cancer and, 278
aged people
　abdominal pain and, 35
　Alzheimer's disease and, 103
　anxiety in, 46
　arthritis and, 106, 107
　BPH and, 129
　bursitis and tendonitis and, 135
　confusion and, 41
　depression in, 46
　dry eyes and, 173
　flu vaccinations for, 186
　glaucoma and, 190
　hearing loss and, 200–1
　high blood pressure and, 23
　high cholesterol and, 217
　insulin resistance and, 28
　knee pain and, 242
　macular degeneration and, 246, 247
　memory loss and, 41
　neck pain and, 257
　pneumonia vaccinations for, 68
　prostate cancer and, 279
　screening tests for, 69
　vision loss and, 58
　vitamin D efficiency in, 151
　weight gain and, 55
aglycones, 218
AIDS, 284, 285
air, clean, **81–2**
air filters, 82
air pollution, 66, **81–2**
air purifiers, **97**
air travel, **84–5**, 91
airconditioning, 177
airway obstruction or infection, 54

alcohol
　acid reflux and, 203
　altitude sickness and, 87
　aspirin and, 71
　cancer and, 129, 133
　cholesterol and, 31, 217
　colorectal cancer and, **149–50**
　constipation and, 42
　coronary artery disease and, 158
　gallstones and, 189
　gout and, 193
　gum disease and, 195
　headache and, 48, 252
　IBD and, 225
　IBS and, 232
　infertility and, 223
　insomnia and, 230
　obstructive sleep apnoea and, 293
　psoriasis and, 280
　rosacea and, 282
　snoring and, 293
　stomach ulcers and, 303
　stroke and, 305–6, 307
　tinnitus and, 312
　travel and, 85, 87, 88
　varicose veins and, 317
　see also beer; wine
alendronate, 264
allergens, 32, 54, 81, **96–7**, 98, 99, **114–15**, 175, 176, 230, 293
allergies, 38, 40, 46, 49, 50, 51, 54, 81–2, **96–9**, 114, 116, 117, 174, **175–6**, 177, 230, 255, 288, 293
allergy-proofed homes, **114–17**
allergy specialists, 117
allicin compounds, 150
almonds, 75, 99, 142, 165, 182, 188, 201, 212, 215, 216, 241, 266, 277
　recipes, **322**, **364**, **370**, **375**

Index

alpha-blockers, 128
alpha-crystallines, 143
alpha-hydroxy acids, 94, 95
alpha linolenic acid, 157
alprazolam, 203
altitude sickness, 87
Alzheimer's disease, 15, 21, 25, 29, 33, 41, **100–3**, 163, 260 *see also* dementia
ambulance, 21
amino acids, 101, 201
amitriptyline, 233, 287
amoxicillin, 301
amyloid precursor protein, 102, 103
amyotrophic lateral sclerosis, 54
anaemia, 46, 199, 239, 251, 255, 301
anal fissures, 36
anaphylactic shock, 54
androgens, 219
andrographis, 146
aneurysms, 35, 48
anger, 32, 48
angina, 39, 102, 159
animals, 73, 162, 293
antacids, 34, 40, 42, 155, 170, 185, 205, 241, 302
anti-anxiety medications, 46
antibacterial wipes, 85, **87**
antibiotic resistance, 15, 88, 94
antibiotic side effects, 37, 38, 43, 47, 135, 185, 205
antibiotics, 47, 53, 57, 59, 85, 88, 90, 94, 95, 232–3, 283, 289, 297, 300, 301, 303, 308, 313, 315
anticonvulsants, 42
antidepressants, 15, 38, 42, 45, 46, 53, 56, 78, 105, 155, 160, 170, 173, 195, 205, 219, 233, 252, 267, 287, 313
antifibrinolytics, 249
antifungal preparations, 57, 311

antihistamines, 45, 46, 47, 58, 97, 155, 170, 173, 199, 230, 293
anti-inflammatories, 52
anti-oxidants, 66, 99, 102, 105, 109, 128, 130, 131, 142, 143, 149, 156, 159, 179, 193, 201, 246, 247, 276, 300
anti-seizure medications, 47
antiseptic cleansers, 89
antispasmodics, 42, 233
antiviral drugs, **186–7, 208–9**
anxiety, 39, 44, 46, 54, 55, 56, 70, **104–5**, 138, 154, 162, 177, 199, 229, 231, 235, 237, 307, 313
aortic aneurysm, abdominal 35
aphthous-stomatitis, 255
appendicitis, 34, 51
appendix perforation, 35
appetite change, **38**, 45, 51, 153, 167
appetite-regulating hormones, 70
apple juice, 241
apples, 99, 165, 169, 185, 215, 216
   recipes, **322, 368, 374**
apricots, 165, 169
   recipes, **320, 364**
arachidonic acid, 248
arm numbness and tingling, 52
armpit stretch (exercise), 259
arsenic, 130
arteries, 22, 23, 25, 27, 30, 31, 32, 33, 72
arthritis, 32, **106–13**, 162, 199, 225 *see also* osteoarthritis; rheumatoid arthritis
asbestos exposure, 245
Asian descent
   BPH and, 129
   glaucoma and, 190
   intra-abdominal fat and, 24
   waistline and, 273
asparagus, 184

aspartame, 252
aspirin, 11, 14, 50
   colon cancer and, 150
   disease prevention and, 71, 100, 117
   dizziness and, 44
   dosage, 71
   headache and, 48
   heart attack and, 39, 71
   menstrual problems and, 249
   migraines and, 51, 257
   side effects, 37, 71, 199, 225, 239, 302, 303, 312
   stomach ulcers and, 302, 303
   stroke and, 71, 306–7
   tinnitus and, 312
asthma, 39, 40, 54, 71, 81, 82, 96, **114–17**, 143, 176, 204, 230
asthma plans, **115–16**
atherosclerosis, 159
athlete's foot, 86, 310
atrial fibrillation, **306**, 307
attention deficit disorder, 230
attitude, 13, 27, 65, 161
Australian Dietary Guidelines, 74
autoimmune disorders, 47, 49
autoimmune nervous system, 275
avian flu, **89**, 90
avobenzone, 290
avocados, 74, 212, **215**, 309, 321
azelaic acid, 283

B

back extension (exercise), 125
back pain, **35**, 52, 53, **118–27**, 271
back rotation (exercise), 124
bacon, 179, 279, 300
bacterial infections, 32, 33, 35, 43, 47, 50, 53, 59, 82, 83, 84, 85, 88, 89, 159, 178, 245, 297, 299, 300, 301, 314
bacterial vaginosis, 57
bagels, 167, 300
baked beans, 212

baked goods recipes, **364–8**
balance, 13, 52
balance exercises, **268–9**
balanced diet, 13, 14, 15
Banana chocolate muffins (recipe), **367**
bananas, 212, **367**
barbecue recipes, **325**
barbiturate side effects, 47
barley, 75, 131, 154, 158, 188, 201, 212, 215, 227, 233, 278, 281, 300, 303, 321
   recipes, **331**
basal cell cancer, 291
Basil pesto (recipe), **334**
beans, 75, 150, 158, 184, 201, 212, 232, 233, 247, 261, 320
   recipes, **331, 334, 338, 348, 352, 363**, 376
bedding covers, 97, 117
beef, **74**, 84, 169, 232, 299
   recipes, **327, 341**
beer, 150, 189, 193 *see also* alcohol
beetroot, 241, 303
   recipes, **331**
beetroot juice, 213
behaviour therapy groups, 62, 63
beliefs, 13, 14, 79, 105
bending, 119
benign prostatic hyperplasia, **128–9**
benzodiazepines, 41, 203
benzoic acid, 254
benzyl peroxide, 94–5
berries, 67, 151, 167, 197
beta amyloid proteins, 100
beta-blockers, 46, 58, 104, 281
beta-carotene, 246
beta-cryptoxanthins, 109, 300
beta-glucan, 215
beta-hydroxy acids, 94, 95
beta-sitosterol, 215
Bifidobacterium, 146, 171, 235

bifonazole, 311
bile acids, 151, 189
binge drinking, 158
biofeedback, 177, 235, 237
biotin, 105
birth control pills *see* oral contraceptives
biscuit tins, 83
biscuits, 75
bisphosphonates, 264
black/bloody stools, 35, **36**, 50
black cohosh, 218
blackheads, 94, 95
bladder cancer, 37, 62, **130–1**
bladder infections, 37
bladder pain/pressure, 53
bleeding disorders, 49, 251
   see also vaginal bleeding or discharge
blepharitis, 173
blind spots, 48, 51
blindness, 23, 72
   see also vision problems
blisters, 49, 53, 85, 86, 208, 209, 286, 287
bloating, 42, 51, 56, 155, 171, 184, 189, 232, 233, 235, 271, 274, 275
blood-brain barrier, 103
blood cancer, 15
blood circulation, 12, 21, 49, 59, 62, 121, 201, 210, 272
blood clots, 22, 23, 25, 29, 31, 33, 39, 48, 54, 71, 84, 157, 158, 193, 195, 249, 251, 270, 273, 304, 306, 307
blood in urine, 37, 53, 56, 131, 241, 279, 315
blood iron levels, 183
blood pressure
   Alzheimer's disease and, 102
   causes of, **23**, 210, **213**
   congestive heart failure and, 152, **153**

   coronary artery disease and, **159**
   danger of, **23**, 25, 72
   definition of, **22–3**
   diet and, 23, 72, **211–12**, 213
   diseases caused by, 21, 22, 23, 48, 52
   exercise and, 23, 65, 72, 212
   high, 11, 12, 13, 15, 21, **22–3**, 25, 29, 48, **72**, 73, 77, 102, 137, 143, 152, **153**, 159, 181, 190, 199, **210–13**, 238, 239, 241, 230, 272, 292, **304–5**, 313
   inflammation and, 32
   insulin levels and, 29
   intra-abdominal fat and, 25
   kidney disease and, 238, 239
   knowing your, **72**
   low, 72
   measurement of, 72
   pre-hypertensive, 22, 68, 72, 213, 305
   PVD and, 272
   sleep deprivation and, 70
   stress and, 13, 23
   stroke and, **304–5**
   tinnitus and, 313
blood pressure monitors, home, 239
blood pressure screening, 68, 69
blood sugar, 12, 13, 24, 25, 28, 29, 38, 41, 45, 52, 59, 66, 68, 69, 70, 75, 76, 79, 90, 95, 129, 142–3, **153**, 164, 166, 167, 181, 182, 191, 195, 198, 204, 238, 247, 272, 308–9, 320 *see also* insulin resistance
blood thinners, 37, 71, 116
blood type and hearing loss, 200
blood vessel malformations, 48
bloody stools, 35, **36**, 38, 50, 56, 148
blueberries, 36, 169, 370
blueberry juice, 315

body mass index, 152, 239, 263, 271
body temperature, **47**, 229
see also fever
bok choy, 130, 246, **344**
bone density, 27, 195, **226**, 264, 265, 266, 267
bone fractures, 27, 35, 226, 264, 265, 266, 267 see also hip fractures
botulinum A, 221, 237
bowel blockages, 25
bowel cancer, 69, **148–51**
brain
　Alzheimer's disease and, 100–1
　anxiety disorders and, 162
　depression and, 26–7
　exercising the, **100–1**
　headaches and, 48
　high blood pressure and, 23, 72
　protein buildup in, 100
　sunlight exposure and, 183
brain-derived neurotrophic factor, 101
brain inflammation, 101
brain injury, 50
brain plaques, 100, 102, 103
brain tumours, 41
brazil nuts, 131, 188, 212, 266, 278
breads, 12, 75, 101, 300
breakfast, **167**, 182, 198, 260–1
　recipes, **322–3**
breast cancer, 62, 68, 71, **132–3**, 183, 218, 270
breastfeeding, 98, 116, 270
breath, shortness of, 39, 40, 44, 45, 51, **54**, 55, 117
breathing exercises, 77, 79, 179
bright light therapy, 228–9
broccoli, 67, 109, 130, 142, 184, 195, 212, 232, 245, 266, 277
bromine, 174
bronchitis, chronic, 15, 40, 47, 54, 81, 143, **178–9**

bronchodilators, 178, 252
brown rice, 75
Brown rice paella (recipe), **335**
bruises, 49, 59
brussels sprouts, 130, 142, 184, 245, 277
buckwheat, 188, 212
bullous pemphigoid, 49
bupropion, 63, 212, 244, 263
burghul, 321
　recipes, **330**, **369**
bursitis, **134–5**
butter, 74, 151, 166, 167, 214, 321

C

cabbage, 84, 130, 184, 232, 245, 277
cadmium exposure, 273
caffeine, 42, 48, 103, 162, 183, 190, 205, 221, 232, 252
cake with raspberries, Rich dark chocolate (recipe), **376**
calcium, 52, 195, 211, 212, 226, 240–1, **264**, **265**, **266**, 274
calcium channel blockers, 15, 42, 153, 155, 170, 205
calcium citrate, 265
calcium oxalate, 266
calcium stones, 240, 241
calf strengthener (exercise), 110
cancer, 320
　appetite changes and, 38
　back pain and, 35
　black or bloody stools and, 36
　bladder, 37, 62, **130–1**
　blood, 15
　bowel, 69, **148–51**
　breast, 62, 68, 71, **132–3**, 183, 218, 270
　cervical, 17, 57, **144–5**, 285
　colorectal, 15, 21, 25, 68, **148–51**, 227
　deaths from, 15
　depression and, 21

endometrial, 57, 145, 251
　environmental causes of, 130, 131
　free radicals and, 66
　gastrointestinal, 56
　insulin levels and, 29
　intra-abdominal fat and, 25
　kidney, 62
　lifestyle and, 11, 12
　liver, 206
　lung, 11, 15, 36, 40, 62, 81, **244–5**
　lymph, 15
　mouth, 62
　obesity and, 67, 133, 151, 260, 271
　oesophageal, 62, 202
　oral, 59, 62
　ovarian, 57, 145, **270–1**
　PCBs and, 82
　prostate, 68, 128, 129, 220, 221, **276–9**
　rectal, 15
　skin, 49, 59, 69, 117, 175, 176, 265, 278, 281, **290–1**
　sleep deprivation and, 70
　smoking and, 62, 145, **244**, 245, 285, 291, 301
　stomach, **300–1**
　stress and, 13, 76
　symptoms of, 27, 29, 33, 35, 36, 37, 38, 47, 48, 50, 57, 59, 182
　throat, 62
　uterine, 57, 218
　vaginal, 57
　VOCs and, 82
cancer drugs/treatments, 37, 38, 43, 45, 53, 59, 132, 183, 313
Candida vulvovaginitis, 308
canned food, 67, 75, 84, 261
canola oil, 75, 157, 166, 173, 189, 214, 217, 225, 253, 306, 321
capsicums, 67, 109, 128, 142, 149, 195, 246, 266, 307

capsicums *continued*
   recipes, **351**
car travel, 88
carbohydrates, 28, **75**, 95, 129, **158**, **247**, 253, 262, 306, 320, **321**
carbon dioxide, 185
carbon monoxide, 62, 156, 306
carbonated drinks *see* soft drinks
cardia cancer, 300, 301
cardiovascular disorders, 21, 54, 65, 72
carotenoids, 217, 300
carotid endarterectomy, 306
carpal tunnel syndrome, 52, **136–41**
carpets, 81, **82**, 96
carrots, 67, 165, 169
   recipes, 334, **361**
casein, 193
cashews, 216
cat allergies, 96, 97, 98
cat stretch (exercise), 127
cataracts, 58, **142–3**
cats, 310
cauliflower, 130, 232, 277
   recipes, 334, **357**
causes of disease, **20–59**
celecoxib, 150, 225, 244
cellulitis, 59
cellulose, 169
cereals, 75, 98, 138, 152, 154, 158, 163, 167, 169, 182, 201, 241, 247, 255, 260, 266, 307
cervical cancer, 17, 57, **144–5**, 285
   vaccines, 17, **144**
cetylpyridinium chloride, 194
chamomile tea, 229
chancroid, 284
chasteberry, 218, 251, 274
cheese, 74, 167, 212, 214, 227, 241, 247, 252, 253, 254, 266, 305, 321

cheese recipes
   breakfast, **323**
   meatless mains, **354–5**, **357**
chemotherapy, 132, 183, 313
cherries, 192–3
chest pain, 39, 44, 45, 50, 51, 54, 55, 59, 156, 159
chest pressure, 39, 50, 54
chewing gum, 185, 203–4
chicken, 74, 101, 138, 169, 192, 214, 261, 262, 279, 297, 298, 299
   recipes, **325**, **331**, **336**, **338**
chicken livers, 151
chickenpox, 49, 286
chickenpox vaccinations, 68
chickpeas, 163, **361**
children
   allergies in, **98**, 116, 176
   asthma in, 114, **116**, 117
   eczema in, 176
   food allergies in, **176**
   hepatitis vaccinations for, 206, 207
   mouth ulcers in, 255
   noise-related hearing loss in, 200
   pets and, 98
   solid food and, 116
chills, 35
chlamydia, 57, 223, 284, 285
chlorhexidine, 89, 194, 254
chlorine, 174
chlorogenic acid, 193
chocolate, 159, 162, 185, 212, 213, 225, 232, 241, 254
   recipes, **367**, **375**, **376**
choking, 54
cholesterol
   Alzheimer's disease and, 101, 102–3
   bad ratio of, **30–1**
   diet and, 30, 31, 66, 74, 75, 214, **215–17**

   HDL, 24, 30, 31, 79, 137, 156, 159, 189, 214, 215, 216–17, 241, 272–3, 305
   high blood pressure and, 22
   high levels of, 13, 15, 21, **30–1**, 78, 101, 102–3, 129, 137, 156, 157, 158, 159, 250, 272–3
   inflammation and, 32
   intra-abdominal fat and, 24
   LDL, 22, 24, 25, 29, 30, 31, 33, 74, 129, 156, 159, 189, 214, 215, 216, 217, 272–3, **305**
   stroke and, **305**
cholesterol ratio, 21, **30–1**, 158, 217, 320
cholesterol stones *see* gallstones
cholesterol targets, **214**
cholesterol tests, 68, 69
chondroitin, **108**
chopping boards, **83**
chronic fatigue syndrome, 46, 183
chronic lower respiratory diseases, 15
chronic obstructive pulmonary disease, 11, 39, 40, 54, **178–9**, 194
cigarettes and cigars, 62, 145, 181, 212, 224, 230, 244, 273, 293
   see also smoking
cimetidine, 116, 204
cinnamon, 254
ciprofloxacin, 135
circulatory problems, 12, 21, 49, 59, 62, 121, 201, 210, 272
circumcision, 284
cirrhosis, 206
citalopram, 233
citrus fruit, 203, 254, 276, 300
clarithromycin, 301
clean air, **81–2**
cleaning products, 82, 91
clothing
   cataracts and, 143

eczema and, **177**
flu protection, **91**
insect-blocking, **86**
skin cancer protection and, **290–1**
thrush and, 308
tinea and, **310–11**
travel and, 86, 88
UTIs and, 315
varicose veins and, 316, **317**
clotrimazole, 308, 311
clots *see* blood clots
cluster headaches, 48, 198, 199
cockroach allergens, 96, **115**
coconut oil, 253
codeine, 155, 205
coeliac disease, 35, 43, 51, 56, 254
coffee, 103, 162, 165, 169–70, 183, 189, 190, 193, 198, 203, 213, 254, 313
cognitive behavioural therapy, 78, 104, 161, 162, 177, **229**, 235, 237
cola drinks, 205, 213, 225, 254
cold intolerance, 38, 55
cold sores, 208, 209
colds, 46, 47, **146–7**
see also influenza
Coleslaw with gado gado (recipe), **360**
collagen, 153
colon disorders, 34
colonoscopy, 148
colorectal cancer, 15, 21, 25, 68, **148–51**, 227
compression stockings, 316, **317**
computer use/ergonomics, 136, 137, 138, 172, 199, 256
concentration, 46, 51, 82, 275
concussion, 50
condoms, 284, 315 *see also* contraception
conflict, 13
confusion, **41**, 47, 48, 58, 73, 153

congestive heart failure, 152–3, 182
conjugated linoleic acid, 151
consciousness, loss of, 48
constipation, 34, **42**, 55, 56, 151, **154–5**, 168, 170, 171, 184, 197, 232, 233, 235
contaminated food, 43, 50, 298
contaminated water, 43, 85, 86, 273
continuous positive airway pressure, 294
contraception, 284, 315
see also condoms; IUDs; oral contraceptives
contraceptive implants, 248
convenience food, 261 *see also* fast food
cookies, Oat and apricot choc-chip (recipe), **364**
copper, 246
corn, 109, 142, 185, 246, 247, 262
recipes, **328**
corn oil, 163, 277, 321
corn syrup, 165, 241, 309
corneal abrasions, 58
corneal injuries, 58
coronary artery disease, 153, **156–9**
corticosteroids, 38, 52, 55, 178, 264
cortisol, 13, 24, 70, 73, 76, 255
cortisone, 226
cough and cold remedies, 38, 46, 289
coughs, chronic, **40**
crabs (cooking), 299
cramps
  menstrual, 248, 250–1
  stomach, 296, 299
cranberries, **314**, 315
recipes, 322, 368, 370
C-reactive proteins, 27
cream, 74

creatinine, 238
Crohn's disease, 35, 36, 43, 47, 51, 56, 185, 224, 225, 226, 227
cruises, 87
curcumin, 291
curries, 203
cycling, 64, 65, 192, 201, 307
cyclizine, 87
cyclomethicone, 282
cysts, 53, 94, 95
cytokines, 27, 33, 195

D

dairy products, 23, 72, **74**, 167, 176, 184, 193, 195, 211, **212**, 214, 226, 227, 232, 245, 252, 264, 266, 274, 305
DASH diet, 72, 211
dates, 185
Dead Sea salts, 280
deafness *see* hearing loss
death
  air pollution and, 81
  COPD and, 178
  depression and, 78
  historic causes of, 15
  hospitals and, 15
  vitamin E supplements and, 277
decluttering, 97, 267
decongestants, 289
DEET, 86
defrosting food, 298
Delhi belly, 86 *see also* diarrhoea
dehumidifiers, 81
dehydration, 41, 44, 50, 84, 199, 227, 241, 299
dementia, 15, 21, 23, 72, 100, 102, 103, 210, 320 *see also* Alzheimer's disease
dengue fever, 86
dental care, 69, 71, 159, 194–5, 236, 237, 245, 254
dental floss, 194, 245, 254
dental plaque, 194, 195

depression
  Alzheimer's disease and, 103
  back pain and, **119–20**
  cancer and, 21, 27, 160
  carpal tunnel syndrome
    and, 138
  congestive heart failure
    and, 153
  danger of, **27**
  definition of, **26–7**
  diabetes and, 27, 78, 160
  diet and, **162–3**
  exercise and, **162**
  fatigue and, 46, 182, 183
  headaches and, 48, 199
  heart disease and, 21, 27,
    78, 160
  loneliness and, 73
  OSA and, 292
  osteoporosis and, **265–6**
  overview of, **26**, **160–3**, 167
  sadness and, 55
  screening for, 68
  shingles and, 286
  sleep problems and, 70, 163,
    228, 231
  stress and, 13–14, 73, 78
  tinnitus and, 313
  treatment for, **78**, **160**, **161**
  weight change and, 55, 56
  see also antidepressants
dermatitis *see* eczema
dermatophytes, 311
dessert recipes, **369–76**
developmental disorders, 82
diabetes, 11, 12, 15, 21, 23, 24, 25,
  27, 26, 29, 33, 38, 42, 45, 46,
  51, 52, 55, 56, 58, 59, 62, 64,
  67, 68, 70, 71, 72, 74, 75, 78,
  86, 101, 103, 136, 137–8,
  142–3, 152, 153, **164–7**, 173,
  181, 182, 183, 190, 191, 194,
  195, 204, 238, 239, 260, 278,
  292, 294, 308

diabetes insipidus, 45
diabetic neuropathy, 52, 59
diabetic retinopathy, 58
diaphragms, 315
diarrhoea, 15, 35, **43**, 56, 84, 85,
  86, 87, 151, 168, 169, 171, 184,
  227, 232, 233, 234–5, 296, 297,
  299 *see also* Delhi belly
diazepam, 203
diclofenac, 249
diet
  acne and, 95
  allergies and, 98
  Alzheimer's disease and, 100,
    101–2, 103
  arthritis and, **109**
  balanced, 13, 14, 15
  blood pressure and, 23, 72,
    211–12, 213
  BPH and, 128, 129
  cancer and, 75, 130, 131,
    132–3
  carpal tunnel syndrome
    and, 138
  cataracts and, 142
  cholesterol and, 30, 31, 66, 74,
    75, 214, **215–17**
  colorectal cancer and, **149**,
    150–1
  congestive heart failure and,
    152, 153
  constipation and, 42, **154**, 155
  coronary artery disease and,
    157–8
  depression and, **162–3**
  diabetes and, **164–7**
  diarrhoea and, 43
  diverticular disease and, **168–9**
  dry eyes and, **173**
  erectile dysfunction and, 180
  fatigue and, 182
  flatulence and, **184**, 185
  gallstones and, 188, 189
  gout and, 192

  gum disease and, 195
  haemorrhoids and, 196, 197
  headaches and, 198
  hearing loss and, 201
  heartburn and GORD and,
    202–3, 205
  IBD and, **224–5**, **226**, **227**
  IBS and, **232**, 241
  inflammation and, 32, 33
  insulin resistance and, 12,
    28, 29
  intra-abdominal fat and, 24, 25
  kidney stones and, 241
  lung cancer and, **245**
  macular degeneration, **246–7**
  menstrual problems and, **250**
  migraine and, 252
  obesity and, 67, 75, **260–2**
  osteoporosis, 264, **266–7**
  PMS and, 274, 275
  PVD and, 273
  prostate cancer and,
    276–8, 279
  shingles and, 287
  stomach cancer and, **300–1**
  stomach ulcers and, **303**
  stroke and, **305–6**, 307
  see also DASH diet
diet pills, 252, 262
dietary goals, **320–1**
dieting, yo-yo, **188–9**
dietitians, 263
digital rectal examinations, 69
dimethicone, 282
diphtheria, 15
  vaccinations, 47
disease causes **20–59**
Disease Prevention Survey, 11,
  12, 13, 17, 61, 64, 73, 78, 79,
  320, 321
disinfection, 83
diuretics, 42, 43, 45, 58, 153,
  155, 170, 173, 193, 238, 241,
  267, 313

diverticular disease, 36, 42, **168–71**
diverticulitis, 35, 168
dizziness, **44**
DMPA injection, 249
DNA, 12, 66, 131, 149
doctors
 asthma plans and, **115–16**
 discussions with, 17, 68
 questions to ask, 17
 screening by, **68**
 support from, 62
 travel preparation and, **85**
 working with, 13, **16–17**
dog allergies, 96, 97, 98
dogs, 162, 310
dong quai, 218
dopamine, 26, 163, 274
Down syndrome, 103
drug use, 207
dry eyes, 58, **172–3**
duodenal ulcers, 302
dust and dust allergies, 54, **81, 96–7**, 98, 99, 116, 117, 175, 176, 177, 178
dyssynergic defaecation, 154
dysthymia, 26

E

E. coli, 43, 50, 84, 315
ear pain, 44
ear problems, 44, 47
 headaches and, 48
 hearing loss, **200–1**, 312, 313
 noise-related, **200–1**, 312, 313
 tinnitus, **312–13**
ecamsule, 290
echinacea, 146
econazole, 311
ectopic pregnancy, 57
eczema, 49, 98, 114, **174–7**
edamame, 129, 165, 241, 261, 277
egg allergies/intolerance, 50, 54
eggplant, 254

eggs, 43, 142, 165, 217, 298
electrolyte solutions, 47
electomyogram biofeedback, 237
emergency phone numbers, 21
emotional therapy, 177
emphysema, 11, 15, 40, 54, 143, **178–9**
encephalitis, 86
endometrial cancer, 57, 145, 251
endometriosis, 223, 249
endorphins, 198, 199, 275
endotoxins, 159
enteritis, 15
environmental allergies, 54
erectile dysfunction, **180–1**
ergonomics, 136, 137, **138**, 199
ergots, 199
escitalopram, 233
esomeprazole, 116, 204, 265, 301
etanercept, 281
ethanol, 87
etonogestrel, 249
European descent
 prostate cancer and, 278
 rosacea and, 282
exercise
 air travel and, 85
 Alzheimer's disease and, 101
 anxiety and, 104
 arthritis and, **106–7, 110–13**, 162
 back pain and, **118, 120–7**
 balance and, **268–9**
 blood pressure and, 23, 65, 72, 212
 bone density and, 226
 BPH and, 129
 breast cancer and, 133
 bursitis and tendonitis and, **134–5**
 carpal tunnel syndrome and, **139–41**
 cholesterol and, 31, **216–17**
 colds and, **146–7**

colorectal cancer and, **148–9**
congestive heart failure and, 152
constipation and, **155**
coronary artery disease and, **156**
depression and, 27, 162
diabetes and, 164, 166
disease prevention plans and, 21
diverticular disease and, 170
emphysema and chronic bronchitis and, 178
erectile dysfunction and, 180
fatigue and, 182, 183
flu and, 187
gallstones and, 189
gout and, 192
haemorrhoids and, **197**
headaches and, 48, 198
hearing loss and, 201
high blood pressure and, 23
IBS and, 234
importance of, 11, 12, 13, 14, 15, 61, **64–5**
inflammation and, 32, 33
insomnia and, **228–9**, 231
insulin resistance and, 28, 29
intra-abdominal fat and, 24, 25
jaw pain and, **237**
knee pain and, **242–3**
macular degeneration and, 247
menstrual cramps and, 250–1
neck pain and, 256, 257, **258–9**
obesity and, 61, **260**, 263
osteoporosis and, **265, 268–9**
PVD and, 273
shingles and, 287
smoking cessation and, **63**
stroke and, 305, 307
warming up, 134
exercise balls, 120
exercise bands, 64
exercise physiologists, 135

exertion headaches, 48
exhaust fans, 81
eye drops, 190–1
eye problems, 48, 58
    cataracts, 58, **142–3**
    dry eyes, 58, **172–3**
    glaucoma, 58, **190–1**
    macular degeneration, 58, 160, **246–7**
    see also vision problems
eye tests, 69
ezetimibe, 15

F

face masks, 91, 179
faecal occult blood tests, 69
faith, 79, 105
fallopian tube infections, 57
falls, **267**
famciclovir, 208, 287
family history, 11–12, 23, 68, 69
family relationships, 13, 27, **73**, 77
famotidine, 116, 204, 265
fast food, 32, 74, 166, 167, 215, 261, 300–1, 305–6 *see also* convenience food
fasting plasma blood sugar test, 69
fat (body) *see* abdominal fat; intra-abdominal fat; obesity and overweight
fat goal, 320, **321**
fatigue, 38, **46**, 48, 55, 56, 70, **182–3**, 238, 239, 292
fats (dietary), 67
    cholesterol and, 30, 31, 214, 215, 216, 217
    colorectal cancer and, 151
    coronary artery disease and, 156
    diabetes and, 166–7
    diverticular disease and, 170
    dry eyes and, **173**
    gallstones and, 189
    IBD and, 224, 225
    inflammation and, 32

    lung cancer and, 245
    menstrual problems and, 250
    migraine and, **253**
    PMS and, 275
    prostate cancer and, 277–8
    stomach cancer and, 301
    stroke and, 305
    swapping bad for good, **75**
    see also hydrogenated fats; monounsaturated fat; polyunsaturated fat; saturated fat
fatty acids, 24, 25, 29, 151, 153, 157, 170, 224–5, 247, 250, 277, 321
feet
    bursitis and tendonitis and, **134–5**
    exercises for, 112
    numbness or tingling in, 52
    pain in, 59, 135
    travel and, 86
    wounds that won't heal on, 59
feminine hygiene products, 309
fever, 34, 35, 44, **47** *see also* body temperature
feverfew, 253
fibre (dietary)
    colorectal cancer and, 148
    constipation and, 42, **154**, 155
    coronary artery disease and, 158
    diverticular disease and, **168–9**, 170
    emphysema and chronic bronchitis and, 179
    fatigue and, **182**
    flatulence and, 185
    gallstones and, 189
    GORD and, 205
    haemorrhoids and, **196–7**
    high cholesterol and, 30, 31, 215, 216
    IBD and, 224, 227
    importance of, 67, **321**

    prostate cancer and, 276
    PVD and, 273
    stomach cancer and, 300
    stomach ulcers and, 303
    see also soluble fibre
fibroids, 57, 248, 251
fibromyalgia, 136, 182, 183
figs, 241, 254, **375**
filaggrin, 177
finasteride, 128, 276
fingers
    carpal tunnel syndrome and, 137
    computer use and, 136
    numbness and tingling in, 52, 137
fish and seafood, 33, 98, 100, 131, 149, 151, 153, **157**, 162–3, 166, 169, 170, 173, 176, 180, 189, 192, 214, 217, 224, 225, 245, 247, 250, 253, 261, 262, 266, 277, 278, 297, 298, 299, 306, 307, 320
    recipes, **344–8**
fish oils, 75, 98, 100, 116, 149, 157, 163, 170, 173, **250**, 306
fist flex (exercise), 139
flame retardants, 81
flashing lights, 48, 51
flatulence, 34, 51, **184–5**, 235
flavonoids, 102, 216, 223, 317
flavonols, 213
flaxseed *see* linseeds and linseed oil
flu, 15, 84, **90–1**, **186–7**
flu injections, 17, 86, 91, 178, 186
fluid retention, 152
fluoxetine, 15, 219, 233, 275
flushes, hot, **218–19**
fluvoxamine, 105
focus, 13
folate/folic acid, 101, 133, 145, 150, 163, 201
food
    balance of, 13, 14, 15

blood pressure and, 72
canned, 67, 75, 84, 261
colourful, **109**
contamination of, 43, 50, 298
cooking of, **299**
cross-contamination of, 298
defrosting of, **298**
disease risk and, **66–7**
eating less, **67**
fat-free, 129, 266
frozen, 67, 261
handling of, **84**
inflammation and, 33
insulin resistance and, 12, 28, 29
intra-abdominal fat and, 24, 25
leftover, 298
low-fat, 72, 74, 129, 165, 166, 193, 211, 212, 214, 226, 241, 245, 264, 266, 274, 305
low-glycaemic, 95, 164, 165, 309
marinating, 298
maroon or black stools and, 36
mouth ulcers and, **254–5**
preparation of, **84**
refrigeration of, 84, **297**, **299**
shopping for, 84, 299
storage of, **84**, 114, 115, 297, 299
stress and, 13
thawing of, 84
washing of, **84**, 297, 299
see also diet; fast food; fortified food; processed foods; refined foods
food additives, 254, 255
food allergies, 43, 50, 51, 96, 98, 99, **176**
food diaries, 176
food goals, 320–1
food intolerance, 35, 43, 50, 51, 176, 184, **232**, 254, 281
food poisoning, 43, 50, 84, 299
food portions, **67**, 220, **261–2**
foot builder (exercise), 112

foot hyperpronation, 135
footwear, 86, 109, 121, 135, **243**, **310–11**, 317
forearm stretch (exercise), 141
foreign objects
    inhalation of, 54
    wounds containing, 59
formaldehyde, 82
fortified food, 266, 274
fractures *see* bone fractures; spinal fractures
free fatty acids, 24, 25
free radicals, 66, 67, 102, 109, 142, 149, 179, 201, 201, 222, 246
friends, 13, 27, 73, 77, 162
frozen food, 67, 261
fructose, 185, 193, 241, 309
fruit, 12, 61, 84
    acne and, 95
    cataracts and, 142
    childhood allergies and, **98**
    colorectal cancer and, 149
    congestive heart failure and, 152
    diabetes and, **164–5**
    diverticular disease and, 169
    flatulence and, 185
    gum disease and, 195
    high blood pressure and, 23, 72, **211–12**
    high cholesterol and, 216, 217
    IBD and, **224**, 225, 227
    IBS and, **233**
    importance of, **66–7**, 320
    inflammation and, 33
    insulin resistance and, 29
    intra-abdominal fat and, 25
    macular degeneration and, 246, 247
    menstrual problems and, 250
    migraine and, 252
    PVD and, 273
    safety of, 299
    shingles and, 287

stomach cancer and, 300, 301
stomach ulcers and, 303
travel and, 86
washing of, 297, 299
fruit goal, 320, **321**
fruit juice, 165, 201, 314, 315
fruit recipes
    baked goods, **364**, **367**, **368**
    breakfast, **322–3**
    dessert, **369**, **370**, **372**, **374**, **375**, **376**
    salad, **325–30**
Fruity bircher muesli (recipe), **322**
fungal infections *see* under name e.g. tinea

G

gall bladder inflammation, 34, 39, 50
gallstones, 34, 50, **188–9**
gamma aminobutyric acid, 104
Gardasil vaccine, **144**
gardening, 64, 65, 162, 265
garlic, **147**, 150, 203
gastric cancer, 301
gastritis, 301
gastrocolic reflex, 155, 170
gastroenteritis, 299
gastrointestinal cancer, 56
gastro-oesophageal reflux disease, 40, 50, **202–5**
generalised anxiety disorder, 105
genetics, 11–12
    acne and, 94, 95
    allergies and, 114
    Alzheimer's disease and, 101, 103
    arthritis and, 106, 109
    asthma and, 114, 117
    back pain and, 121
    bone density and, 264
    breast cancer and, 133
    colorectal cancer and, 148, 151
    COPD and, 179

genetics *continued*
  coronary artery disease and, 156
  Crohn's disease and, 225
  depression and, 26, 163
  diabetes and, 164, 167
  gallstones and, 189
  hearing loss and, 200
  high cholesterol and, 217
  IBD and, 225, 226
  insulin resistance and, 28
  kidney disorders and, 37
  kidney stones and, 241
  knee pain and, 242
  obesity and, 263
  ovarian cancer and, 270
  PMS and, 274
  prostate cancer and, 278
  psoriasis and, 281
  rosacea and, 283
  shingles and, 287
  ulcerative colitis and, 225
  varicose veins and, 316, 317
genital herpes, 53, 208
genital sores, 53
genital warts, 53, 285
germs, **82–4**, **88–9**
ghrelin, 70, 167
ginger, 50, 253
ginkgo biloba, 71
glaucoma, 58, **190–1**
glomerular filtration rate, 238
glucocortoids, 226
glucosamine, **108**
glucose *see* blood sugar
gluten intolerance, 43, 56, 184, 185, 254, 281
goat's cheese, 74
gonorrhoea, 53, 57, 284, 285
GORD *see* gastro-oesophageal reflux disease
gout, **192–3**
grapefruit, 84, 276, 307
grapefruit juice, 241
grapes, 66, 84, 99, 185

green bean recipes, **334**, **352**, **363**
green tea, 276–7
GSM mobile network international emergency numbers, 21
guaifenesin, 178, 289
guided imagery, 191
gum disease, 28, 32, 33, 159, **194–5**, 239, 245
gym work, 64, 65

H

H2 blockers, 116, 185, **204**, 265
habits, 15
haemorrhagic stroke, 23
haemorrhoids, 36, **196–17**
hair growth, excessive, 55, 57
hair loss, 38, 45, 46, 55, 56, 273, 278
halfway sit-up (exercise), 125
hallucinations, 47
ham, 74, 158, 169, 211, 300
hamburgers, 245, 247, 297
hamstring builder (exercise), 112
hamstring stretch (exercise), 122
hand problems
  carpal tunnel syndrome and, **136–41**
  numbness or tingling in, 52, 137
hand sanitisers, 147, 187, 207
hand washing, 87, 89, 90, 91, **146**, 187, 207, 296, 297, 298, 301
  see also hygiene
handbags, 121, 257
hay fever, 96, 99, 114
hazelnuts, 142, 277
HDL cholesterol, 24, 30, 31, 79, 137, 156, 159, 189, 214, 215, 216–17, 241, 272–3, 305
head injuries, 41, 102
head tilt (exercise), 259
head tip (exercise), 258

headaches, **48**, 51, 58, 63, 76, 111, **198–9**, **252–3**
healthcare system, 14–15, 16
hearing loss, **200–1**, 312, 313
hearing tests, 69
heart arrhythmias, 44, 54, 157
heart attack, 12, 16, 21, 23, 25, 27, 31, 33, 39, 44, 50, 54, 62, 71, 72, 73, 74, 102, 104, 152, 153, 156, 158, 193, 210, 211, 214, 272, 273
heart disease, 11, 12, 13, 15, 21, 24, 27, 46, 55, 59, 62, 67, 70, 71, 72, 73, 75, 78, 101, 102, 132, **156–9**, 181 191, 194, 213, 214, 216, 217, 218, 260, 273, 292, 293, 321
heart failure, 15, 45, 51, 71, **152–3**, 182, 210
heartburn, 34, 40, 185, **202–5**
heat exhaustion, 47, 88
heatstroke, 47, 88
heel raise (exercise), 268
Helicobacter pylori, 33, 300, 301, 302, 303
HEPA filters, 81, 97
hepatitis, **206–7**
herbal tea, 75, 91
herbs and supplements, 71, 218, 313
herniated discs, 52
herpes, 53, 208, 209, 284
herrings, 173, 300
hiccups, 239
high blood pressure *see* blood pressure
high cholesterol *see* cholesterol; HDL cholesterol; LDL cholesterol
hip bridge and roll down (exercise), 126
hip flexor builder (exercise), 111
hip fractures, 64, 265, 266 *see also* bone fractures

hip replacements, 106
hip strengthener (exercise), 268
hip stretch (exercise), 268
HIV/AIDS, 47, 53, 284, 285
hives, 54, 99
hobbies, 120, 136, 183, 200
home environment, **81–4**, 91, 96, 121, 177, 179, 228, 267, **296–7**, 298
homocysteine, 101, 201
hormone replacement therapy, **132**, 133, **218**
hormones
　acne and, 94, 95
　appetite-stimulating, 167
　breast cancer and, 132–3
　carpal tunnel syndrome and, 136
　depression and, 27
　imbalances in, 45, 56
　insulin resistance and, 28
　menstrual problems and, 248, 249, 251, 255
　obesity and, 151
　reproductive, 129, 222, 271, 277, 279
　sleep deprivation and, 70, 229
　stress, 13, 24, 26, 27, 70, 73, 76, 104, 105, 164, 213, 223, 229, 255
　thyroid, 38, 46, 55, 183
　walking and, 104
horse chestnut, **316**
hospital
　dangers of, 14, 15
　deaths in, 15
　infections acquired in, 15, **89–90**
　medications and, 15
　staph infection prevention and, **89–90**
　super bugs and, 15
hot flushes, **218–19**

hotcakes with lime cardamom fruit salad, Ricotta (recipe), **323**
human adenovirus-36, 263
human papillomavirus, 144, 145, 285
humidifiers, 289
humidity, 81, 177, 179
'hunger headaches', 198
hydrogenated fats, 30, 31, 32, 33, 74, 75, 98, **214–15**
hydrometers, 81
hygiene, **310–11**, 314
　see also hand washing
hypercalcaemia, 42
hyperglycaemia, 45
hypertension see blood pressure
hyperthyroidism, 38, 45
hyperventilation, 54, 104
hypnotherapy, 234
hypoallergenic covers, 97, 117
hypoallergenic cleansers and moisturisers, 283
hypothyroidism, 38, 42, 46, 55, 56, 136, 137, 183
hysterectomy, 221

I

ibuprofen, 47, 48, 53, 71, 90, 100, 135, 199, 225, 239, 248, 249, 302, 303
ice-cream, 214, 245, 247
identical twins, 12
imipramine, 233
immune globulin, 206
immune system, 13, 32, 70, 96, 98, 99, 107, 109, 114, 116, 117, 132, 146, 147, 159, 187, 195, 224, 227, 255, 266, 281, 285, 286, 287, 299
immunoglobulin A, 187
immunomodulator cream, **176**
immunotherapy, 96, 116, 176
impaired fasting glucose, 142

impetigo, 49
impotence see erectile dysfunction
incontinence, **220–1**
indapamide, 238
indigenous people, 23, 68, 206
indomethacin, 281
indoor environment see home environment
infertility, 55, 57, **222–3** see also reproductive disorders
inflammation, **32**, 70, 71
inflammatory bowel disease, 143, 151, **224–7**
inflammatory compounds, 24, 25
infliximab, 281
influenza, 15, 84, **90–1**, **186–7**
influenza injections, 17, 80, 91, 178, 186
inhalers, **116–17**, 178, 252
inner strength, 16
innersoles, 109, 135
inositol, 105
insect-blocking clothing, **86**
insect repellent, **86**
insoluble fibre, 233
insomnia, 70, 76
　depression and, 163, 228
　diabetes and, 167
　exercise and, **228–9**, 231
　hyperthyroidism and, 38, 45, 56
　increased appetite and, 38
　PMS and, 274
　prevention strategies, **228–31**
　thirst and, 45
　see also sleep disorders; snoring
insulin, 28, 29, 103, 151, 158, 164, 167
insulin production, 26, 28
insulin receptors, 29
insulin resistance, 12, 21, 25, **28–9**, 33, 137, 165, 166, 167, 189, 241, 309, 321 see also blood sugar
insulin response, 12

international emergency numbers, 21
intestinal pain, 56
intestinal scars, 42
intestinal tumours, 42
intra-abdominal fat, 12, 13, 21, **24–5**, 28, 32, 33, 76 *see also* abdominal fat
iPods, 200
iron supplements, 36, 42, 170, 205
irritable bowel syndrome, 35, 42, 43, 51, 184, 185, **232–5**
ischaemic stroke, 23
isoflavones, 218, 277
isothiocyanates, 130, 245
isotretinoin, 95
IUDs, 57, 248, 249 *see also* contraceptives
IVF, 223

J

jaundice, 207
jaw pain, **236–7**, 312
jogging, 21, 265
joint inflammation, **134–5**
joint injuries, 106, 107
joint pain, 67, 108, 135, **192–3**, 260
junk food, 13

K

Kangaroo meatloaf with Asian flavours (recipe), **339**
kava, 105
Kegel exercises, 220
keratin, 310
ketoconazole, 311
key steps, **60–79**
kidney beans, 212, 376
kidney cancer, 62
kidney disease/disorders, 15, 37, 46, 47, 53, 72, **238–9**, 241
kidney failure, 23, 45, 54, 72, 193
kidney health tests, 69

kidney stones, 35, 37, 53, 239, **240–1**
kilojoule consumption, 13, 24, 135
kitchen equipment, **82–3**, 298
kitchen sinks, 82
kitchen sponges, **82**
knee arthritis, 107, 108, 109
knee bend (exercise), 268
knee pain, **242–3**
knee-to-chest stretch (exercise), 123
kumara, 99

L

lactalbumin, 193
lactic acid, 94
Lactobacillus acidophilus, 171, 235
Lactobacillus bulgaricus, 297
Lactobacillus casei, 297
Lactobacillus gasseri, 146, 171
lactoferrin, 151
lactose intolerance, 35, 43, 51, 184, 185, 227
lamb, 169, 232
lansoprazole, 204
laryngitis, 205
lasagne with mushrooms and silverbeet, Wholemeal (recipe), **354–5**
laundry (washing), **83–4**, 89, 91
lavender, 229
laxatives, 43, 233
LDL cholesterol, 22, 24, 25, 29, 30, 31, 33, 74, 129, 156, 159, 189, 214, 215, 216, **217**, 272–3, 305
lead, 36, 273
learning problems, 100
left ventricular hypertrophy, 153
leg length, 243
leg problems
  numbness and tingling, 52
  pain, 59, 272
  PVD, **272–3**

varicose veins, **316–17**
wounds that won't heal, 59
legumes, 67, 75, 101, 150, 151, 154, 169, 180, 192, 205, 227, 250, 303, 309, 321
lentils, 150, 163, 165, 201, 261
  recipes, **356**
leptin, 70, 151
lesions and skin rashes, **49**
lettuce, 84, 299, 303
leukaemia, 15
levamisole, 255
levonorgestrel, 249
licorice, 36
lifestyle factors, 11–12, 21, 42
lifting, 119
ligaments, torn, 242
light sensitivity, 48, 51, 173, 253
light therapy, 95, 228–9
lighting, 267
linoleic acid, 151
linseeds and linseed oil, **128–9**, 157, 170, 173, 182, 196–7, 225, 253, 321, 370
lithium, 55, 281
liver cancer, 206
liver disease/problems, 24, 25, 46, 49, **206–7**, 218
liver failure, 45, 51, 206
lobster, 299
loneliness, 13, 73, 77, 183
longevity, 12, 73
loperamide, 233, 235
low-glycaemic diet, 95, 164, 165, 309
luggage, 88
lung cancer, 11, 15, 36, 40, 62, 81, **244–5**
lung disease/problems, 33, 39, 55, 59, 62, 178, 179
lupus, 47, 143, 173, 183, 239
lutein, 128, 142, 246
lymph cancer, 15
lymphoma, 136, 137, 176

M

macadamia nuts, 138
Macaroni cheese with vegetables (recipe), **357**
mackerel, 153, 157, 277
macrophages, 242
macular degeneration, 58, 160, **246–7**
magnesium, 201, 211, 212, 213, 274
magnesium silicate, 271
major depression, 26
malaria, 85, 86
mammograms, 69, **133**
mandarines, 246
mangos, 109, **346**
mannitol, 185, 232
margarine, 74, 98, 157, 215, 217, 247
mattress covers, 97, 116, 117, 176
mattresses, 118, 256
meals, **66–7**
   see also breakfast; food portions
meat (red), **74**, **149**, 151, 179, 166, 169, 180, 192, 214, 224, 225, 245, 253, 262, 279, 297, 298, 299, 300–1, 305, 320, 321
   recipes, **339–42**
   see also beef; lamb; pork; processed meats
meat thermometers, 84, 297
medial-knee arthritis, 109
medication interactions, 71
'medication overuse headaches', 199
medications
   hospitals and, 15
   side effects of, 14–15, 37, 38, 40, 41, 42, 43, 44, 45, 46, 47, 49, 50, 53, 55, 56, 58, 59, 63, 71, 135, 143, 150, 154, **155**, 170, 173, 175, 176, 177, 183, 185, 193, 195, 198, 199, 203, 204, **205**, 225, 230, 239, 241, 244, 264, 267, 281, **302–3**, 312, 313

   travel and, 85, 86, 87
   see also under type e.g. antidepressants
meditation, 13, 14, 42, 55, 56, 77, **79**, 185, 213
Mediterranean diet, 98, 180
mefenamic acid, 249
melanoma, 49, 61, 291
melatonin, 70, 183, 229
memory loss, 21, 25, **41**, 100, 102, 103, 153
men
   Alzheimer's disease and, 103
   bladder cancer and, 130
   blood in urine and, 37
   BPH and, **128–9**
   cluster headaches and, 48
   diabetes and, 103
   erectile dysfunction and, **180–1**
   heart failure and, 152
   high blood pressure and, 23
   incontinence in, 220, 221
   infertility and, **222–3**
   intra-abdominal fat and, 24, 166
   osteoporosis and, 264, 267
   prostate cancer and, 68, 128, 129, 220, 221, **276–9**
   prostate enlargement, 37, 239, 276
   screening tests for, **69**
   skin cancer and, 290
   STIs and, 284, 285
   waistline measurements of, 24, 137, 166
meningitis, 47
meningococcal disease, 49, 86
menopause, 48, 58, 132, 133, 136, 173, 199, 218, 221, 264
menstrual problems, **248–51**
menstruation trigger, 48
mental challenges, 21, 41
mental health, 78

metabolic syndrome, 129, **137–8**, 165, 166, 167, 241
methicillin-resistant *Staphylococcus aureus* *see* MRSA
metoprolol, 104
metronidazole, 283, 301
miconazole, 308, 311
migraines, 48, 51, 199, **252–3**
milk, 43, 74, 193, 212, 241, 253, 254, 266, 274
milk allergies/intolerance, 50, 184, 186, 227
milk of magnesia, 233
mind-set, 65
mindfulness-based stress reduction, 77, 281
minerals, 211, **212**, 321
Minestrone with basil pesto (recipe), **334**
mint, 203
miscarriage, 57, 223
misoprostol, 303
moles, 49
mononucleosis, 47
monounsaturated fat, 30, 180, 215, 216, 277, 321
mood, 26, 27, 162, 163, 234, 274, 275
mopeds, 88
morning sickness, 50
morphine, 155
mosquitoes, 86
motion sickness, 85, 87
motivation, 16
motor cycles, 88
mould, **81–2**, 96, 99
mouse allergens, **114**
mouth cancer, 62
mouth sores, 59
mouth ulcers, 49, **254–5**
mouthwashes, 194, 254
moxifloxacin, 135
MP3 players, 200

MRSA, 15, 88–9, 90
MSG, 252
muesli, Fruity bircher (recipe), **322**
muffins, Banana chocolate (recipe), **367**
multiple myeloma, 136
multiple sclerosis, 183
muscle aches, 46
muscle mass, 64
muscle relaxation, progressive, 229, 234
muscle strengthener (exercise), 140
muscular dystrophy, 54
mushroom contamination, 50
mushrooms and silverbeet, Wholemeal lasagne with (recipe), **354–5**
music, 79, 230–1, 294–5
mussels, 201, 255, 299
myeloma, multiple, 136
myristyl nicotinate, 291

N

nappy changes, **83**
naproxen, 225, 248, 249, 302
narcotic pain relievers, 38, 41, 56
nasal sprays, 147, 289
nasal strips, 294
nasal washes, 97, 99
nature, 79
nausea and vomiting, **50–1**, 296, 297, 299
naval pain, 34, 51
nebulisers, 289
neck exercises, 256, 257, **258–9**
neck injuries, 52
neck pain, 48, **256–7**
neck rotation (exercise), 258
neck stiffness, 47
negative attitude, 161
nephritis, 15

nerve injuries, 52
neuromonics, 312
neurotransmitters, 26, 163, 275
niacin, 101, 291
nicotine, 156, 272, 303, 306
nicotine addiction, 62–3
nicotine-replacement therapy, **62–3**, 130, 244
night sweats, 218, 285
night-time cough, 40
night vision, 58
nitrates, 179, 300
nitric oxide, 23, 181, 205, 303
nitroglycerin, 39, 44
nitrosamines, 300, 301
nizatidine, 204
NOCs, 149
noise-related hearing loss, **200, 201**, 312, 313
non-cardia cancer, 300, 301
non-Hodgkin's lymphoma, 136, 137
noodles, 185
noradrenaline, 26, 27
norepinephrine, 262
norfloxacin, 135
noroviruses, 84, 87, 296, 299
nortriptyline, 233
NSAIDs, 150, 225, 239, **249**, 302, 303
numbness or tingling, 48, **52**
nut allergies, 54
nut recipes
  baked goods, **364**, 368
  breakfast, **322**
  desserts, **369**, **370**, 372, 374, **375**
  meatless mains, **352**
  salad, **326**
nuts, 75, 101, 142, 157, 166, 171, 180, 189, **216**, 217, 224, 227, 247, 252, 266, 277, 305, 309, 321

O

oat bran, 201, 212
Oat and apricot choc-chip cookies (recipe), **364**
oats, 75, 158, 188, 215, 300
  recipes, **322**, **364**, **368**, **370**
obesity and overweight, 11
  Alzheimer's disease and, 101, 260
  arthritis and, 106
  asthma and, 115
  BPH and, 129
  breast cancer and, 133
  carpal tunnel syndrome and, 138
  cataracts and, 143
  cholesterol and, 30, 217
  colorectal cancer and, 151
  congestive heart failure and, 152
  diabetes and, **164**, 167, 260
  diverticular disease and, 171
  exercise and, 61, **260**, 263
  food and, 67, 75, 260–2
  gallstones and, 188
  gout and, 192
  gum disease and, 195
  heartburn and GORD and, 202
  high blood pressure and, 23, **210**
  hot flushes and, 219
  incontinence and, 220, 221
  infertility and, 222
  insomnia and, 228
  insulin resistance and, 12, 28
  kidney disease and, 239
  kidney stones and, 241
  knee pain and, 242, 243
  macular degeneration and, 247
  ovarian cancer and, 271
  prevention strategies, **260–3**
  psoriasis and, 280
  PVD and, 273

sleep deprivation and, 70
snoring and, 292, 293, 295
varicose veins and, 316–17
obstructive sleep apnoea, 25, 46, 72, 182, 213, 239, **292–3**, 294, 295
ocular lubricants, 172
oesophageal cancer, 62, 202
oestrogen, 128, 129, 132, 133, 145, 218, 219, 223, 250, 251, 252, 264, 267, 271, 274, 275
oils, 75, **214–15**
see also under name e.g. olive oil
oily fish, 100, 109, 117
olive oil, 74, 75, 98, 151, 166, 180, 189, 217, 224, 245, 253, 261, 277, 306, 321
olives, 309
omega-3 fatty acids, 100, 153, 157, 163, 170, 173, 176, 224, 247, 250, 277, 320, 321
omega-6 fatty acids, 163, 247
omeprazole, 116, 204, 265, 301
onions, 99, 128, 149, 203, 252
opioids, 155, 170, 199, 205
optic nerve damage, 190, 191
oral cancer, 59, 62
oral contraceptives, 145, 173, 199, **248**, **249**, 252, 270, 275, 315
see also birth control pills; contraception
oral herpes, 209
orange juice, 142, 241, 266, 274
oranges, 109, 158, 169, 300, 307
organisation, **61**
orthotics, 135, 243
oseltamivir, 91, 186, 187
osteoarthritis, 106, 107, **108**, **109**, 243 *see also* arthritis
osteoporosis, 27, 33, 35, 53, 226, **264–9**
ovarian cancer, 57, 145, **270–1**
ovarian cysts, 53
ovarian infections, 57

overactive bladder *see* incontinence
ovulation migraines, 48
oxalic acid, 240, 241
oxidative stress, 149
oxidised LDL, 30, 33
oxycodone, 155, 205
oysters, 278, 299

P

paella, Brown rice (recipe), **335**
pain
abdominal, **34–5**, 42, 50, 51, 56, 57, 151, 168, 171, 184, 227, 233, 235, 241, 251, 270, 271
arthritis, 107, 108, 109
back, **35**, 52, 53, **118–27**, 271
blood in urine and, 37
burning, 39
carpal tunnel syndrome and, 137
cervical cancer and, 145
chest, **39**, 44, 45, 50, 51, 54, 55, 59, 156, 159
constipation and, 42
diabetes and, 59
diverticular disease and, 168, 171
ear, 44
eye, 48, 58
faith and, 79
foot, 59, 135
gallstone, 188, 189
gout, 192, 193
haemorrhoid, 196
heartburn, 202
inflammatory bowel disease, 224
intestinal, 56
irritable bowel syndrome, 232, 233, 234, 235
jaw, **236–7**, 312
joint, 67, 108, 135, **192–3**, 260
kidney stone, 240, 241

knee, **242–3**
leg, 59, 272
menstrual, **248–9**, 250, 251
migraine, **252–3**
neck, 48, **256–9**
pelvic, 57, 145, 271, 284
PMS, 274, 275
post-exercise, 48
shingles, 286, 287
sinusitis and sinus infection, 288, 289
stomach ulcer, 302, 303
urination and, **53**
vaginal discharge and, 57
see also headaches
pain relievers, 42, 52, 56, 58, 90, 155, 170, 199, 205, **225**, **248–9**, **252**, 253, **302–3**
see also under name e.g. paracetamol
paint, 82
palm kernel oil, 75
palm oil, 75, 253
pancreatic disease, 39
panic attacks/disorder, 39, 44, 54, 104, 105
pantoprazole, 204
pantries, 84
Pap smears, 68, 69, **144**
paracetamol, 47, 48, 90, 91, 225, 302
parasites, 43, 131
Parkinson's disease, 42, 181, 230
paroxetine, 15, 219, 233
passive smoking, 116, 159, **178–9**, 244, 245, 247
pasta, 75, 262
recipes, 352, **354–5**, 357
pathological processes, **21–59**
patience, 78
PCBs, 82
peaches, 109, 169, 185
recipes, **325**
peak flow meters, 115, 117

peanut allergies, 99
peanut butter, 105
peanuts, 241
    recipes, **358**, **360**, **370**
pears, 158, 185, 216, 233, 303
    recipes, **326**, **374**
peas, 109, 150, 158, 169
pecans, 216
pelvic floor muscle exercises, 220
pelvic inflammatory disease and, 34
pelvic pain, 57, 145, 271, 284
pelvic tilt (exercise), 123
peppermint, 183
peppermint oil, 233, 234
Pepto-Bismol, 86
peripheral vascular disease, 23, 59, **272–3**
personal trainers, 65, 134, 135, 219
pesticides, 81, 96, 116
pet allergies, 96, 97, 98
pet dander, 54, 96
pets, 73, 293, 310
pharyngitis, 255
phone posture, 257
photodynamic therapy, 58
phytochemicals, 67
phyto-oestrogens, 128, 218
picaridin, 86
Pilates, 120
pillows, 97, 117, **256**, 295
pimecrolimus cream, 176
pimples, 94
    see also acne
pineapple, 84, 149
pinpoint rashes, 49
pipe smoking, 62
    see also smoking
pistachios, 216, **369**
pizza, 203
plaque, 15, 22, 25, 27, 33, 72, 100, 102, 156, 157, 159, 180, 181, 214, 217, 272, 273, 304, 305, 307

platelet counts, 49
plums, 185
pneumococcal disease vaccine, 17, 91
pneumonia, 15, 17, 39, 47, 54, 194
pneumonia vaccinations, 47, 68, 86, 91, 178
poison, 36
    see also food poisoning
poisons information, 21
pollen, 54, 98, 99, 175, 177
pollution, 66, 81–2, 96, 117
polychlorinated biphenyls, 82
polycystic ovary syndrome, 55, 57, 223
polysomnography, 239
polyunsaturated fat, 277–8
pomegranate juice, 102
popcorn, 171
pork, 169, 232, 261
pork with pomegranate sauce, Roasted (recipe), **342**
porridge, 154, 158, 182, 215, 227, 303, 307
positional vertigo, 44
positive attitude, 13, 27, 65, 161
positive relationships, 13
post-herpetic neuralgia, 286
postnasal drip, 40
posture
    back pain and, 118–19
    carpal tunnel syndrome and, 136
    neck pain and, **256**, 257
    sitting, 118
    tinnitus and, 313
potassium, 23, 205, 211, 212
potassium citrate, 240, 241
potassium levels, 52
Potato salad with salmon (recipe), **347**
potatoes, 12, 75, 169, 185, 198, 212, 254, 247, 262
potential, 13

prawns, 217, 261, 299
    recipes, **335**, **346**
prazosin, 128
prediabetes, 164, 167
prednisone, 226, 302, 303
pregnancy, 136
    bleeding during, 57
    childhood allergy and, **98**
    childhood asthma and, 116
    childhood eczema and, 176
    constipation and, 42
    haemorrhoids and, 197
    morning sickness and, 50
    nausea and vomiting and, 50
    quitting smoking during, 63
    varicose veins and, 316, 317
    weight gain during, 263
pre-hypertension, 22, 68, 72, 213, 305
premenstrual dysphoric disorder, 274, 275
premenstrual syndrome, **274–5**
prepatellar bursitis, 134
presbyopia, 58
probiotics, 98, 146, **170–1**, 176, 226, 235, 297
problem solving, **160–1**
processed foods, 12, 158, 163, 198, 211, **214–15**, 300, 309, 320
processed meats, 74, 75, 149, 158, 169, 179, 211, 225, 252, 279
progesterone, 223, 251
progestin, 145, 218, 248, 249, 275
progressive muscle relaxation, 229, 234
Propionibacterium acnes, 94
propranolol, 104, 252
prostaglandins, 248, 249, 250, 251, 253
prostate cancer, 68, 128, 129, 220, 221, **276–9**
prostate enlargement, 37, 239, 276

prostate specific antigen test, 69, 276, **278–9**
prostatic hyperplasia, **128–9**
protective clothing *see* clothing; shoes
protein(s), 70, 151, 182, 192, 198, 262, 309, 320
proton-pump inhibitors, 116, **204**, 205, 265, 301, 302
prunes, 155, 216
PSA test, 69, 276, **278–9**
pseudoephedrine, 155, 170
psoriasis, 77, **280–1**
psoriatic arthritis, 281
psychogenic polydipsia, 45
psychotherapy, 161, 313
psyllium, 227
pulmonary hypertension, 54
pulmonary inflammatory disease, 57
pumpkin, 212
pumpkin seeds, 173, 188, 201, 212
punctal plugs, 172
purines, 192, 193
purpose, sense of, **79**
PVD *see* peripheral vascular disease

Q

qigong, 186
quadriceps toner (exercise), 111
quercetin, 99
quinines, 313
quinoa, 75
   recipes, **328, 351**
quiz, health habits, **18–19**

R

rabeprazole, 204
radiation, 32
radon, **244–5**
raisins, 212
raloxifene, 132, 264
ramipril, 153

ranitidine, 116, 204, 265
rashes *see* eczema; skin disorders
raspberries, Rich dark chocolate cake with (recipe), **376**
'rebound congestion', 289
'rebound headaches', 199
recipes
   baked goods, **364–8**
   breakfast, **322–3**
   chicken, **335–8**
   desserts, **369–76**
   fish and seafood, **344–8**
   meat, **339–42**
   meatless main, **351–8**
   salad, **325–30, 331**
   side, **360–3**
   soup, **331–4**
rectal cancer, 15
red clover, 218
red meat *see* meat (red)
refined foods, 158, 300, 320, 321
'reflex nasal congestion', 288
refrigeration (food), 84, **297, 299**
relationships, 13, 27, **73**, 77
relative risk reduction, 61
relaxation, 13, 14, 25, 55, 56, 70, 77, 104, 162, 177, 191, **198–9**, 204, 209, 213, 231, 234–5, 253, 255, 257, 281
religion, 79, 105
reproductive disorders, 81
   see also infertility
reproductive hormones, 129, 222, 271, 277, 279
resistance training, 107
resorcinol, 94
respirators, 179
restaurant dining, 67, 215, 261
resveratrol, 247
retina injuries, 58
retinoid products, 94, 95, 283
rheumatoid arthritis, 32, 47, 107, 109, 136, 137, 143, 173, 243 *see also* arthritis

rhubarb, 241, **372**
rib pain, 35
rice, 12, 75, 138, 154, 158, 185, 215, 247, 261, 262, 307, 321, 358
   recipes, **335**
Rich dark chocolate cake with raspberries (recipe), **376**
Ricotta hotcakes with lime cardamom fruit salad (recipe), **323**
rifaximin, 85
risedronate, 264
risk defined, **61**
Roasted pork with pomegranate sauce (recipe), **342**
rocket, 67, **348**
rockmelon, 84
rosacea, 173, **282–3**
rye intolerance, 281

S

Saccharomyces boulardii, 171
sadness, 55, 56, 68
safety, **88**
safflower oil, 163, 247, 278, 321
St John's wort, 71
salad leaves, 67, 145
salads, 67, **325–30**, **346**, **348**, **361**
salami, 74, 158, 169, 179, 211, 279
salicylic acid, 94
saline nasal sprays, 147
saline rinses, 97, **288**
salmon, 100, 109, 116, 117, 151, 153, 157, 162–3, 173, 212, 255, 266, 273, 277, 278, 300, 321
   recipes, **344, 347**
salmonella, 83, 84
salt (sodium), 23, 52, 72, 85, 158, 210–11, 213, 300, 305, 313
sardines, 109, 116, 117, 151, 153, 157, 173, 195, 212, 266, 277, **347**

saturated fat, 13, 23, 28, 29, 30, 31, **74–5**, 131, 156, 157, 166, 167, 189, 212, **214**, 215, 224, 245, 247, 253, 272, 301, 305, 320, 321
saunas, 147
schistosomiasis, 131
sciatica, 52
scleroderma, 173
scones, Wholemeal oat and fruit (recipe), **368**
screening tests, **68–9**
   see also under name e.g. mammograms
seafood see fish and seafood
seasonal affective disorder, 26, 160
seatbelts, 88
sedatives, 56, 58, 173, 203, 205, **230**, 267, 293
sedentary lifestyle, 12, 13, 24
seeds, 171, 227
seizures, 63
selenium, 131, 149, 223, **278**
senility, 15
   see also dementia
sense of purpose, 79
septoplasty, 294
serotonin, 26, 27, 162, 163, 199, 253, 262, 275
serotonin-reuptake inhibitors, 233
sertraline, 233
sex hormones see reproductive hormones
sexual intercourse
   thrush and, 309
   UTIs and, 315
   vaginal bleeding or discharge and, 57
sexually transmissible infections, 53, 57, 145, 207, 208, 223, **284–5**
shellfish allergies, 54, 99
shellfish contamination, 50
shingles, 17, 49, 68, **286–7**

shoe orthotics, 135, 243
shoes, 86, 109, 121, 135, 243, 310, 311, 317
shopping, 84, 299
shortness of breath, 39, 40, 44, 45, 51, **54**, 55, 117
shoulder pain, 48, 257
shoulder shrug (exercise), 113, 259
shoulder strengthener (exercise), 113
sibutramine, 262
side leg raise (exercise), 268
side recipes, **360–3**
side tip (exercise), 259
sildenafil, 180, 181
silent heart attacks, 153, 159
silverbeet, 246, **354–5**
singing, 294–5, 307
sinusitis and sinus infections, 40, 62, 96, 179, 199, **288–9**
sitz baths, 196
Sjögren's syndrome, 173
skim milk, 74, 109, 131, 151, 165–6, 167, 182, 212, 264
skin cancer, 49, 59, 69, 117, 175, 176, 265, 278, 281, **290–1**
skin disorders, **49**
   see also acne; eczema; psoriasis; rosacea; shingles
skin ulcers, 49
sleep
   back pain and, 119
   fatigue and, 182
   key steps to, **70**
   recommended hours of, 13, 33, 70
sleep apnoea see obstructive sleep apnoea
sleep disorders, 46, 70, 73
   see also insomnia
sleep schedules, 228
sleeping environment, 228
sleeping pills see sedatives
smoked foods, 300

smoker's lung see chronic obstructive pulmonary disease
smoking
   arthritis and, 107
   aspirin and, 71
   back pain and, 121
   bladder cancer and, 130
   blood pressure and, 23, 27, 72, 212
   cataracts and, 143
   cervical cancer and, 145, 285
   cholesterol and, 30, 31, 215
   chronic cough and, 40, 62
   COPD and, 178–9
   coronary artery disease and, **156–7**, 159
   dry eyes and, 173
   emphysema and chronic bronchitis and, 178
   erectile dysfunction and, 180–1
   glaucoma and, 191
   hearing loss and, 200–1
   heartburn and GORD and, 203
   hospital stays and, 90
   IBD and, 224
   infertility and, 222
   inflammation and, 32, 33
   insomnia and, 230
   knee pain and, 242
   lung cancer and, **244**, 245
   macular degeneration and, 246, 247
   obesity and, 263
   osteoporosis and, 266
   passive, 116, 159, **178–9**, 244, 245, 247
   psoriasis and, 280
   PVD and, 272
   quitting, 61, **62–3**
   skin cancer and, 291
   snoring and, 293
   STIs and, 285
   stomach cancer and, 301

stomach ulcers and, 303
stroke and, 306
weight gain after quitting, 55
see also cigarettes and cigars; pipe smoking
smoking-cessation support groups, 62
smoothies, 266, 314
snacks, 55, 67, 75, 85, 129, 182, 169, 198, 201, 211, **216**, 226, 247, 266, 277, 305
sneezing, 187
snoring, 25, 70, 212–13, 231, 239, **292–5**
soap, 174
social interactions/relationships, 13, 14, 27, **73**, **77**, 105, 161
social isolation, 13, 73
socks, 310
soda water, 165, 185
sodium *see* salt (sodium)
sodium lauryl sulfate, 254
soft drinks, 75, 165, 185, 193, 205, 213, 225, 241, 313
soluble fibre, 30, 31, 216, 227, 233, 276, 303 *see also* fibre (dietary)
sorbitol, 185, 232
sorbolene cream, 174
sore throats, 82
sound sensitivity, 48, 51
soup recipes, **334**, **361**
soy products, 129, 151, 157, 163, 193, 201, 212, 215, 218, 232, 241, 261, 266, 277
speech problems, 44, 58
spinach, 36, 67, 84, 99, 101, 109, 128, 142, 145, 163, 188, 201, 212, 241, 246, 266, 267, 303
recipes, **356–8**
spinal fractures, 266, 267
spirits, 150, 189
sport, 65, 102, 180
squamous cell cancer, 291

squash, 65
stanols, 217
staphylococcus infections, 15, 43, 50, 83, **88–90**
statins, 14, 103, 143, 150, 244, 305
steam inhalations, 289, 293
step stools, 121
steroids, 45, 59, 115, 117, **174**, 190, 289, 302, 303
sterols, 217
stinging nettle capsules, 99
stomach bugs, **296–9**
stomach cancer, **300–1**
stomach flu, 43, 87, 296
stomach ulcers, 32, 71, **302–3**
stools
    black or bloody, 35, **36**, 50, 56, 148, 151, 197, 239, 301, 303
    colorectal cancer and, 148, 151
    diverticular disease and, 168, 171
    haemorrhoids and, 196
storage
    food, **84**, 114, 115, 297, 299
    toothbrush, 83
strawberries, 66, 109, 142, 241, 307
    recipes, **372**
strength training, 64–5, **107**
strep throat, 47
Streptococcus thermophilus, 297
stress
    acne and, 94
    cancer and, 13, 76, 145
    carpal tunnel syndrome and, 138
    cervical cancer and, 145
    chronic levels of, 13–14, 24, 26, **76–7**
    colds and, 147
    constipation and, 42
    coronary artery disease and, 159
    depression and, 13–14, 26, 27, 163
    diabetes and, 164

eczema and, 177
family and friends and, 13
glaucoma and, 191
headaches and, 48
heartburn and GORD and, 204
herpes simplex and, 209
high blood pressure and, 13, 23
high cholesterol and, 216
IBD and, 226
IBS and, 234
immune system and, 13
infertility and, 223
inflammation and, 32
intra-abdominal fat and, 24
jaw pain and, 237
mental challenges and, 21
mouth ulcers and, 255
neck pain and, 256, 257
psoriasis and, 281
rosacea and, 282
shingles and, 287
shortness of breath and, 54
social interaction and, 73, 79
tinnitus and, 313
weight change and, 55, 56
see also anxiety
stress hormones, 13, 24, 26, 27, 70, 73, 76, 104, 105, 164, 213, 223, 229, 255
stress-relief techniques, 13, 42, 55, 56, **76–7**, 79, 138, 199
stroke, 11, 12, 15, 16, 21, 23, 25, 27, 31, 33, 41, 44, 48, 52, 58, 62, 64, 70, 71, 72, 104, 132, 156, 211, 218, 219, 272, 273, 292, **304–7**
submucous resection, 294
sucralfate, 303
sugar, 12, 29, 189
suicidal thoughts, 27, 55, 56
sulforaphane, 277
sunburn, 85, 86, 174
sunflower oil, 163, 247, 278, 321
sunflower seeds, 99, 142

sunlamps/sunbeds, 175, 281, 291
sunlight exposure
    arthritis and, 107, 109
    asthma and, 117
    colorectal cancer and, **151**
    fatigue and, 183
    melanoma and, 61
    osteoporosis and, 264–5
    prostate cancer and, **278**
    psoriasis and, 280, 281
    rosacea and, **283–4**
    skin cancer and, **290–1**
sunscreen, 86, 88, 209, 264, 281, 282–3, **290**
super-bugs, 15
sweet corn *see* corn
sweet potato, 99, **358**
sweeteners, 232
swimming, 21, 191, 192, 242, 307
swine flu, 90
symptoms, **34–59**
    see also under disorder e.g. arthritis
syphilis, 53, 284

T

tadalafil, 180, 181
tahini, 142, 188, 212, 266, 277
tai chi, 186, 213, 216, 231, 287
talcum powder, 270
Tamiflu, 91, 186
tamoxifen, 132
tamsulosin, 128
tattoos, 207
tazarotene, 95
tea, 99, 105, 165, 169–70, 203, 221, 254, 276–7, 313
temporal arteritis, 48
temporomandibular joint disorders, **236–7**, 312
tendonitis, **134–5**
tennis, 65
tension headaches, 48, 76, 198–9
terazosin, 128

terbinafine, 311
testosterone, 128, 129, 133, 267, 276, 277, 279
tetanus vaccinations, 47, 86
tetracycline, 283
thirst, excessive, 42, 45, 51, 55, 56, 59, 167
throat cancer, 62
thongs, 310
thrush, 57, **308–9**
thyroid hormone replacement, 38, 46, 55
ticks, 86
tinea, **310–11**
tingling or numbness, 48, **52**
tinnitus, **312–13**
tissue factor, 33
titanium oxide, 283, 290
tobacco *see* smoking
tofu, 157, 193, 212, 277
Tofu in peanut sauce with sweet potatoes and spinach (recipe), **358**
tolnaftate, 311
    recipes, **363**
tomatoes, 36, 66, 84, 254
    recipes, **363**
toothbrushes(ing), **83**, 194, 245
toothpaste, 254, 255
total cholesterol, **214**
toxic gases, 81
toxins, 32
trace elements, 223, 278
traffic accidents, 88
traffic exhaust, 117
tranquillisers, 205
trans fats, 75, 116, 166, 214–15, 320
transient ischaemic attacks, 41, 44, 52, 58, 304
trauma, 105, 163, 257
travel
    accidents and injuries and, **88**
    constipation and, 42

diarrhoea and, 43, 85, 86
    disease free, **84–7, 88–91**
tretinoin, 95
triazolam, 203
trichomoniasis, 57, 284, 285
triclosan, 254
tricyclic antidepressant, 287
trigeminal nerve system, 253
triglycerides, 29, 75, 137, 143, 156, 157, 158, 214, 217, 241, 305–6
tropical oils, **75**
trout, 116, 153, 157, 162, 173, 277
tubal ligation, 270–1
tuberculosis, 15
tumours, 41, 42, 48, 54
tuna, 130, 153, 157, 162
    recipes, **347, 348**
tunnel vision, 190, 191
turkey, 74, 261, 279, 298
turmeric, 291
twins, 12, 263

U

ulcerative colitis, 35, 36, 43, 47, 51, 56, 185, 224, 225, 226, 227
ulcers, 51
    abdominal pain and, 35
    burning pain and, 39
    intestinal, 15
    mouth, 49, **254–5**
    skin, 49
    stomach, 32, 71, **302–3**
    upper gastrointestinal tract, 36
ultraviolet light, 175, 278, 282, 290, 291
unsaturated fats, 217
upper gastrointestinal tract ulcers, 36
uric acid, 192, 193
uric acid stones, 240
urinary incontinence, **220–1**
urinary tract infections, 15, 34, 47, 53, 221, 241, **314–15**

urination frequency, 42, 44, 45, 51, 53, 55, 56, 59, 128, 129, 131, 167, 241, 271, 279, 315
urination pain, **53**
urine, blood in, **37**, 53, 56, 131, 241, 279, 315
uterine cancer, 57, 218
uterine fibroids, 57, 248, 251
uterine infections, 57

V

vaccines
    adults and, 17
    cervical cancer, 17, **144**
    chickenpox, 286
    fever after, 47
    flu, 17, 91, 178, 186
    hepatitis, **206–7**
    HPV, 285
    meningococcal, 86
    pneumococcal disease, 17, 91
    pneumonia, 47, 68, 86, 91, 178
    shingles, 17, 68, **286**, 287
    tetanus, 47, 86
    travel and, 85, 86
    yellow fever, 86
    see also immunotherapy
vacuuming, 81, 96, 97
vaginal bleeding or discharge, 53, **57**, 145, 309
vaginal cancer, 57
vaginal douches, 315
vaginal rings, 248
vaginosis, bacterial, 57
valaciclovir, 208–9, 287
vardenafil, 181
varenicline, 63, 244
varicella zoster virus, 286, 287
varicose veins, **316–17**
vegetable goal, 320, **321**
vegetable recipes
    chicken, **335–8**
    dessert, **376**

fish and seafood, **344–8**
meatless mains, **351–8**
salad, **325–31**
sides, **360–3**
soup, **331**, **332**, **334**
vegetables
    acne and, 95
    bladder cancer and, 130
    BPH and, 128
    cataracts and, 142
    cervical cancer and, 145
    childhood allergies and, **98**
    colorectal cancer and, 149
    congestive heart failure and, 152
    constipation and, 154
    diabetes and, **164**
    emphysema and chronic bronchitis and, 179
    'fast food', 261
    flatulence and, 184, 185
    hearing loss and, 201
    high blood pressure and, 72, **211–12**
    high cholesterol and, 216, 217
    IBD and, 224, 227
    importance of, 55, 61, **66–7**, 75
    inflammation and, 33
    insulin resistance and, 29
    lung cancer and, 245
    macular degeneration and, **246**, 247
    menstrual problems and, 250
    osteoporosis and, 266, 267
    PMS and, 275
    prostate cancer and, 277
    PVD and, 273
    safety and, 299
    shingles and, 287
    stomach ulcers and, 303
    travel and, 86
    washing, 84, 297
    weight loss and, 261, **262**

vegetarian diet, 157, 169, 250, 275, 276
venlafaxine, 219
verapamil, 198
vertigo, positional, 44
Viagra, 180, 181
viral hepatitis, **206–7**
viral infections, 43, 47, 49, 82, 84, 85, 87, 88, 178, 208, 209, 297, 299 *see also* under infection e.g. colds
virtual colonoscopy, 148
vision problems, 23, 44, 48, **58**, 72, 160, 173
    see also blindness; cataracts; eye problems; glaucoma; macular degeneration
visualisation, 55, 56
vitamin A, 95, 283
vitamin B, 101, 133, 138, 145, 163, **201**, 255
vitamin B_6, 50, 101, 275
vitamin B_7, 105
vitamin B_{12}, 52, 145, **201**, 253, 255
vitamin C, 109, 128, 142, 146, 195, 205, 223, 246, 266, 300, 307
vitamin D, **107**, **109**, 149, 151, 166, 226, 243, **264–5**, 274, 278, 279
vitamin E, 71, 99, 142, 216, 219, 223, 245, 246, 250, 277
vitamin K, 267
VOCs, 81, 82
volunteering, 77, 79, 120
vomiting and nausea, **50–1**, 296, 297, 299
von Willebrand's disease, 251

W

waiting lists, 17
walking, **64–5**, 85, 101, 104, 119, **146–7**, **155**, **156**, 164, 166, 182, 191, 192, 212, 242, 265, 307

walking shoes, 243
walnuts, 75, 157, 165, 170, 173, 216, 225, 253, 254
　recipes, 322, **326**, **352**, **367**, **368**
warfarin, 71, 306
washing *see* laundry (washing)
water aerobics, 65
water consumption, 75, 85, 86, 154, 165, 168, 185, 197, 226–7
water contamination, 43, 85, 86, 273
watermelon, 109, 299
weight *see* obesity and overweight
weight gain, unintentional, 45, 46, **55**, 70
weigh loss support groups, 262
weight loss, unintentional, 12, 29, 45, 46, 47, **56**, 59, 151
weights, 64
wheat bran, 241
wheat dextrin, 227
wheat intolerance, 176, 184, 232, 254, 281
wheatgerm, 99
whiplash injury, 256, 257
white blood cells
　cholesterol and, 30, 31
　high blood pressure and, 22
　inflammation and, 33
white foods, 75, 164, 198, 205, 247, 300, 309, 321
white noise, 229
whiteheads, 95
wholegrain recipes
　baked goods, **364**, **367**, **368**
　breakfast, **322**
　chicken, **335**, **338**
　desserts, **369**, **370**, **372**
　fish, **348**
　meat, **339**, **341**
　meatless mains, **351–8**
　salad, **328**, **330**, **331**
　sides, **360**
　soup, **331**, **332**
whole grains, 29, 72, 75, 95, 98, 142, 152, 154, 158, 163, 164, 165, 169, 180, 182, 198, 205, 215, 224, 227, 241, 247, 260, 261, 266, 273, 300, 305, 307, 309, 320, **321**
Wholemeal lasagne with mushrooms and silverbeet (recipe), **354–5**
Wholemeal oat and fruit scones (recipe), **368**
willpower, 61, 65
wind *see* flatulence
wine, 102, 150, **158**, 189, 193, 317
　see also alcohol
women
　acne treatment for, 95
　alcohol intake and, 133
　arthritis and, 106, 108, 109
　breast cancer and, 62, 68, 71, **132–3**, 183, 218, 270
　cervical cancer and, 57, **144–5**, 285
　colorectal cancer and, 150, 151
　dry eyes and, 173
　fatigue and, 183
　heart failure and, 152
　high blood pressure and, 213
　hot flushes and, **218–19**
　infertility and, **222–3**
　intra-abdominal fat and, 24, 166
　menstrual problems, **248–51**
　migraine and, 48
　osteoporosis and, 264, 265, 266, 267
　ovarian cancer and, 57, 145, **270–1**
　ovarian cysts and, 53
　PMS and, **274–5**
　screening tests for, **69**
　skin cancer and, 290
　STDs and, 284, 285
　unintentional weight gain in, 55
　urinary incontinence in, 220, 221
　urinary infections in, 314
　vaginal bleeding or discharge and, 53, **57**, 145, 309
　waistline measurements of, 24, 137, 166, 188
　see also pregnancy
work stations, 119, 199
wound healing, poor, 38, 55, 56, **59**
wrist extender (exercise), 140
wrist numbness and tingling, 52
wrist splints, 137

Y

yeast breads, 252
yeast infections, 53, **308–9**
yellow fever vaccine, 86
yoga, 55, 56, 77, 104, 138, 213, 216, 219, 234–5, 255, 307
yogurt, 99, 131, 165, 167, 176, 193, 212, **226**, 227, 235, 240, 241, 264, 274, 297, 308
yo-yo dieting, **188–9**

Z

zanamivir, 91, 186, 187
zeaxanthin, 109, 142, 246
zinc, 246
zinc oxide, 283, 290
zolpidem, 230
zucchini, 142, 334